PSYCHOSOCIAL NURSING
FOR GENERAL PATIENT CARE

3rd Edition

Linda M. Gorman, APRN, BC, MN, CHPN, OCN
Palliative Care Clinical Nurse Specialist
Cedars-Sinai Medical Center
Los Angeles, California

Assistant Professor
University of California, Los Ang
Los Angeles, California

Donna F. Sultan, RN, MS
Mental Health Counselor, RN
West Valley Mental Health Center
Los Angeles County Department of Mental Health
Los Angeles, California

F. A. DAVIS COMPANY • Philadelphia

BP45

F. A. Davis Company
1915 Arch Street
Philadelphia, PA 19103
www.fadavis.com

Printed in the United States of America

Last digit indicates print number: 10 9 8 7 6 5 4 3 2

Publisher, Nursing: Joanne Patzek DaCunha, RN, MSN
Director of Content Development: Darlene D. Pedersen
Project Editor: Padraic Maroney
Art and Design Manager: Carolyn O'Brien

As new scientific information becomes available through basic and clinical research, recommended treatments and drug therapies undergo changes. The author(s) and publisher have done everything possible to make this book accurate, up to date, and in accord with accepted standards at the time of publication. The author(s), editors, and publisher are not responsible for errors or omissions or for consequences from application of the book, and make no warranty, expressed or implied, in regard to the contents of the book. Any practice described in this book should be applied by the reader in accordance with professional standards of care used in regard to the unique circumstances that may apply in each situation. The reader is advised always to check product information (package inserts) for changes and new information regarding dose and contraindications before administering any drug. Caution is especially urged when using new or infrequently ordered drugs.

Library of Congress Cataloging-in-Publication Data
Gorman, Linda M.
  Psychosocial nursing for general patient care / Linda M. Gorman, Donna F. Sultan. — 3rd ed.
     p. ; cm.
  Includes bibliographical references and index.
  ISBN-13: 978-0-8036-1784-1
  ISBN-10: 0-8036-1784-4
  1. Psychiatric nursing—Handbooks, manuals, etc. 2. Nursing—Social aspects—Handbooks, manuals, etc. I. Sultan, Donna. II. Title.
  [DNLM: 1. Nursing Care—psychology—Handbooks. 2. Nurse-Patient Relations—Handbooks. 3. Nursing Assessment—Handbooks. WY 49 G671p 2008]
  RC440.G659 2008
  616.89′0231—dc22
                                                                              2007040704

12/2/09

Preface

Having worked in a variety of specialty areas over the years as staff nurses, clinical nurse specialists, educators, therapists, and managers, we realize that nurses aspire to become highly proficient in their area of practice. But psychosocial skills are often more difficult to perfect. Very often nurses feel inadequately prepared to deal with complex behaviors and psychiatric problems on top of the demands of providing physical care for the patient and family. Even nurses who practice in the psychiatric setting find themselves dealing with unique situations that challenge their level of expertise. And yet, a large percentage of a nurse's time is spent dealing with these issues.

Psychosocial Nursing for General Patient Care bridges the gap between the information contained in the large, comprehensive psychiatric texts and the information needed to function effectively in a variety of healthcare settings. The clinician can refer to this book to find the information to effectively handle specific patient problems. The nursing student can use this book as a supplement to other texts and will be useful throughout nursing school curriculum.

The concise, quick reference format used throughout this book allows the nurse to easily find information on a specific psychosocial problem commonly seen in practice. In addition to common psychosocial problems, psychiatric disorders are explained and discussed. Each chapter is organized to provide easy access to information on etiology, assessment, age-specific implications, nursing diagnosis and interventions, patient/family education, interdisciplinary management including pharmacology, and community based care. The fast-paced healthcare environment we are all experiencing demands quick assessment and treatment plans that are realistic, cost-effective, and outcome driving. The information contained in this book is readily applicable to all patient care settings.

Each psychosocial problem includes a section on common nurses' reactions to the patient behaviors that may result from the problem. Nurses often think they should only have acceptable and "proper" emotional reactions to their patients. Nurses may deny certain feelings and have unrealistic expectations of themselves. These factors impact how the nurse then responds to the patient's problems. The more aware the nurse becomes of how one reacts to the patient's behaviors, the easier it will be to accept one's own feelings and understand how these feelings affect the patient and influence interventions.

In this third edition we have added two new chapters that reflect concerns faced by many nurses. The Homeless Patient with Chronic Illness reflects the increasingly frequent encounters that nurses in all areas of the country are facing. Disaster Planning and Response–Psychosocial Impact provides the nurse with tools to prepare for the emotional impact of a natural or man-made disaster. Throughout this third edition we have updated information on patient safety, pharmacologic interventions, and psychiatric diagnoses and treatment. We continue to include information that will apply to the inpatient hospital setting, long-term care, and outpatient care.

We wish to thank our contributors Yoshi Arai and Margaret Mitchell who revised their chapters from the second edition. We also thank our new contributors Bill Whetstone and Carl Magnum. Particular thanks go to our editors Annette Ferrans and Joanne DaCunha of FA Davis. This was our third collaboration with Joanne and she remains a dynamic force that keeps us on track.

For those of you familiar with our earlier two editions, you will notice the name of author Marcia L. Raines, RN, PhD is missing. Marcia died in 2006 after a long illness. Marcia was the consummate nurse who strove for excellence throughout her career. She started as a psychiatric nurse, became a clinical nurse specialist, was an educator and administrator, and faculty member and chair of a university school of nursing. She inspired countless nurses over the years with her wise and gentle approach. Working with her on the previous two editions was always a joy because of her genuine love of the work and her enthusiasm to produce an outstanding book. Marcia wrote many of the original chapters from the first and second edition including chapters on anxiety, sexual dysfunction, confusion, pain, and sleep. We have strived to carry on in her memory but know the nursing world has lost a great one. This edition is dedicated to Marcia.

Linda M. Gorman
Donna F. Sultan

Contributors

Yoshinao Arai, RN, MN, CNS
Senior Mental Health Counselor, RN
Los Angeles County Department of Mental Health
Los Angeles, California

Carl Magnum, RN, MSN, PhD(c), CHS, FF
Assistant Professor of Nursing
Emergency Preparedness Coordinator
The University of Mississippi Medical Center
Jackson, Mississippi

Margaret L. Mitchell, RN, MN, MDIV, MA, CNS
Senior Mental Health Counselor, RN
Los Angeles County Department of Mental Health
Los Angeles, California

William R. Whetstone, RN, CNS, PhD
Professor, Nursing
Clinical Nurse Specialist, Adult Psychiatric Mental Health Nursing
California State University, Dominguez Hills
Carson, California

Reviewers

Michael Beach, MSN, APRN, BC, ACNP, PNP
Instructor
University of Pittsburgh
Pittsburgh, Pennsylvania

Dorie V. Beres, PhD, MSN, ANP-C
Associate Professor and Coordinator
Vitterbo University
La Crosse, Wisconsin

Earl Goldberg, EdD, APRN, BC
Assistant Professor
LaSalle University
Philadelphia, Pennsylvania

Barbara A. Jones, RN, MSN, DNSc
Professor
Gwynedd-Mercy College
Gwynedd Valley, Pennsylvania

Nancy L. Kostin, MSN, RN
Associate Professor
Madonna University
Livonia, Michigan

Karen P. Petersen, RN, CCRN, MSN
Nursing Instructor
Chemeketa Community College
Salem, Oregon

Glenda Shockley, RN, MS
Director of Nursing
Connors State College
Warner, Oklahoma

Margaret A, Wetsel, PhD, MSN
Associate Professor
Clemson University
Clemson, South Carolina

Ellen F. Wirtz, RN, MN
Faculty
Chemeketa Community College
Salem, Oregon

Contents

SECTION I– Aspects of Psychosocial Nursing

SECTION II– Commonly Encountered Problems

SECTION III– Special Topics

SECTION I   Aspects of Psychosocial Nursing

1 Introduction to Psychosocial Nursing for General Patient Care

Learning Objectives

- Define psychosocial nursing care.
- Describe the impact of patient behavior problems in a managed-care setting.
- Describe the role of patient education in psychosocial care.
- Name the resources the nurse can use when planning for patients across care settings.

Every day, nurses are confronted with patient problems and crises that fall in the realm of the psychosocial, and they must find a way to deal with them. The Agency for Healthcare Research and Quality found in 2004 that one in four stays in U.S. hospitals for patients 18 and over involved depressive, bipolar, schizophrenia, and other mental disorders or substance abuse. Nurses often must care for patients with:

- Intense emotional responses to illness
- Personality styles that make care difficult
- Psychiatric disorders
- Stresses and family problems that affect patients' reactions to illness or hospitalization

Nurses can be proficient in managing patients' physical health problems and yet be less prepared to manage emotional problems. The ability to recognize behaviors that suggest psychosocial problems and to develop skills to manage them effectively not only improves the patients' chances of healing but can also reduce frustration for nurses.

Psychosocial care emphasizes interventions to assist individuals who are having difficulty coping with the emotional aspects of illness, with life crises that affect health and health care, or with psychiatric disorders. For example, problems with depression, anger, substance abuse, or grief can influence a patient's response to illness or to the interventions of the health-care system. In psychosocial care, the nurse focuses on the effects of stress in psychological or physiological illness and on the intrapsychic and social functioning of individuals responding to stress.

The nurse has a responsibility to facilitate each patient's adaptations to his or her unique stresses by helping and supporting the person in his or her environment, level of wellness, and adjustment to the illness or condition. Identifying the patient's coping responses, maximizing strengths, and maintaining integrity will help the nurse meet this responsibility.

NURSES' POSSIBLE REACTIONS

A factor whose importance cannot be overlooked in psychosocial care is awareness of one's own reactions to patient behaviors. These reactions will influence the nurse-patient relationship, assessment findings, and selection of potential interventions. They can help or hinder the relationship. Recognizing the influence of these reactions can help the nurse to:

- Increase awareness of the reactions that influence objectivity
- Identify reactions frequently experienced by other nurses to ease feelings of guilt and resentment
- Increase understanding of colleagues' reactions to enhance the work environment
- Facilitate self-support by reducing self-criticism and reinforcing skills
- Select better assessment tools to identify patients' dilemmas and responses
- Recognize how personal reactions to patients can influence assessment, planning, and effective interventions

In coming chapters, "Possible Nurses' Reactions" will be presented as boxed text, so that you can easily find and refer to it.

THE ROLE OF PSYCHOSOCIAL NURSING IN MANAGED-CARE SETTINGS

Patients with psychosocial and psychiatric problems often require many more resources than patients without such problems. A patient's emotional reactions can increase his or her length of stay in the hospital or under a nurse's care, can contribute to the patient's not complying with care, and can drain physical and emotional resources. Once these patient problems are identified, the nurse needs to use skills to meet the patient's needs while making judicious use of available resources.

In the managed-care system, controls are exerted over access, use, quality, and effectiveness of health services. Managed care is now the dominant form of health care in the United States (Shoemaker & Varcarolis, 2006). It has led to shortened hospital stays and limitations in available resources. Outpatient programs and home health care are now being used more to address problems in place of inpatient care. To work within this system, the nurse must quickly identify the patient's needs, establish a realistic plan of care, implement interventions, and evaluate outcomes, all within a predetermined length of time. Psychosocial and psychiatric patient problems complicate the demands made on the nurse in an already stretched health-care environment and can negatively affect patient outcomes. When the nurse has skills readily at hand to identify problems and intervene effectively, patient outcomes can be improved and nurse satisfaction will be enhanced.

Managed care has also intensified the focus on outcome-based interventions to address key problems within a shorter timeframe. Clinical pathways or clinical practice guidelines are often used to drive this process. These pathways are evidence-based approaches to plans of care, and their focus is on outcomes. Psychosocial and psychiatric problems often have to be addressed to keep on target with the pathway.

PATIENT SAFETY

The incorporation of methods to improve patient safety is an important consideration for all levels of patient care today. The Joint Commission on Accreditation of Healthcare Organizations (JCAHO) has spearheaded a national movement, which includes avoiding the use of abbreviations that can be confused with one another, using universal protocol to prevent surgical error involving "wrong site, wrong procedure, and wrong person," and the development of National Patient Safety Goals (JCAHO, 2007). Psychosocial care incorporates these patient safety measures as a routine part of practice by maintaining open communication with the patient and health-care team.

LIFE SPAN ISSUES

Although each individual is unique, we all share certain patterns and common links throughout the life cycle. Psychosocial development proceeds through a series of stages and crises. Each phase of the life span presents new challenges, experiences, and problems. Many psychosocial problems have their origins in developmental crises that remain unresolved or that are resolved with negative outcomes. Problems such as depression and grief affect individuals differently in each stage of life. Childhood, adolescence, and old age are times of particular vulnerability to psychosocial dysfunction. Look for this heading in the coming chapters indicating discussions of life span issues.

Interventions in this book are geared to adults, but many of them can be adapted to the care of children. To adapt an intervention to a pediatric population, the nurse must consider children's developmental and cognitive levels, and incorporate them in the care plan as well as consult specialists in pediatrics, if necessary.

COLLABORATIVE MANAGEMENT

Our complex health-care system relies on a variety of health-care professionals to meet patients' needs. Obviously, the nurse does not work in a vacuum but must participate in the interdisciplinary team and be aware of other disciplines as resources for psychosocial intervention. The nurse also needs to know when work needs to be shared or delegated through referrals. For example, social workers may be helpful because they are often familiar with psychotherapists and community support groups for emotional problems. The nurse should be aware of agency policies regarding referrals to psychotherapists. Some may require a doctor's order.

Other resources include physicians, advanced practice nurses, pharmacists, clergy, dietitians, and others, depending on the specialty and setting. Knowing when and how to access them and work effectively with them will improve patient outcomes and enhance the working environment. Collaborative management is addressed throughout the book in terms specific to the topic discussed in each chapter.

WHEN AND WHO TO CALL FOR HELP

Many difficult, challenging situations require a number of complex skills. While continuing to gain knowledge in identifying psychosocial issues and intervening in cases in which patients require psychosocial care, nurses also need to recognize their own limitations and be able to recognize patient behaviors that may precede or currently signal a dangerous or emergency situation. Knowing when to seek out resources and who to call for help are essential factors in providing quality, cost-effective care.

When and who to call for help will also be set inside a box in coming chapters so that you can easily reference it.

PATIENT EDUCATION

Patient education is an important component of psychosocial care. Nurses are required to incorporate appropriate patient education in their practice. To provide adequate education, the nurse needs to be aware of how psychosocial issues influence learning. For example, assessing the patient's anxiety level or disturbed thoughts will influence the timing of teaching as well as the type of information the nurse tries to convey. Patient education can enhance the patient's independence and control, involvement of the patient and his or her family in the treatment plan, and help prepare the patient for possible emotional changes, coping skills needed, and responses to medications. Patient education can be influential in reducing length of stay and helping patients to take more responsibility for their own care.

Many factors can affect effective patient education, including patients' cultural beliefs and language, as well as knowledge of and access to computer technology.

CHARTING TIPS

Changes in patients' emotional responses and behaviors, and their responses to interventions and education are significant and must be noted in the medical record. The increased use of computerized documentation can present new challenges to nurses who are trying to identify and record behavioral problems succinctly.

Charting tips are given in each chapter for specific situations and are identified with a chapter heading.

COMMUNITY-BASED CARE

Many patients require care that crosses settings, for instance from hospital-based care to home nursing care. In most cases, acute hospital care is now a small part of the treatment plan and eventually ends. To ensure continuity of care, planning for the next level of care should begin as early as possible. While the patient is in the acute setting, this planning needs to begin on admission. Long-term care, outpatient rehabilitation, other outpatient programs, and home health care are now used for many patients. Nurses in all these settings must also consider planning for the next level of care.

Home health agencies may have nurses with psychiatric backgrounds on staff. Box 1–1 lists possible interventions by psychiatric home care nurses. These nurses can be helpful in evaluating patients' responses to psychotropic medications, confusion, psychotic behavior, and suicide risk. Patients may need referrals to other types of care, such as psychiatric hospitalization or convalescent care, and

---

BOX 1–1
Interventions by Psychiatric Home Care Nurses

- Crisis intervention
- Suicide risk assessment
- Management of psychiatric medications and blood level monitoring
- Administration of long-acting injectable psychiatric medications
- Counseling and education
- Assessment of patient and family coping
- Safety assessment

assistance with financial support. Other professionals such as social workers, case managers, and counselors can help ensure safe and effective home care. Other resources including support groups, hotlines, and even telemedicine increase access to care. For a patient to be eligible for psychiatric home care, usually the patient has to be homebound, have a psychiatric diagnosis, and have a need for the skills of a psychiatric nurse (Shoemaker & Varcarolis, 2006).

PATIENT PRIVACY AND RIGHT TO CONFIDENTIALITY

Patient rights are becoming increasingly emphasized in all health-care settings. These rights generally include autonomy, informed consent, treatment with dignity and respect, and confidentiality. The Health Insurance Portability and Accountability Act (HIPAA) enacted in 2003 established a number of mechanisms to maintain privacy, including the requirement that health-care professional obtain permission from the patient to share information with persons who are not directly involved in the patient's care, and that medical records be viewed only by people directly involved in patient's treatment. The American Nurses' Association Code of Ethics also requires a nurse to protect confidential information.

DSM-IV-TR

The American Psychiatric Association (APA) has developed a classification system for mental disorders. It is the most widely accepted system in the United States today and is published and revised periodically as the Diagnostic and Statistical Manual. The fourth edition was published in 1994 and is referred to as DSM-IV. In 2000, the APA published a revised version called DSM-IV-TR, meaning text revision that is also referenced in this book. These references provide clinicians with guidelines, specific criteria, and accepted terminology. Throughout this book, you will see references to the criteria published in DSM-IV and DSM-IV-TR. These criteria are used to prevent negative labeling or incorrect categorization of patient behaviors as psychiatric disorders.

OVERVIEW OF THE BOOK

Chapters 2 through 6 cover basic skills and emphasize aspects of Psychosocial Nursing including assessment and culturally sensitive care. Chapters 7 through 18 address Commonly Encountered Problems. Nursing interventions are provided for major nursing diagnoses. Chapters 19 through 21 cover Special Topics, including care of patients who belong to special populations, care in the face of disaster, and medications that the nurse may be using to manage behavioral symptoms.

Many of the topics addressed in this opening chapter appear in the coming chapters, so readers should quickly be able to discern the pattern of approach and will be able to use this book not only as a textbook but also as a reference in their future care of patients with psychosocial problems.

2 Psychosocial Response to Illness

Learning Objectives

- Describe the role of self-esteem, body image, powerlessness, and guilt in the patient's emotional response to illness.
- Describe the role of Maslow's Hierarchy of Needs in explaining a patient's response to illness.
- Define defense mechanisms and give examples of each.
- Describe commonly used coping mechanisms.

Psychological impact is present in any illness. Illness threatens the individual and evokes a wide array of emotions, such as fear, sadness, anger, depression, despair, and loss of control. Each individual who faces an illness responds differently according to personality, previous life experiences, and coping style. Extreme denial, noncompliance, aggression, and threats of suicide are some of the more maladaptive responses that the nurse may face in caring for ill individuals. Most often these responses are temporary and subside with time. However, they can also be chronic maladaptive behavioral responses that the patient uses whenever he or she experiences a stressful situation. There is often no way of knowing on first meeting a patient whether his or her response is temporary or habitual.

All behavior is an attempt to communicate needs. To determine a person's underlying motivation, identifying the need can be a first step to understanding. Maslow's Hierarchy of Needs (1954) provides a framework within which to begin examining the motivation a person may have for a behavior (Fig. 2–1). Maslow identified five levels of needs. Each type of need, starting at the most basic physiological level, must be met before one can move on to the next level.

Professional nursing uses a holistic framework by which it views the individual and his or her environment in its entirety. The influence of the mind as well as the body is recognized in the development of and response to illness. It is known that the response to stress involves the immune and neuroendocrine systems. Emotional response to stress suppresses the immune system, stimulates the cardiovascular system, and alters secretions of hormones that influence the body's response to the illness.

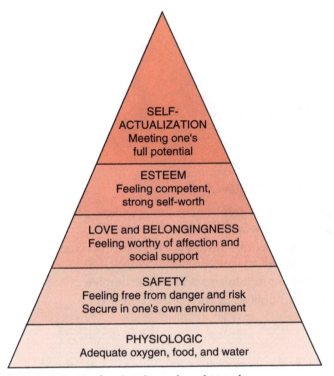

FIGURE 2–1. Maslow's Hierarchy of Needs.

Stress cannot be avoided. It is a normal part of living. It does not matter if a stressor is pleasant, such as an upcoming holiday, or unpleasant, such as illness, disability, or hospitalization. What is critical is the individual's perception of the intensity of the stressor requiring readjustment and his or her capacity to adjust to it.

KEY ISSUES IN RESPONSE TO ILLNESS

Altered Self-Esteem

Self-esteem is the individual's personal judgment of his or her own worth. The roots of self-esteem are in early parental and social relationships as well as in the person's perception of goal attainment and his or her own ideal. Maslow places self-esteem at a very high level, indicating that this need can be accomplished only when the more basic needs are fulfilled. Self-esteem increases as the individual achieves personal goals. High self-esteem indicates that the individual has accepted his or her good and bad points and knows that he or she is loved and respected by others. High self-esteem also implies a sense of control over personal destiny. Feeling good about one's self influences many aspects of life, including dealing with others, managing conflict, standing up for one's own beliefs, taking risks, and believing in one's ability to handle adversity.

Throughout life, both internal and external factors influence self-esteem. For instance, falling in love or graduating from school promotes positive self-esteem, whereas illness can represent a threat to self-esteem. Illness and disability often require a person to alter or even abandon personal goals and may strongly influence the person's view of himself or herself. Some people are able to adjust readily and create new, more realistic goals with little impact on self-esteem. Others may struggle with the changes and be unable to regain the previous level of self-esteem. Serious illnesses such as prostate or breast cancer, heart disease, or stroke not only require adaptation of personal goals but often distort the deeper sense of self. This is a major contributor to depression. But the desire to maintain a strong sense of self is a powerful drive, and over time many people adapt to changes in health.

Altered Body Image

Body image is the mental picture a person has of his or her own body. It significantly influences the way a person thinks and feels about his or her body as a whole, about its functions, and about the internal and external sensations associated with it. It also includes perceptions of the way others see the person's body and is central to self-concept and self-esteem. Often a person's belief about his or her body mirrors self-concept. This is evident when an individual seeks out cosmetic surgery to alter his or her appearance. However, when the self-concept is poor, even cosmetic surgery may not change the person's body image. This person may continue to struggle with low self-esteem even though the physical "imperfections" are changed.

A person's body image changes constantly. Illness, surgery, and weight loss or gain can have a major influence on the view of self. Amputation, colostomy, and dependence on equipment such as dialysis are examples of obvious external changes that influence body image. Some conditions such as a myocardial infarction may not cause obvious external body changes, but the individual may now view his or her body as weak or damaged. Altered body image can contribute to lowered self-esteem and, possibly, depression.

Powerlessness

Powerlessness is a perceived lack of personal control over certain events and over one's self. Individuals need to maintain a sense of power and control over their destiny and environment. Loss of this sense of control can negatively affect an individual's view of his or her effectiveness. Illness consistently forces the individual to face his or her powerlessness over a situation.

Entry into the health-care system adds to this sense of powerlessness. Now, in addition to facing the feeling of helplessness over the illness, the person is being subjected to following the orders of strangers, complying with others' schedules, and losing privacy. When an individual is hospitalized and gives up his/her clothes and puts on a hospital gown, a sense of powerlessness within this new role can occur quite quickly. Resisting a doctor's orders and even refusing pain medication suggest that the patient is attempting to maintain some sense of control and fight off feelings of powerlessness. Helping these patients to maintain some sense of power and control is an important nursing intervention. Individuals who chronically view themselves as helpless may be more prone to depression and vulnerable to victimization by others who try to control them.

Loss

Actual or potential loss is any situation in which something a person values is rendered or threatened to be rendered inaccessible. Loss occurs throughout life as we experience changes in relationships, inability to reach an expected goal, and disappointment in others. Any time we have an emotional investment in someone or something, we are vulnerable to losing it. This includes loss of a body part or body function. All losses in life can contribute to loss of hopes, dreams, and goals and require some period of grieving as the individual adapts to the new situation. The degree of response to the loss depends on the amount of value the individual places on whatever is lost. Eventually the individual will go on to develop new attachments and goals. Maladaptive responses to loss can include anger, guilt, depression, and, possibly, suicidal thoughts.

Hopelessness

Hope is fundamental to life. No matter how bad the situation may be, the ability to hope for improvement will help an individual get through it. Hopelessness is the sustained subjective state in which an individual sees no alternatives or personal choices available to solve problems or to achieve desired goals. Lack of hope can develop from an overwhelming loss of control and is related to a sense of despair, helplessness, apathy, and depression.

The person without hope is unable to mobilize enough energy to even establish personal goals and may be unable to recognize or accept help or new ideas. Serious illness alone usually does not cause hopelessness. Usually deep personal feelings of loss, depleted emotional reserves, and an overwhelming sense of powerlessness also contribute. To regain a sense of hope, the individual needs to view the situation differently, alter negative goals and expectations, and, possibly, create new ones. For example, a terminally ill patient, rather than hoping to cure the illness, may need to refocus on achieving a pain-free state or making contact with family members. For some individuals, hopelessness can lead to discovery of alternatives that will add meaning and purpose to life. Spiritual crises may be related to hopelessness as well.

Guilt

Guilt is self-blame and regret for some real or perceived action. It is a painful emotion that can negatively influence feelings, behaviors, and relationships with others. Conflicts within relationships can occur when an individual feels guilty about resentment that his or her needs are not being met.

Nurses frequently observe behavior in patients or their families that seems to be motivated by guilt. Family members may display guilt behaviors when they suddenly become very involved in the care of an ill patient they have not seen in years. Examples of this may include hovering over this patient or making numerous demands on the staff. Self-blame is another frequent behavior motivated by guilt. For example, a wife may blame herself for not taking her husband to the doctor sooner or a patient may blame himself for the stress his illness is causing his wife. Survivor guilt is often seen in people who survive traumatic events in which others are killed or injured.

Anxiety

Anxiety is a universal, primitive, unpleasant feeling of tension and apprehension. It may be an early warning signal of possible danger. Anxiety is an important motivator of behavior that makes people act or change to reduce the uncomfortable feelings of tension. Low to moderate levels of anxiety can enhance learning and action. More severe anxiety may be reduced by using defense or coping mechanisms as the unconscious self tries to protect us from this discomfort.

DEFENSE MECHANISMS

Defense mechanisms protect the individual from threats, feelings of inadequacy, and unacceptable feelings or thoughts. They are unconscious mental processes used to reduce anxiety and conflict by modifying, distorting, and rejecting reality (Table 2–1). Because they are unconscious, the individual is not aware of how these mechanisms affect thoughts, feelings, and behavior. In some ways, they are used to alter reality to make the situation more acceptable. Without these mechanisms, the threatening feelings might overwhelm and paralyze the individual and interfere with daily living. Essential, adaptive defense mechanisms help to lower anxiety so that goals can be achieved. We could not survive without them. However, when they are used too extensively, they can contribute to highly distorted perceptions and interfere with normal functioning and interpersonal relationships. Excessively distorted defense mechanisms can be characterized as psychiatric disorders.

An individual's repertoire of defense mechanisms is learned through childhood experiences. Each time a defense mechanism reduces uncomfortable anxiety feelings, it provides positive reinforcement.

COPING MECHANISMS

Coping mechanisms are usually conscious methods that the individual uses to overcome a problem or stressor. They are learned adaptive or maladaptive responses to anxiety based on problem-solving, and they may lead to changed behavior. They involve higher levels of emotional and ego development than defense mechanisms. However, overuse of coping mechanisms such as overeating or smoking can create problems. In addition, unconscious mechanisms can also play a role in using or selecting a specific coping mechanism. Inappropriate

TABLE 2–1
Common Defense Mechanisms

Defense Mechanism	Definition	Example
Denial	Attempt to remove an experience or a feeling from consciousness	After a diagnosis of terminal condition, the patient does not exhibit any expected emotional reaction and states that diagnosis is not true.
Displacement	The belief that one would be in great danger if true feelings about someone were known to that person, which causes the individual to discharge or displace feelings onto a third person or object	A family member is angry at the patient for not taking better care of himself and feels too guilty to express this to the ill person. Instead, he expresses anger at the nursing staff for giving inadequate care.
Identification	Accepting the other person's circumstances as though they were one's own	A man's wife died a very painful death from cancer. When he is diagnosed with cancer, he experiences extreme anxiety because he has accepted his wife's experiences as if he had lived them.
Intellectualization	Separating emotion from an idea or thought because emotionally it is too painful	A patient discusses the physiology of his leukemia at length without any emotional reaction.
Isolation	Blocking out feelings associated with an unpleasant or threatening situation or thought	A nurse caring for a critically ill patient who is the same age provides care without experiencing the emotions related to tragedy of the patient's situation.

Defense Mechanism	Definition	Example
Projection	Transferring or blaming others for one's own unacceptable ideas, impulses, wishes, or feelings	After a myocardial infarction, a patient relates that his wife is coping poorly with his condition. This patient's anxiety may be too great and threatening to face, so he places his own fears onto his wife.
Rationalization	Substituting acceptable reasons for the true reasons for personal behavior because admitting true reasons is too threatening	Smoker continues to smoke despite physician's warning because he knows many people who smoke and have no ill effects.
Reaction formation	Actions that are opposite of the true, unacceptable feelings that the person is experiencing	A woman has negative feelings about her pregnancy but then lavishes constant attention on her newborn.
Regression	Reverting to earlier patterns of development as a way to reduce anxiety and demands on one's self	During serious illness, a patient exhibits behavior more appropriate for a younger developmental age, such as excessive dependency.
Repression	Forcibly dismissing unacceptable thoughts, feelings, impulses, or memories from consciousness	A person is unable to recall feelings of hostility toward a sibling or specific memories from childhood.
Sublimation	Expressing repressed urges or desires in socially acceptable ways	An angry person writes a poem about his reactions to his feelings.

coping mechanisms can be readily changed because the patient is usually aware of using them.

Some common coping mechanisms include:

- Talking problems out with others and gaining new insights by other people's view or approach to the problem
- Expressing intense emotion by crying, yelling, or laughing

- Seeking comfort from friends, favorite foods, cigarettes, treasured objects, or consciousness-altering substances
- Using humor to discharge tension in a way that avoids fully acknowledging a difficult situation
- Exercising or performing manual labor to relieve tension
- Problem-solving using a series of strategies and step-by-step approaches to the resolution of a problem
- Sleeping to avoid problems or escape
- Avoiding upsetting situations, for example, by feigning illness, to avoid a confrontation

CONCLUSION

Nurses will encounter in their patients a wide range of psychosocial responses to illness.

Understanding these types of responses and knowing what to expect can help the nurses to better care for their patients.

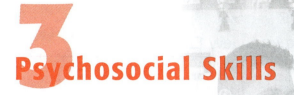

3 Psychosocial Skills

Learning Objectives

- Describe the key components of a psychosocial assessment.
- Describe how and when to use a mental status examination.
- List the forms of therapeutic communication.
- Describe the impact of the psychosocial skills of role modeling, role playing, and acceptance.

Providing psychosocial care requires a combination of astute psychosocial assessment skills, experience in performing mental status examinations, and using therapeutic communication.

PSYCHOSOCIAL NURSING ASSESSMENT

To develop a thorough nursing diagnosis as well as goals and interventions, psychosocial information must be part of every patient assessment. The presence of psychosocial problems in a patient has an influence on the diagnosis arrived at and on the course of treatment chosen. With a thorough assessment, the nurse can determine the patient's needs, problems, and potential problems, and identify patients who are at a higher risk for developing more serious problems. Information to be gathered in a psychosocial assessment includes the patient's socio-cultural background, emotional and biologic aspects of current problems, history, spiritual and philosophical beliefs, and family issues.

To perform a thorough psychosocial assessment, the nurse uses many skills. The first is the ability to establish a rapport with the patient. Showing an interest in what the patient is saying, asking appropriate questions, and making observations help to put the patient at ease and enable him or her to divulge personal information. Box 3–1 offers suggestions for creating an appropriate interview environment.

The psychosocial assessment focuses on the effect of the illness on the patient and family rather than on physical symptoms. This assessment begins the process of identifying key nursing diagnoses. In addition, it provides important information for the patient's treatment plan. The assessment should include the following:

BOX 3–1
Creating an Appropriate Interview Environment

- Create a quiet, private space.
- Minimize interruptions if possible.
- Maintain appropriate eye contact.
- Sit at eye level with the patient.
- Ask open-ended questions to encourage the patient to talk.
- Avoid writing a lot of notes during the interview.
- Demonstrate an interest in the patient's concerns.
- Ask the patient's permission to be interviewed.
- Indicate acceptance of the patient by avoiding criticism, frowning, or demonstrating shock.
- Avoid asking more personal questions than are actually needed.
- Determine whether the family can provide information if the patient is unable to communicate.
- Maintain confidentiality.
- Be aware of your own biases and discomforts that could influence the assessment.
- Keep the focus on the patient.

Lifestyle information: Determine whom the patient lives with as well as the patient's significant relationships, available support people, marital status, occupation, religion, and other important components of the patient's lifestyle.

Normal coping patterns: Identify which coping mechanisms the patient uses when under stress and which he or she used during past illnesses or hospitalizations. Questions that can be asked include the following: What happened the last time the patient was under severe stress? How is the patient currently coping? What helps in stressful situations?

Understanding of current illness: Ask the patient about his or her understanding of the diagnosis or reason for seeking medical attention. Determine how the patient views the illness affecting his or her life.

Personality style: After interacting with the patient, identify any important personality traits that may affect his or her care or compliance, such as a tendency to be dependent, hostile, dramatic, or critical.

History of psychiatric disorder: If the patient is currently taking medications for psychiatric problems, be sure to ask why he or she is taking them. Consider asking if the patient has experienced any psychiatric symptoms, such as depression. If his or her behavior indicates a psychiatric disorder, explore this further. Have a list of screening questions for alcohol use if needed (see Box 13–1).

Recent life changes or stressors: Determine if there have been any major changes or traumatic events recently (especially in the last year). Keep in mind that these changes may be both positive and negative, such as moving to a new house or area, a death in the family, a job or role change, or recent birth of a child.

Spirituality: Determine the role of spirituality and religion. Use of the HOPE assessment includes questions as follows: H–sources of hope, strength, comfort; O–Role of organized religion for patient's P–personal spirituality practices; and E–effects on medical care and end of life decisions (Anandarajah & Hight, 2001).

Major issues raised by current illness: Determine how this illness has affected the patient's lifestyle or sense of self, including areas such as self-esteem, body image, loss of intimacy, role changes, and change in family dynamics.

Mental status examination: Perform the mental status examination to help identify dysfunction in emotional, cognitive, or behavioral spheres.

THE MENTAL STATUS EXAMINATION

The mental status examination is used to determine whether or not there are abnormalities in the patient's thinking and reasoning ability, feelings, or behavior. It is fundamental in all areas of medicine (Varcarolis, 2006). Nurses often perform quick mental status examinations every time they see their patients without realizing they are doing it. Changes in a patient's appearance, memory, emotions, or thinking can be observed while the nurse is making quick rounds or having a social conversation with the patient. A more formal mental status examination can be part of a psychosocial assessment in a new patient, or it may be done when changes in the patient's condition are seen.

The mental status examination includes observations and questions in the following categories: appearance, behavior, and speech; thoughts; mood and affect; ability to perform abstract reasoning; memory; intelligence; concentration; orientation; judgment; and insight (Table 3–1 and Fig. 3–1).

To gather a comprehensive evaluation, review all the categories of the examination. Congruence or discrepancies between sections may reveal important information. Note inappropriate responses as well as the absence of the usual anticipated responses. For example, a patient may relate that the physician says her cancer has metastasized too much to consider surgery (thought). This clear and coherent thought, expressed in a droning, monotonous voice (speech) without any apparent intensity, distress, or expression of emotion (mood) may suggest that the patient is denying her illness. A patient who is experiencing an extreme stress response to his or her illness may be unable to verbalize any expected concerns (thoughts) but may become increasingly anxious or depressed (mood and/or emotions) with increasing restlessness (behavior). Choosing an

TABLE 3–1

Mental Status Examination and Related Definitions

Category	Description	Related Definitions
Appearance	Describe what patient looks like including dress, posture, grooming.	
Behavior	Describe behavior, motor activity, mannerisms.	*Catatonic:* Remaining totally immobile *Posturing:* Assuming inappropriate or bizarre positions *Compulsions:* Insistent, repetitive unwanted actions
Speech	Describe how patient speaks; list barriers to communication.	*Perseveration:* Mechanical repetition or words, thoughts *Pressured:* Highly accelerated rapid speech *Loose associations:* Absence of logical connections between thoughts *Flight of ideas:* Rapidly jumping from one thought to another with minimal links *Tangential:* Talking around main point *Word salad:* Unconnected words and phrases without meaning or logic *Thought blocking:* Stopping suddenly in the middle of verbalizing a thought and staring into space *Neologism:* Making up new words only speaker understands

Category	Description	Related Definitions
Mood/affect	Describe the emotions that are apparent from facial expressions, motor behavior, words used.	*Labile:* Emotions that change quickly and unpredictably *Flat affect:* No demonstration of any feeling *Blunted affect:* Constricted display of emotions *Anhedonia:* Absence of any pleasure *Inappropriate affect:* Emotions displayed not fitting with topic discussed *Ambivalence:* Contradictory feelings experienced simultaneously
Thoughts	What are themes in conversation? Does patient make sense? Is patient preoccupied with certain thoughts?	*Hallucinations:* Sensory perceptions (auditory, visual, gustatory, olfactory, tactile) without external stimuli, e.g., hearing nonexistent voices. *Illusions:* Misinterpretations of real external sensory stimuli, e.g., seeing a ghost in a shadow *Delusions:* False, fixed beliefs not alterable by logical explanations *Obsessions:* Unwanted, distressing recurring thoughts *Phobia:* Irrational fear of a specific situation, accompanied by avoidance of the phenomenon feared *Depersonalization:* Sense of not being real; sense of being detached from one's body or self *Magical thinking:* Believing that thinking about something happening is the same as doing it

Continued

TABLE 3–1

Mental Status Examination and Related Definitions—*cont'd*

Category	Description	Related Definitions
		Grandiosity: Exaggerated beliefs in own worth and/or abilities *Paranoia:* Unwarranted belief that others have harmful intentions to person
Ability to abstract	Describe the patient's ability to define similarities between objects or explain a proverb.	*Concrete description:* See objects in very definite simple ways, e.g., sees an apple and an orange as "round" rather than the overall category "fruit" *Abstract ability:* Can generalize the meaning of a concept and find meaning in symbols, e.g., "still water runs deep" means that quiet people have depth rather than lakes are deep bodies of water
Memory	Describe patient's ability to repeat the names of 3 objects immediately after being told and again in 5 minutes.	
Intelligence	Describe patient's level of knowledge, language, understanding of instructions.	
Concentration	Describe patient's ability to focus on a single thought without becoming distracted.	*Serial 7s:* Test to determine the patient's ability to concentrate by having him or her continually subtract from 100 by 7 (93, 86, etc.)

Category	Description	Related Definitions
Orientation	Describe patient's awareness of person and surroundings. A person is fully oriented when he or she is aware of person, place, time and situation.	*Orientation to person:* Knows his or her name *Orientation to place:* Knows where he or she is (Ask for specific location.) *Orientation to time:* Knows the date, day of week, year; most serious impairment is if the patient cannot identify year *Orientation to situation:* Knows what is wrong with him or her, why he or she is receiving care, the circumstances of current situation
Judgment	Describe patient's ability to use common sense to make reasonable decisions.	
Insight	Determine patient's understanding of factors contributing to his or her condition.	

appropriate nursing diagnosis will depend on integrating all these observations along with knowledge of the patient's usual responses to stress.

Changes in mental status are often caused by alterations in the psychological or physical state. For example, behavioral changes such as confusion, depression, delirium, or even psychosis may be signs of drug toxicity, electrolyte imbalance, or intracranial bleeding (Table 3–2).

THERAPEUTIC COMMUNICATION

Therapeutic communication, the essence of the helping relationship, occurs when the nurse communicates with the patient in a manner that facilitates acquiring information about and understanding of the patient's concerns and problems. It is the art of reaching a person by means of verbal and nonverbal messages. Acceptance, respect, honesty, trust, concern, protection, and support must all be present for communication to be therapeutic. Therapeutic communication allows the patient to share feelings, feel accepted, and look at problems from a new perspective. It should not be confused with counseling, which focuses on interpreta-

Mental Status Examination Answer Sheet

Circle the correct words or fill in the blanks.

Appearance
Neat   clean   disheveled   poor grooming   erect posture
good eye contact   inappropriate makeup _____

Behavior
Calm   appropriate   restless   agitated   compulsions
unusual actions _____

Speech
Appropriate   pressured   loose association   loud
soft   mute   _____

Mood
Appropriate   labile   flat   depressed   worried
anxious   angry   hopeless _____

Thoughts
Appropriate   low self-esteem   suicidal ideations   hallucinations
delusions   phobias _____

Ability to abstract
Impaired   Yes   No

Memory
Impaired recent memory   Yes   No
Impaired past memory   Yes   No
Number of objects able to remember after 5 minutes _____

Estmated intelligence
Below average   average   above average

Concentration
Able to focus   easily distractible _____
Able to subtract backwards by 7's from 100 correctly until the number _____

Orientation
Person _____ Time   _____
Place   _____ Situation _____

Judgment
Realistic decision-making   Yes   No

Insight
Good   fair   poor

Summary of Impressions:

FIGURE 3–1. Mental Status Examination Answer Sheet.

tion and the process of communication rather than the content. The patient should also be able to expect that confidentiality will be maintained (Tables 3–3 and 3–4).

TABLE 3–2

Mental Status Changes Caused By Electrolyte Imbalance

Electrolyte Imbalance	Possible Cause	Mental Status Changes
Calcium (Blood Level: 8.5–10.5 mg/dL)		
Hypercalcemia	Hyperparathyroidism Bone metastasis (breast, lung cancer)	Loss of energy Depression Confusion Lethargy
Hypocalcemia	Hypoparathyroidism due to calcium defi- ciency, lack of dietary vitamin D, or iatrogenic causes	Reduced concentra- tion and intellectual function Emotional lability Depression Psychosis (if surgical excision of a parathy- roid gland) Irritability Seizures
Sodium (Blood Level: 135–145 mEq/L)		
Hypernatremia	Dehydration caused by excessive water loss (diarrhea, vom- iting, diuresis) Restricted fluid intake Diabetes insipidus	Irritability Hallucinations Hyperactive intellectual function Stupor
Hyponatremia	Severe dietary sodium restriction Addison's disease Excessive water intake SIADH (syndrome inappropriate anti- diuretic hormone)	Depression Lethargy Withdrawal Anorexia

Continued

TABLE 3–2

Mental Status Changes Caused By Electrolyte Imbalance—*cont'd*

Electrolyte Imbalance	Possible Cause	Mental Status Changes
Phosphorus (Blood Level: 2.6–4.5 mg/dL)		
Hypophosphatemia	Gram-negative septicemia Alcohol withdrawal Intravenous hyperalimentation Low dietary intake	Apprehension Irritability Numbness Stupor
Potassium (Blood Level: 3.5–5 mEq/L)		
Hyperkalemia	Renal disease Potassium-sparing diuretics Increased IV intake	Weakness Dysphagia
Hypokalemia	Renal disease Cushing's syndrome Potassium-wasting diuretics Vomiting Diarrhea	Mood and personality change Tearfulness Hopeless Helplessness Fatigue
Base Bicarbonate (Blood Level: 24 mEq/L, pH 7.38)		
Alkalosis	Prolonged vomiting Status asthmaticus Renal failure Diabetes mellitus with ketosis	Decreased intellectual function Drowsiness Confusion Delirium

Source: Adapted from Barry, P. (1989). *Psychosocial nursing assessment and intervention* (3rd ed). Philadelphia: Lippincott-Raven; Mulvey, M. A. (2004). Fluid and electrolytes: balance and distribution. In S. C. Smeltzer & B. G. Bare (Eds.), *Brunner & Suddarth's textbook of medical-surgical nursing* (10th ed) (pp. 249–294). Philadelphia: Lippincott Williams & Wilkins.

Because nonverbal language is such a major part of any communication, the nurse needs to be aware of how his or her body language may enhance or inhibit therapeutic communication. Studies consistently support the concept that the way in which we communicate is much more powerful than the content of our words. Nonverbal communication includes eye contact, body movements, facial expressions, gestures, and posture. Facial expressions are probably one of the most important sources of communication. Posture can communicate interest, tension, or boredom. A person's walk can convey anxiety or confidence. Eye contact can be comforting and supportive or invasive and threatening. Gestures such

TABLE 3–3

Therapeutic Communication Techniques

Technique	Definition	Example
Empathy	The helper becomes keenly attuned to the patient's feelings to understand them fully while maintaining a sense of one's own separateness	In response to a patient's recounting the recent loss of a baby, the nurse says, "You must have felt very disappointed."
Open-ended questions	Questions structured to encourage the patient to share information and feelings	"How did you feel when the doctor told you of your diagnosis?"
Closed-ended questions	Information-gathering questions that require only a one-word or very brief answer	"Where does it hurt?"
Active listening	Accepting what the speaker has said, analyzing it, and reflecting back your understanding of what was heard	"From what I understand, you are planning to stop coming to counseling."
Clarification	Increasing the understanding of what the patient is trying to communicate	"I'm not sure I understand what happened next. Could you go over it again?"
Silence	Allowing time for the patient to gather thoughts and ponder a topic without interruption (This can communicate acceptance and concern.)	
Reflection	Verbally giving back the feeling part of the patient's communication to help focus on the feeling tone	"You sound very worried about the test results."

Continued

TABLE 3–3

Therapeutic Communication Techniques—*cont'd*

Technique	Definition	Example
Nonverbal communication	Overt behavior that indicates listening and attention	Maintaining eye contact, leaning forward, keeping facial expressions appropriate for the emotions being expressed, keeping a comfortable distance.
Congruent communication	Body language, facial expression, and verbal content all expressing the same thing	Nurse's physical appearance, voice, and emotional reaction all communicate that she or he is listening, accepting, concerned, and understanding.

as placing a hand on the patient's arm during intense emotions can be very supportive, especially in contrast to standing away from the patient with your arms crossed in a judgmental way.

OTHER PSYCHOSOCIAL SKILLS

In addition to therapeutic communication, nurses use a variety of other skills to help patients find new ways of coping with illness and the problems it causes. Many of these skills are used without the nurse's even being aware of using them. Perfecting the following techniques can greatly enhance your ability to meet the psychosocial needs of your patients.

Acceptance: Demonstrating an interest in a patient's behavior and feelings communicates to the patient that he or she is valued. You can demonstrate acceptance of the patient by listening to him or her even if you disagree with the ideas being communicated. It is important not to criticize or judge the patient. Acceptance reinforces self-esteem.

Reassurance: Providing support by giving your attention to matters that are important to the patient reinforces emotional security and helps reduce the patient's anxiety. With less anxiety to deal with, the patient can spend more time on effective problem solving and healing. However, nurses should

TABLE 3–4
Barriers to Therapeutic Communication

Technique	Possible Result	Example
Giving advice	Inhibits communication and sharing feelings. Patient may think you are not listening.	"You should go back to school."
False reassurances	May communicate that you do not fully understand the patient's feelings.	"I'm sure you'll do just fine."
Judgmental	Patient will sense your disapproval.	"How can you still smoke when your husband has lung cancer?"
Leading statements	Inhibits communication by possibly imposing feelings on the patient that he or she may not have.	"I'm sure you must have felt depressed after the divorce."
Multiple questions	Patient may not know what to answer first.	"Whom do you live with? Is that the way you want to live?"
Why question	May inhibit communication by threatening the patient. Often we may not know why we do the things we do or feel the way we do.	"Why do you feel that way?"
Parroting	Continually repeating what the patient says may appear to be too mechanical and frustrate the patient.	*Patient:* "I'm worried about the test results." *Nurse:* "You're worried about the test results?"

avoid giving false reassurance. If something unexpected occurs after the nurse has reassured the patient, for instance, that everything will be all right, it can reinforce a sense of distrust in the nurse.

Enhancing self-esteem: Increased self-esteem gives the patient a sense of control and hope. This will help reduce anxiety and give the patient more time for problem solving and healing. Techniques to reinforce positive self-esteem include focusing on patient's positive traits and accomplishments, providing opportunities for the patient to demonstrate skills and abilities successfully, and providing emotional support and reassurance.

Expression of feelings: Providing an environment in which a patient can feel safe and comfortable to express emotions, including sorrow or anger, and to verbalize disagreement, fear, and disappointment is essential for both enhancing a therapeutic relationship and allowing the patient to solve problems.

Role modeling: The nurse can exhibit more socially acceptable ways of performing a certain role or demonstrating a certain behavior. When the patient sees how effective these behaviors are, he or she can more easily understand how to use them and emulate the behaviors. For example, the nurse can communicate assertively with a family member who may be intimidating the patient. When the patient sees how that family member responds to assertive behavior, he or she may adopt that method of interaction. The nurse also provides a role model for adopting a healthy lifestyle by eating healthy foods, exercising, and not smoking.

Role playing: Role playing is acting out other methods of response to a situation. It can be done to increase one's own or another's understanding of the other's point of view or to practice appropriate responses, such as assertiveness. This is done with a supportive person playing the part of someone you want to communicate with in a new way.

Stress management: Accepting stress as a fact of life and managing it using specific, tested techniques can reduce feelings of anxiety. The techniques are meant to promote a feeling of calm and a sense of control over the situation. Common stress management techniques include physical interventions such as taking deep breaths, exercising, and avoiding caffeine and psychological interventions such as counting to 10, avoiding additional stressors, maintaining a positive attitude, and seeking out emotional support.

Assertiveness: Assertiveness is the use of behavioral techniques that allow the individual to stand up for his or her rights without infringing on the rights of others. To gain expertise in using assertive behavior, role-playing, and practicing with others is useful. You may try role-playing assertive responses to common situations in a supportive environment, such as asking for a refund or telling a colleague that you are not satisfied with the quality of work performed.

Limit setting: Limit setting is a form of behavior modification rather than a punishment and is used for times when acceptance of the patient's behavior is no longer appropriate. To set limits on behavior, you need to clearly define the desired behaviors and the consequences of not conforming to them. Then you must be prepared to follow through with the stated consequences. If appropriate limits are not set to control the patient's inappropriate behavior, it can escalate and possibly lead to injury and resentment from those who feel manipulated by the patient. Setting limits may be required to ensure patient safety (Manos & Braun, 2006).

De-escalation: De-escalation techniques are also used to reduce anxiety and slow down the emotional response to it, such as aggressive behavior. Useful techniques include removing the patient from volatile situations and using appropriate medication and physical restraints.

Confrontation: At times it is necessary to make direct statements that challenge the patient's behavior or beliefs. Confrontation is a verbal message designed to help the other person recognize inconsistencies or inappropriate behavior. It can assist the patient in gaining insight. However, it can also be so threatening that it could precipitate a crisis situation, so be sure to consult with specialists before using this method.

Empathy: Communicating an understanding of how the client feels indicates that the nurse shares the feelings. Empathy differs from sympathy in that empathy does not indicate sharing of personal feelings.

Silence: Sometimes saying nothing for a few moments can communicate more than words. This can convey support, acceptance, and concern and give the patient time to compose himself or herself.

Relaxation techniques: The nurse can use a variety of techniques, including deep breathing, imagery, and muscle relaxation. See Box 3–2 for more details.

ASSESSING USE OF COMPLEMENTARY AND ALTERNATIVE THERAPIES

Americans are using complementary and alternative therapies in increasing numbers. The National Center for Complementary and Alternative Medicine (NCCAM) reports that more than one third of U.S. adults uses complementary and alternative medicine (2004). The federal government established NCCAM (nccam.nih.gov) as a clearinghouse for information on products so consumers and health-care professionals can easily access the latest scientific and medical literature on the various substances. The American Hospital Association (2005) reports that to meet this growing need, the number of hospitals with complementary and alternative medicine programs doubled between 1999 and 2005. Complementary approaches are defined as those used in addition to conventional treatment. Alternative ones are used in place of conventional therapies. See Box 3–3 for a listing of commonly used approaches. Many of these are used to treat emotional problems such as anxiety and depression.

BOX 3–2
Relaxation Techniques

Relaxation techniques can include any of the following:

- *Deep Breathing:* Take in several slow deep breaths by inhaling through your nose and exhaling slowly through your mouth. As you exhale, focus on relaxing your shoulders. Each time you take a deep breath, repeat a calming word to yourself such as "peace" or "one."
- *Muscle Relaxation:* After taking two slow deep breaths, raise your shoulders for 2 to 3 seconds and then let go. Do this two to three times. Then make a fist, hold it for 2 to 3 seconds, and then let go. Each time you let go, think of another part of your body becoming more relaxed. Imagine yourself going limp like a rag doll. You can continue to tense and relax other muscle groups in your body.
- *Imagery:* After taking several slow deep breaths and relaxing your muscles, create a pleasant image in your mind that you associate with relaxation. It can be a comforting memory or an image such as a garden or floating on a raft in the sunshine. Let your mind wander to whatever you find relaxing.

  Tips on enhancing relaxation:
- Create a quiet environment.
- Sit in a comfortable chair.
- Give yourself permission to take this time for yourself.
- Devote enough time for practice.
- Every time your mind wanders to distracting thoughts, focus on your breathing.
- Practice regularly (relaxation is not always easy and often must become a learned skill).
- Consider the use of audio or video tapes or downloadable sources of relaxation information

BOX 3–3
Complementary and Alternative Approaches

Acupressure—Using massage on traditional acupuncture points.

Acupuncture—Using thin needles at designated points along meridians to balance the flow of energy. Used to treat uncomfortable symptoms and some conditions.

Alternative nutrition—Use of food to heal and maintain optimal health (e.g., macrobiotic diet).

Aromatherapy—Therapeutic use of odors from plant oils to treat illness and promote relaxation.

Biofeedback—Using electrical devices to record changes in body function to achieve relaxation and/or muscle control.

Chelation therapy—Investigational therapy using the man-made amino acid, EDTA, to treat some conditions like heart disease

Chiropractic—Form of healthcare that focuses on the relationship between body structure–primarily the spine–and function

Energy medicine—Use of energy fields such as magnetic fields or biofields (energy fields that some believe surround and penetrate the human body).

Folk remedies—Alternative health practices and therapies based on health beliefs and practices within cultural groups.

Guided imagery—Using the conscious mind to create images to evoke physiological changes and promote healing and relaxation.

Healing touch—Healing method based on concept of human energy fields.

Herbal medicine—Use of plants for healing purposes.

Homeopathy—Therapy based on concept of "like cures like." Uses minute amounts of drug that normally would produce the same symptoms as the illness being treated.

Hypnotherapy—Creating a state of heightened awareness in which suggestions to improve health are made and are likely to be followed.

Light therapy—Use of alternative light (e.g., colored light, ultraviolet light) to treat various disorders.

Magnet therapy—Using electromagnetic frequencies emitting from the body to treat illness.

Massage—Manipulation of tissues and muscles to promote relaxation and healing.

Megavitamin therapy—Using higher doses of vitamins than usually recommended to prevent or cure illness.

Meditation—Ancient art of focusing one's attention on a single sound or image to promote relaxation and health.

Naturopathy—A system of healing that views disease as a manifestation of alternation in processes that interfere with the body's healing

Reiki—A form of energy medicine where practitioner through his/her hands transmits life force energy (Ki) for healing

Yoga—A philosophy and exercise system that combines movement and positions to promote health.

Source: National Center for Complementary and Alternative Medicine. Available at nccam.nih.gov

Health-care professionals need to incorporate assessment of complementary and alternative therapies in their care. Eisenberg (1998) found that fewer than 40 percent of patients tell their health-care provider about products they are using. Patients often do not tell their provider that they are using herbs or megavitamins because they believe the products are harmless or think their health-care provider will discourage the use of such products.

The Food and Drug Administration now tracks the adverse drug reactions of herbal products, and the public needs to be aware of possible drug interactions or negative effects. Impurities, lack of regulation in dosing, and lack of knowledge about interactions with other prescribed medications can create complications. For example, St. John's wort, which is often used for depression, interacts with some HIV protease inhibitors, making them less effective.

The increased use of these herbal products reflects the public's wish for more control, incorporation of cultural values, and hope in their care. Nurses, as patient advocates, need to be sensitive to these approaches and incorporate them in the plan of care when possible. Routine questions about use of herbs and supplements should be part of the routine nursing assessment.

4

Nurses' Responses to Difficult Patient Behaviors

Learning Objectives

- List qualities expected in a "good" patient.
- Describe how the concept of a "difficult patient" reflects both the patient's behavior and the nurse's interpretation of that behavior.
- Identify the process of evaluating what patients may be communicating by difficult behavior.
- List types of nurses' responses that may impair awareness of the dynamics of problematic patient behavior.
- List resources available in most health-care agencies for psychosocial support.

Nurses often see patients behaving at their worst. Fear, stress, pain, and other discomforts all contribute to patients not being at their best, and the nurse is frequently dealing with these responses. The nurse-patient relationships may change as the patient's health-care needs change, requiring different types of involvement. Optimally, each nurse should respond positively to each patient, but human nature makes that all but impossible. The next best strategy, then, is to learn the most effective ways to deal with patients who are "difficult," usually defined by the amount of trouble and distress that the staff experiences in managing them.

Manos and Braun (2006) define the difficult patient as one whose behavior is an obstacle to the provision of good nursing care. These patients often exhibit problem behaviors such as anger, regression, and out-of-control or manipulative behaviors (Fincannon, 1995). Nursing interventions may make the problem worse if staff members are unable to differentiate their responses to the behavior from their response to the person. If you think of these patients as having "difficult-to-care-for behaviors" rather than as being "difficult patients," you may find that your frustration and also the staff's frustration decreases and more effective care strategies can be identified. Sometimes the patient uses objectionable behaviors, with or without being aware of it, to regain personal equilibrium and to reduce anxiety and fears and maintain control. Thus, although these behaviors may cause stress for the staff, they work "just fine" for the patient. In addition, some patients are totally unaware that they are affecting the staff negatively. Nurses who learn effective skills to deal with these problem behaviors may experience a sense of enhanced competence, and improved patient outcomes will follow.

NURSE-PATIENT INTERACTIONS

The nurse-patient interaction is based on the continuous flow of communication between the nurse and patient with input from both. The nurse's therapeutic use of self is the basic tool that enhances the interaction. Communication skills, an awareness of how personal responses can influence the patient, and a good knowledge base combine to enhance a positive nurse-patient interaction.

Difficult patient behaviors can negatively influence the nurse-patient interaction and, possibly, the quality of nursing care. Whenever a relationship is disrupted, the nurse needs to identify the source of the problem. Does it originate in the patient, in the nurse, or in both? For example, a demanding patient who constantly rings the call bell may be communicating the fear that she will not recover and is seeking reassurance that someone will respond if she needs it. If the nurse interprets this behavior to mean that the patient feels that the nurse is doing his or her job poorly, he or she may become resentful and angry. The nurse needs to assess the situation objectively to determine if the patient is truly looking for reassurance or if the nurse is just not as tolerant as usual because of the workload. Responding without assessing the situation could inhibit favorable nurse-patient interactions and negatively affect the patient's outcome. To be effective, the nurse must treat the behaviors as symptoms and assess their cause. The nurse needs to explore his or her own attitudes and reactions, which may be unwittingly initiating or perpetuating the undesired behavior. Better understanding can lead to a greater acceptance of both the patient's and the nurse's feelings to create a more positive cycle of nurse-patient interactions. Table 4–1 compares the ways in which assessment and appropriate interventions can significantly alter patient outcomes.

Sometimes the only effective way to change a patient's behavior is for the nurse to change his or her response. If there is still no resolution of the situation, the nurse should seek the advice or interventions of other available resources to help understand the patient's behavior and the nurse's response to it, and then select more effective interventions. If the patient continues to manifest difficult behaviors despite all efforts, the nurse should focus on self-awareness to remain objective.

ROLE EXPECTATIONS

Clarifying the nurse's intertwining role expectations of the patient in the sick role and himself or herself as the helper can provide a useful perspective. Keep in mind that nurses have chosen their roles as helpers but most patients have not deliberately chosen to become patients. A nurse may have chosen this profession for the personal satisfaction and self-esteem resulting from attaining a high level of

TABLE 4–1

The Nursing Process with Difficult Patient Behaviors

Assessment Step	Positive Cycle	Negative Cycle
Assessment	Nurse assesses patient's and his or her own understanding of what is happening. Nurse evaluates if he or she is stereotyping or reacting personally. Nurse gets assistance and support.	Patient does not explore issues. Patient responds only to surface level of communication. Patient reacts personally. Nurse complains to staff about patient.
Intervention	Nurse responds accurately and with empathy to patient.	Nurse avoids or rejects patient. Nurse is unable to control patient's behavior.
Patient outcome	Patient feels heard, accepted, and understood, resulting in less anxiety. Difficult behavior decreases. Patient can participate more fully in health care.	Patient feels alienated with escalation of undesirable behaviors. Potential exists for negative health outcome.

expertise. The patient, on the other hand, may feel that his or her self-esteem is threatened by entering the health-care system. The patient is expected to adapt to the routines and expectations of others. Some patients cannot accept this new role and may revert to using dysfunctional behaviors.

Optimally, "good" patients are consistently cooperative, comply with the nurse's instructions and agency rules, are pleasant, polite, and respectful, show improvement, and appreciate the nurse's help. These patients ensure that the nurse meets his or her own role expectations; that is, the nurse feels helpful, effective, and accepted and valued by both patients and colleagues. "Difficult" patients produce the opposite effect. The nurse can experience frustration, anxiety, feelings of incompetence, lowered self-esteem, and a sense of being out of control.

Nurses must objectively evaluate some common myths about these role expectations. A prevalent one is that nurses can control their patients' behavior to conform to expectations. They cannot. They can encourage, suggest, negotiate, and set limits. Only in very rare situations such as when a patient poses a threat of imminent danger to himself or herself or to the staff can the nurse force a patient into expected behaviors. A nurse who believes that he or she can control a patient's behavior is creating a setup for failure.

Many nurses believe that only certain feelings toward patients are acceptable. Because nurses are human, they respond with a whole range of human emotions, including empathy, sympathy, disgust, love, hate, and, possibly, sexual feelings. Experiencing all feelings is acceptable. Displaying these feelings to patients may not be. The nurse must use professional judgment in determining which feelings are helpful to display to the patient and which are not. Responding genuinely to the patient with realistic concern is usually appropriate. If the nurse determines that it would not be appropriate to display other feelings, he or she may want to find suitable ways to express them. Often, just acknowledging the feelings to a trusted colleague can be beneficial.

Once the nurse has learned to accept and tolerate a broader range of human responses within himself or herself, he or she will develop more tolerance for formerly forbidden feelings displayed by patients. The nurse will be less likely to blame or avoid patients who stir up disturbing feelings. Often, before engaging with patients to work on problems, the nurse needs to work with ways to accept and assimilate personal experiences. Throughout this book, common nurses' reactions are listed as a way to help the reader identify them.

The following recommendations are listed to assist nurses in maintaining professional distance while remaining available to patients:

- Listen to what the patient is really asking. People have a need to be heard. When a patient tells a nurse about his or her concerns and problems, he or she may simply need someone to listen and understand his or her feelings and suffering and to feel less alone. The nurse may erroneously believe that he or she has to do something or give advice.
- Assess the patient's ability to use comments or receive information about more negative emotions like anger before sharing them and risking alienating the patient. Occasionally, however, it may be therapeutic to share even very negative feelings if this is done in a calm, matter-of-fact tone, without accusation. For example, when working with a very provocative patient, point out that this behavior elicits angry responses and pushes others away. The patient may not be aware of the cause and effect. Bringing it to his or her attention may lead to a fruitful discussion of the true fears underlying the behavior and ways of developing a realization of why others often react negatively.
- If a nurse determines that, even with the advice of specialists, he or she would not be able to work with the patient without bias, then alternate arrangements for patient care need to be made.

PATIENT ISSUES

Covert Communication

Consciously or unconsciously, patients often communicate their real needs and wishes indirectly, possibly because they are not aware of their fears. If the nurse does not analyze the patient's communication, the nurse may select ineffective interventions because he or she is dealing only with what the patient said, not what the patient really meant. Once the real concerns are identified, more effective interventions can be used. For example, the noncompliant patient may be indirectly expressing fear or a need for more reassurance or help. If fear is the underlying issue, interventions directed toward reassuring the patient will be the most successful.

Transference

This is a common issue with difficult-to-care-for patients. Sometimes even without being aware of it, the patient transfers early childhood perceptions, feelings, and experiences onto people with whom he or she is currently interacting. The patient may take positive or negative experiences with parents, teachers, siblings, or other significant people in his or her life and connect them to the nurse if there are similarities between them, either superficial or substantial. This usually occurs on an unconscious level, but the patient then feels, expects, and responds as if the nurse were that other person. For example, if the patient sees the nurse as his loving but somewhat controlling mother, he may respond with dependence tinged with resentment along with magical expectations of the nurse's effectiveness, reflecting earlier responses to his mother. If the nurse is viewed as a hostile, attacking parent, the patient may become hostile and defensive for self-protection.

Other examples of patient behaviors suggesting transference include a preoccupation with a particular nurse, a desire to be the nurse's only patient, jealousy if the nurse spends time with other patients, and recurrent attempts to provoke a specific emotion from the nurse. A common warning sign of transference is when a patient displays a strong attachment to a single staff member.

If you suspect that the patient is using transference, use the following guidelines:

- Find out if the patient is responding in similar ways to other staff members.
- Determine, if possible, whether the patient acts in similar ways toward other individuals in his or her personal life.
- Ask other staff members to provide support for the patient and a more balanced viewpoint.
- Avoid increasing the patient's dependency on you.
- Consult with a supervisor or specialist to determine the appropriateness of gently confronting the patient with these issues.
- Set limits on the patient's behavior. Do not allow the patient to obtain special privileges.
- Do not personalize any hostility.

NURSING ISSUES

Usually, not all nurses have the same amount of difficulty dealing with a patient who displays problematic behaviors. Each nurse responds to the behavior based on individual expectations of correct and proper patient behavior, previous experience working with a particular type of patient behavior, and the degree of success he or she has had in dealing with a similar situation. Personal value systems, coping mechanisms, styles of communication, conflicts, and "pet peeves" also play a role. A caring approach while maintaining professional boundaries is generally the goal for the nurse/patient relationship (Manos & Braun, 2006). The following issues may contribute to a deteriorating nurse-patient relationship.

Identification

The nurse may identify with a patient because of similarities such as age, gender, and social interests, and then superimpose his or her own conflicts, values, and expectations onto the patient. So when the nurse seems to be responding to the patient, he or she is actually responding to himself or herself. A classic example of identification is a young female nurse who is caring for a critically ill woman her own age. The nurse sees herself in the patient and begins feeling intense sadness for all the things she (the nurse) has not yet accomplished in life. The nurse may do things for the patient that she would want done for herself, regardless of their significance for this patient.

Countertransference

Countertransference is a conscious or unconscious emotional response to the patient based on the nurse's own inner needs rather than the patient's. It occurs when the nurse transfers significant positive or negative early childhood figures and conflicts onto the patient. This may present problems if the nurse does not recognize what is happening and therefore chooses interventions based on faulty assessment findings. For example, a nurse whose father physically abused her may find herself reacting with fear or rage toward a particular male patient and initially may not understand why. If she does not recognize what is triggering her response, she may conclude that the problem is with the patient's behavior rather than her response to the patient.

For both countertransference and identification, the nurse must recognize both personal feelings and the patient's behavior, speech, or attitudes that contribute to the discomfort, and then determine whether the difficulty lies with the patient's behavior or stems from the nurse's own distorted or exaggerated response to it. It is always important for nurses to compare their own reactions to their usual way of responding and question other nurses to determine whether they have a similar reaction to the patient. If other staff members have not had the same reaction to the patient, the nurse may want to examine his or her personal feelings more closely. Box 4–1 lists guidelines to identify countertransference.

Judgmental Attitude

Judging another's behavior by personal values can significantly influence the nurse-patient relationship. Patients can usually sense these attitudes and may

BOX 4–1
Identifying Countertransference

- Repeatedly experiences affectionate feeling toward certain patients
- Experiences depressed or uneasy feelings during or after interactions with certain patients
- Permits or even encourages resistance in the form of acting out
- Persistently attempts to impress a patient
- Cultivates a patient's continued dependence on nurse
- Is sadistic or unnecessarily sharp with a particular patient
- Experiences a strong need to care for patient
- Experiences conscious satisfaction from patient's praise, appreciation, and evidence of affection
- Constantly argues with the patient
- Rigid about the structure of the nurse/patient relationship
- Has an intense reaction to the patient
- Instantly likes or dislikes patient
- Does not trust anyone else to care for patient
- Feels intimidated by or is angry with the patient

Source: Adapted from Lewis, A. & Levy, J. (1992). *Psychiatric liasion nursing.* Reston, VA: Reston Publishing; Leach McMahon, A. (1997). The nurse-client relationship. In J. Haber, B. Miller, A. Leach McMahon, & P. Price-Hoskins (Eds.), *Comprehensive psychiatric nursing* (5th ed) (pp. 143-161). St. Louis: Mosby.

withhold important information for fear of being judged. The nurse may be unable or even unwilling to refrain from judging immediately but needs to be aware of these attitudes to diminish their impact on the patient.

Rescue Feelings

The nurse may believe that he or she is the only person who really understands the patient and will be the one to save or cure a patient. This usually involves some internal needs of the nurse that are often reinforced by the patient. Secrets and secret alliances may result. Nurses should keep in mind, however, that becoming a rescuer undermines the patient's responsibility for his or her own health care.

Losing Credibility

Stating facts such as "85% of patients have no complications with this type of surgery" is very different from telling a patient that he or she will not have any problems with upcoming surgery. In this example, if problems do occur after the nurse has stated that they would not, the nurse will lose credibility, and the patient may stop sharing further concerns because the patient no longer feels confident in the nurse's opinions or information. Reassurance should be based on proper information and facts. Being evasive or dishonest also destroys credibility.

Labeling

Labeling, or referring to the patient by his or her diagnosis, problem ("he's just a junkie"), or even room number, diminishes the value of the person. Almost without realizing it, once a label is used, nurses will begin to focus on the label and place less value on the patient's underlying needs and feelings. Optimal patient care requires that those needs and feelings be recognized and honored.

STRATEGIES FOR SURVIVAL

Some overall recommendations can help nurses to cope better with difficult patient behaviors. Table 4–2 offers some general guidelines for selecting effective interventions. Personal survival strategies also need to include strategies to maintain objectivity and prevent burnout. These can include using relaxation and stress management techniques and assertiveness training, as well as developing a professional support group to share concerns and help with problem-solving. Developing a sense of team cooperation also lessens the chances of a single nurse being called upon to meet everyone's needs. Attending classes and reading about managing commonly seen difficult patient behaviors gives the nurse more effective tools as well. Maintaining a satisfying personal life is also very important. Nurses tend to give of themselves as much in their personal life as they do at work. To prevent becoming burned out, you need to create a balance in life. Developing supportive relationships and participating in enjoyable activities can decrease the pressure to have patients behave in ways that meet your own personal needs. Adequate rest and exercise and good nutrition are also extremely important.

IDENTIFYING PSYCHOSOCIAL RESOURCE PERSONNEL

Many times, outside assistance is needed in addition to the nurse's own personal strategies. A first step is to identify the sources of help that are available in your agency. Depending on the institution, any or all of the following may be available:

- Social workers
- Advanced Practice Nurses
- Nurse Educators or managers
- Psychiatric liaison staff
- Psychiatrists or psychologists, including those specializing in chemical dependency, rehabilitation, or pain
- Chaplains
- Psychotherapists or staff members from other agencies who are familiar with the patient and his or her problem and previous treatment

TABLE 4–2

Staff Responses to Difficult-to-Care-for Patients

Staff Responses	Intervention
Feeling inadequate to respond effectively to patient's symptoms	Lower emotional reactivity.
Feeling angry when patient gets angry	Maintain objectivity.
Fear of the patient who exhibits bizarre or unpredictable behavior or who is confused, psychotic, or exhibits other psychiatric symptoms	Provide staff education on identifying and handling patients.
Identifying with patients who are the same age or race or who share similar life experience	Use empathy rather than sympathy to protect self and yet not harm patient.
Frustrated because there is not enough time or energy to work with patient	Share workload evenly.
Concern over being manipulated by patient's demands	Schedule consistent staffing.
Labeling patients rather than their behavior in an attempt to achieve an emotional distance	Foster staff value system that precludes patients labeling.
Uncomfortable with certain personal topics related to family dynamics or personal history	Support staff through discussion and education.

Source: Reproduced with permission of Fincannon, J. L. (1995). Analysis of psychiatric referrals and interventions in an oncology population. *Oncology Nursing Forum 22(1),* 87.

MENTAL HEALTH CONSULTATION

Sometimes agencies request outside consultation from mental health professionals for staff support and education, management of a crisis such as patient suicide, problem-solving for difficult patient behaviors, or improving workplace communications. The consultant may be a mental health clinical nurse specialist, psychologist, psychiatrist, or social worker with consultation experience. This specialist needs to have experience and skill in providing consultation, as well as some understanding of the type of problems the staff is encountering. The consultant may be from within or outside the agency. Staff attitudes can significantly influence whether this option can be used. Facilitative attitudes encourage use of these resources. These include:

- Feeling comfortable identifying problem areas and learning needs
- Recognizing that requesting assistance for areas outside personal knowledge or expertise is a sign of strength, not of weakness, and is necessary for professional development
- Approaching the consultant as a resource and role model
- Anticipating the opportunity to gain insight

Hindering attitudes discourage or prevent use of resources. These include:

- Fearing exposure of inadequacies or embarrassment about not having all the answers
- Underestimating the specialized skill or knowledge needed to work with patients' problems
- Viewing patients' difficult-to-manage behaviors as deliberate or willful
- Calling the consultant too late and then challenging him or her to "fix" everything
- Harboring a prejudice against or fear of psychiatry
- Not maintaining confidentiality of group process

If the staff is meeting with the consultant as a group, the group leader will usually establish the ground rules for staff participation at the first meeting. If multiple sessions are planned, it will be necessary for all involved staff members to make a commitment to attend all of the sessions. The administration needs to ensure adequate resources for coverage to ensure patient safety and reduce the level of staff discomfort about leaving their patients to attend the meetings. All members need to be aware of the objectives of these meetings. Hidden agendas, such as finding out who the troublemaker is, must be avoided.

Even though today's health-care environment is facing tremendous economic pressures, mental health consultation has been recognized as providing a cost-effective way to enhance problem solving, reduce workplace stress, and, potentially, increase productivity. For example, anger in staff members that has been expressed by chronic lateness or increased sick time can be explored through consultation. This resource should, therefore, not be overlooked.

5 Crisis Intervention

Learning Objectives

- Identify variables that influence the response to a crisis.
- List interventions the nurse can use to reduce the impact of a crisis for a patient.
- Describe key questions to ask a patient experiencing a crisis.

All people experience crises. Crisis is a state of disequilibrium resulting from a stressful event or perceived threat to one's self when usual coping mechanisms are ineffective and lead to the individual's experiencing increased anxiety. Nurses see patients and families in a crisis state as part of their daily routine.

It is impossible to predict what events will trigger a crisis in an individual. A breakup of a relationship or a minor car accident may cause a crisis situation for one person but not another. Certain events, such as the death of a spouse, trigger a crisis in everyone. A diagnosis of serious illness, recurrence or metastasis of cancer, and terminal illness all present the likelihood of a crisis (Van Fleet, 2006).

Many factors influence how an individual responds to a specific situation and whether a crisis will ensue. Unresolved losses, coping with other stressful events at the same time, or being excessively tired or in pain, which may reduce one's ability to cope, increase the risk of a person's viewing the situation as a crisis. Personal issues, such as low self-esteem, difficulty with anger, or need to control, may also cause an event to become a crisis in a vulnerable individual. With or without intervention, a crisis usually resolves in 4 to 6 weeks because it is much too difficult for the individual to maintain the high level of tension and distress. The person develops some type of coping mechanism to get through the situation, changes the goal, or redefines the problem.

A crisis represents both danger and opportunity. A person is at risk for emotional breakdown, but the period of vulnerability can also stimulate personal growth and strength. Crisis intervention is short-term active support that focuses on immediate problem solving and re-establishing emotional equilibrium to facilitate a positive and adaptive resolution. See Table 5–1 for the most common types of crises.

TABLE 5–1

Types of Crises

Types of Crises	Examples
Maturational—Crisis in response to facing a new developmental phase	Young adult leaving home for the first time, birth of a child
Situational—An unanticipated, external event triggers a strong response	Loss of a job, death of a loved one
Adventitious—Crisis of disaster	Natural disaster, terrorism

NURSES' REACTIONS TO PATIENT CRISIS

The ways in which a nurse responds to a patient in crisis are as varied as the ways in which the patient will respond because nurse and patient are influenced by the same factors. Some common responses may be:

- Feeling anxious or unsure about how to proceed
- Becoming overinvolved and attempting to take over for the patient, possibly causing the patient to become dependent on the nurse
- Viewing the patient's crisis as insignificant
- Taking on some of the patient's anxiety
- Setting unrealistic expectations or goals

Because health-care personnel can be exposed to traumatic events, critical incident debriefing may be needed (Everly, Lating, & Mitchell, 2000). This gives the staff a safe and controlled environment to debrief after a difficult situation. Examples might include suicide of client or staff members or another type of traumatic event including violence against an employee.

ASSESSMENT

Aguilera (1998) identified three factors to determine the development of a crisis. They include:

Perception of the event: Successful resolution is more likely if the stressor is seen in a realistic rather than in a distorted way. For example, two students may get a C grade on an examination. One student may see this as an indication of the need to study harder and may realize that it is only a part of the final picture for the school year. The other student may view the grade as a personal failure, reflecting his low self-esteem and feelings of worthlessness.

Situational support: Lack of available resources or personal support systems, in addition to the specific situation, could be the factor that changes the situation into a crisis. In contrast, having someone to whom to turn to vent grief or frustration can increase one's ability to cope.

Adequate coping mechanisms: Having proven mechanisms to deal with anxiety can prevent the situation from escalating into a crisis. If the individual has never used effective coping mechanisms or the mechanisms are not currently available, the situation could escalate into a crisis. For example, an individual who uses smoking or running as a mechanism to reduce stress may have a crisis response to being hospitalized in an intensive care unit because he will not be able to smoke or run.

To effectively assess the patient's response, follow these guidelines for conducting a crisis interview:

- Identify the precipitating event and determine its meaning.
  - What has happened in the past few days or hours?
  - If the patient describes an ongoing problem, what is different about the problem today from yesterday? Be specific.
  - What does the event mean to the patient?
  - What is the patient most worried about in relation to the event?
  - What are some of the consequences of the event?
  - Does the patient see this event as influencing his or her future?

- Evaluate the patient's support system.
  - With whom does the patient have a close relationship?
  - To whom does the patient talk when he or she has a problem?
  - Are these people available now?
  - Have these resources helped in the past?
  - Whom does the patient trust?
  - Are any other resources available in the patient's life such as a clergy member or a counselor?

- Evaluate previously used effective coping mechanisms.
  - What does the patient normally do to cope with stress?
  - What is he or she doing now to cope with this situation?
  - If this has not helped, does the patient have any idea why not?
  - What has helped in the past in similar situations?

INTERVENTIONS

Crisis intervention is short-term problem-oriented support that ideally allows the individual to advance to a higher level of functioning as he or she develops new insights, strengths, and coping mechanisms. At the minimum, the individual will return to the precrisis level of functioning. The crisis is considered unresolved if the person functions at a lower level after the crisis, for example, by abusing substances, communicating ineffectively with family or loved ones, or exhibiting signs of depression or psychosis.

When facing a crisis, consider the following interventions:

- Make an accurate assessment of the precipitating event, the patient's perception of the event, and the available support systems and coping mechanisms. Also assess the patient's safety.

- Provide only small amounts of information at a time, and be prepared to repeat the information several times. Focus on concrete actions rather than vague ones.

- Communicate in a supportive, nonjudgmental way. Use gentle physical contact, as appropriate. Use calming hand gestures, a calm voice, and an unhurried manner.

- Help the patient to confront the reality of the event. This should be done slowly at first, such as gently bringing the patient back to a discussion of a car accident. More concrete, specific wording may be needed. This process may need to be repeated.

- Help the patient focus on one "here-and-now" problem at a time rather than jumping from one possible problem to another. For example, a man who is frantic about his continuing pain may begin thinking about what will happen if the pain never stops. This will only escalate his anxiety. Rather, help him stay focused on dealing with the pain he is having now.

- In some situations, you may need to direct the person as to what to do next. His or her ability to make even the smallest decision may be compromised due to the overwhelming anxiety the crisis is producing.

- Encourage the patient to express his or her emotions in a socially acceptable manner.

- Assist with problem solving. This may include brainstorming all possible options and helping the patient narrow these down to the ones that can be used now. Focus on one or two possible options to give the patient a sense of control without overwhelming him or her with multiple options.

- Encourage the people in the patient's support system to become involved. Be sure to obtain the patient's permission before notifying family and friends to ensure that the patient maintains control of the situation. Be creative in identifying sources of support.

- Reinforce the patient's self-esteem by acknowledging how difficult the situation is and saying that you understand he or she is doing all that is possible to cope with it. Provide positive feedback.

- Reinforce effective coping mechanisms such as deep breathing, exercising, or making prioritized lists.

- Identify other resources in the agency that could provide assistance. Avoid being the only staff member assisting this patient.
- Assess the need for medications to reduce anxiety.

Occasionally, a patient's response to a crisis requires more intense intervention, including psychiatric treatment or hospitalization. The nurse needs to recognize signs of patient decompensation that go beyond the usual symptoms of a crisis. For example, suicidal behavior, evidence of psychotic thoughts, or violent behavior that could endanger others must be identified and resources for intervention obtained. If these signs occur, be sure to obtain a consultation for specialized assistance.

6

Cultural Considerations: Implications for Psychosocial Nursing Care

Learning Objectives

- Explain the concept of culturally sensitive psychosocial nursing care.
- Discuss factors to consider when assessing culture and ethnicity in patients and their families.
- Consider treatment approaches to patients in various cultural and ethnic groups.
- Describe guidelines for using interpreters and what to do when an interpreter is not available.

Culture is a system of beliefs, behaviors, and symbols that are learned, shared, and passed on through generations of a social group. Culture influences what people perceive, it guides their interactions, and it can change over time. Culture describes a particular society's entire way of living. Ethnicity is a somewhat narrower term: it relates to people who identify with each other because of a shared heritage.

CULTURALLY COMPETENT NURSING CARE

The need to incorporate culturally competent care is more important than ever as the U.S. population continues to be increasingly diverse. More than 11% of the population is foreign born, and the primary language of about 20% is one other than English (U.S. Census Bureau, 2005).

Culturally competent nursing care is defined as being sensitive to issues related to culture, race, religion, gender, sexual orientation, and social or economic class. Cultural competence implies not only awareness of cultural differences but also the ability to assess and intervene appropriately and effectively. Cultural competence in nursing care requires more than simply acquiring knowledge about other ethnic or cultural groups. It is a complex combination of attitudes and skills as well as knowledge (Campinha-Bacote, 1994).

Cultural information by itself can interfere with care if nurses use it in a "cookbook" manner. Inappropriate use of cultural information can lead to stereotyping patients by making assumptions based on limited information. Because stereotyping comes from jumping to conclusions based on insufficient data or experience with a cultural group, it is important to suspend judgment as long as possible (Lipson & Steiger, 1996). Cross-cultural misunderstandings surrounding end of life care are increasing as differences in attitudes exist toward truth telling, life-prolonging technology, and decision-making styles between patients, families, and health-care providers (Kagawa-Singer & Blackhall, 2001).

Cultures can be compared using six phenomena that vary with application and use, yet are seen across all cultural groups (Giger & Davidhizar, 1995; 2004). These phenomena are:

1. *Communication:* This refers to all verbal and nonverbal behavior in the presence of another. Communication has its roots in culture. Cultural mores, norms, ideas, and customs are all expressed through communication. The nurse who cares for diverse patients must have an understanding of the client's needs and expectations as expressed through their communication and culture.

2. *Space:* This element of culture refers to territoriality, density, and distance. It relates to how space is controlled, used, and defended. Three interpersonal dimensions of space in Western culture have been identified: the intimate zone (0–18 inches), the personal zone (18–36 inches), and the social zone (3–6 feet).

3. *Social organization:* Cultural behaviors are acquired through social interactions in groups such as families, religious groups, and ethnic groups. This process of learning cultural values is called acculturation.

4. *Time:* Awareness of time is learned gradually. Some cultures place great importance on punctuality and efficiency, whereas others ignore the clock. Time orientation, meaning present-, future-, or past-oriented perceptions, influences many aspects of a culture.

5. *Environmental control:* This element has to do with the degree to which individuals perceive they have control over their environment. Persons from various cultures have different beliefs about how much they can influence events in their lives, some being more fatalistic and others more active. To provide culturally appropriate care, nurses should respect the individual's unique beliefs while understanding how these beliefs can be used to promote health in the patient's environment.

6. *Biological variations:* This element refers to biological differences in people from various racial and ethnic groups, such as body size and shape, skin and hair color, physiologic responses to medications, susceptibility to disease, and nutritional preferences. A new field called ethnopharmacology is addressing different responses to medications.

Acknowledging that people from different cultures and ethnic groups perceive these phenomena in different ways can help the nurse understand variations in patients' behavior, values, and expectations.

A cultural assessment helps the nurse gather and use other information related to culture that is vital in providing culturally sensitive care. The nurse must be aware that beliefs about health and the causes of illness, appropriate care, and who should provide that care, can differ among cultures. It is important for the nurse to listen to what the patient believes, what has been done in the past, and even to consult with the patient's cultural healers (perhaps a spiritualist, curandero, shaman, or medicine man).

The nurse must realize that mental illness is unacceptable in some cultures. People who believe that expressing emotions is unacceptable present unique problems in a psychiatric setting. Nurses need to work slowly to establish trust and rapport with patients from other cultures. In some cases, it may be necessary to follow the health-care practices that the client views as essential, as long as they do not harm the patient. For example, letting family members bring in special foods, inviting a folk healer to the hospital, or making time for a spiritual reading serve as an important acknowledgment of the patient's traditions (Townsend, 2006).

CULTURAL ASSESSMENT

A thorough cultural assessment may take several hours. The list of questions in Box 6–1 can provide a brief but helpful focus for a relevant cultural assessment. Answers to these questions do not guarantee culturally competent care, but nevertheless good care cannot be provided without specific cultural and ethnic information (Lipson, Dibble & Minarik, 1996). When patient and health-care professionals are from different cultures, questions must be asked that respectfully acknowledge differences and build trust.

CULTURAL INFLUENCE ON MENTAL HEALTH BELIEFS

Culture can significantly influence communication, particularly when the cultures of the nurse and patient are vastly different and not understood by each other. Culture is defined as a configuration of learned behaviors and beliefs that are shared and transmitted in a society and by a particular group of people. The values, beliefs, traditions, attitudes, and prejudices that each of us brings from our culture and past experiences influence all interactions with others. Ethnocentrism is defined as the belief that one's own cultural beliefs and health-care practices are superior to those of other cultures. To provide quality care to all individuals, nurses must be sensitive to patients' cultural differences and as aware as possible of their own cultural beliefs and behaviors.

Rather than stereotyping individuals into specific cultural classes, nurses should approach each patient as an individual who holds very personal attitudes,

---

BOX 6–1
Cultural Assessment—Questions to Ask

- Where was the patient born? If an immigrant, how long in this country?
- What is the patient's ethnic affiliation, how strong is the ethnic identity?
- Who are the patient's major support people? Does patient live in an ethnic community?
- Who in the family takes responsibility for health concerns and decisions?
- Any activities in which the client may decline to participate because of culture, religious taboos?
- Any special food preferences, food refusals because of culture, religion?
- What are the primary and secondary languages, speaking and reading abilities?
- What is patient's religion, its importance in daily life, current practices?
- What is the patient's economic situation, is income adequate for needs?
- What are the patient's health beliefs and practices?
- What are patient's perceptions of health problem and expectations of health care?

---

beliefs, and values that are influenced by his or her culture and environment. (See Box 6–2 for ways of enhancing cultural sensitivity.)

Culture often influences what a patient believes about his or her illness, its causes, and when and from whom to seek care. Although you may not be able to be aware of the specific beliefs of every culture, having some general information about the culture and ethnicity of patients for whom you frequently care for is important. Incorporating some questions in the assessment on culture and observing for influences can help you become more familiar with these cultures (Purnell & Paulanka, 1998).

BOX 6–2
Enhancing Cultural Sensitivity

- Know your own attitudes, values, and beliefs.
- Be aware of your own ethnocentrism.
- Be aware of your own prejudices that may influence your assessment.
- Maintain an open mind and seek out more information about your patient's culture, beliefs, and values.
- Communicate your interest about the patient's beliefs and values.
- Approach each patient as an individual. Avoid assuming people from one cultural background all hold the same beliefs.

Questions to be included in the assessment may include, "What do you believe caused your illness?" and "What other treatments for the illness have you pursued?" Recognize the impact of these beliefs on the patient's ability to accept the illness and his or her response to it. For example, in cultures that view men as always being strong, even a mild illness could contribute to depression (Spector, 1996).

Be sensitive to each individual's beliefs about his or her illness and its causes, and design your care to incorporate these ideas. For example, in a culture in which the oldest woman plays a pivotal role in the family, the grandmother may be the one the patient consults on decisions about surgery, discharge planning, and follow-up care. She would need to be incorporated into the treatment planning in order for this patient to receive the best follow-up care. If a patient believes in folk healers or cures, don't ridicule or judge his or her beliefs. Rather, acknowledge the beliefs, and incorporate them into the treatment plan if possible. For example, if a Chinese patient is taking herbs to cure his diabetes, it is more beneficial to discuss the possible impact of these herbs on blood sugar than to ignore their use or forbid the patient to use them (Lipson, Dibble & Minarik, 1996).

Respect the role of the family in the patient's treatment. In some cultures, the family is responsible for protecting the patient, especially when the patient is the parent. In their role, family members may want to protect the patient from bad news. This may be contrary to your own belief in patient autonomy and, therefore, may lead to conflicts between the health-care providers and the family. Of course, the patient must be in agreement with involving the family. Also be aware that in psychiatric settings, different approaches may be used to preserve patient autonomy and confidentiality.

Psychiatric professionals have recognized that some symptoms commonly seen in mental illness, such as delusions or hallucinations, could represent a culturally appropriate behavior. For example, being possessed by an evil spirit could be a delusion or a culturally sanctioned experience of an altered state of consciousness. Be careful not to judge individual cultural variations as psychopathology. It is helpful to discuss these issues with other health-care providers from diverse cultural or ethnic groups who can increase your understanding of behaviors and beliefs outside your own experiences (Townsend, 2006). The Diagnostic and Statistical Manual of Mental Disorder, fourth edition, revised (DSM-IV-TR, 2000) identifies behaviors (culture-bound syndromes) associated with various cultures that may be mistaken for psychiatric symptoms. This can be a useful reference.

CULTURAL AND ETHNIC INFLUENCE ON COMMUNICATION

Verbal and nonverbal communication patterns are closely tied to cultural beliefs and practices. Eye contact, hand gestures, facial expressions, and personal space, as well as how words or slang are used and what can be discussed, are defined by our culture and environment. For many people, eye contact indicates honesty, openness, and alertness. However, people in some cultures do not value eye contact and, in fact, even avoid it. For example, in some Asian cultures, eye contact is viewed as impolite and an invasion of privacy. It is especially inappropriate with authority figures, such as doctors and nurses. Judging a patient's response based on eye contact without understanding this difference can lead to an invalid assessment finding (Luckmann, 1999).

Some nonverbal behaviors such as facial expressions, hand gestures, and social distance vary among cultures. For example, it may be important to know that lack of facial expression in some Asian groups is not an indication of lack of feeling or that an Arab family member who stands very close is not threatening but rather standing at the distance considered appropriate in their culture. Addressing a patient, especially an elderly one, by his or her first name may suggest a lack of respect, or even seduction, in many Asian and Latin cultures. Also, some patients may be extremely uncomfortable when asked intimate, very personal questions, no matter how accepting and professional the nurse may be. If this information is vital to patient care, efforts need to be made to explain how the information will be used (Schuster, 2000).

COMMUNICATING THROUGH AN INTERPRETER

Language differences pose a barrier to even the most basic communication and cultural assessment. Caring for a patient who does not speak the same language as you can cause anxiety, frustration, fear, and a sense of helplessness on your part as well as the patient's. It may cause resentment because of the extra time and work that are needed. Some nurses try to compensate for their perceived deficiency by concentrating on performing tasks rather than on the patient's concerns. Although it is not usually possible to learn the language of every potential patient, it would be beneficial to learn the language spoken by a majority of the patients you care for. If you cannot speak the language, use an interpreter as much as possible.

There may be a family member who can translate, and you may need to provide accommodations if this person needs to stay with the patient. When using a family member to translate, keep in mind that, because of the emotional ties or role conflicts and lack of medical vocabulary, the person may base messages to both patient and provider on his or her own perception of the situation and may withhold vital information because it may embarrass or overwhelm the patient. For example, if the family member does not want the patient to know about the seriousness of his or her condition, he or she may not relay all the information to the patient. In addition, patients may feel too embarrassed to disclose key information in the presence of their relatives, especially if it is of a sensitive nature. Using family members as interpreters is probably best when basic communication is needed rather than when critical conversations are needed for diagnosis, treatment, and psychosocial assessments (Luckmann, 1999).

Check with your institution to see if an interpreter is available. The Civil Rights Act of 1964, the 1973 Rehabilitation Act, and the more recent Americans with Disabilities Act (ADA) have established the federal standards that ensure that communication does not interfere with equal access to health care for all people. Therefore, all health-care institutions must establish systems for identifying available language interpreters, as well as interpreters trained in sign language, telecommunication device for the deaf (TDDs), closed-caption decoders for television, and amplifiers on the phones. Many institutions have access to telephone interpretation services, such as the AT&T Language Line. This nationwide, 24-hour service provides interpreters for about 170 languages. Although this service cannot take the place of a trained interpreter at the bedside, it does allow patients to communicate their history and symptoms to health-care providers, especially in emergencies.

Interpreters can be professional interpreters or employees of the institution who have other duties. If you are using employees who are not trained interpreters, evaluate their ability to understand the information you wish to have translated and how much time they have to provide the service. If the interpreter has limited medical knowledge or knowledge of the patient, it may be difficult to ensure effective communication.

In the home, family members and neighbors are usually the only resource unless nurses who speak the language are available. In addition to being aware of agency resources for interpreters, the nurse should become familiar with key words that can be useful in assessing patients who speak another language. A language board containing key words in the languages most frequently used in your agency can be a very effective, time-saving tool.

When using an interpreter, keep the following points in mind:

- Address the patient directly rather than speaking to the interpreter. Maintain eye contact with the patient to ensure the patient's involvement.
- Do not interrupt the patient and interpreter. At times, their interaction may take longer because of the need to clarify, and descriptions may require more time because of dialect differences or the interpreter's awareness that the patient needs more preparation before being asked a particular question.
- Ask the interpreter to give you verbatim translations so that you can assess what the patient is thinking and understanding.
- Avoid using medical jargon that the interpreter or patient may not understand.
- Avoid talking or commenting to the interpreter at length; the patient may feel left out and distrustful.
- Be aware that asking intimate or emotionally laden questions may be difficult for both the patient and the interpreter. Lead up to these questions slowly. Always ask permission to discuss these topics first, and prepare the interpreter for the content of the interview.
- When possible, allow the patient and interpreter to meet each other ahead of time to establish some rapport. If possible, try to use the same interpreter for succeeding interviews with the patient.

- If possible, request an interpreter of the same gender as the patient and of similar age. To make good use of the interpreter's time, decide beforehand which questions you will ask. Meet with the interpreter briefly before going to see the patient so that you can let the interpreter know what you are planning to ask. During the session, face the patient and direct your questions to the patient, not the interpreter. After the session, review the questions and answers with the interpreter to check any remaining concerns (Luckmann, 1999).

- Anticipate when emotional, difficult topics will be addressed and prepare the interpreter ahead of time for this, for example, a discussion of code status. If not well prepared or well trained, an interpreter can identify with a patient and this could influence the interpretations as well as contribute to the interpreter's discomfort (Norris et al, 2005).

GUIDELINES FOR WORKING WITHOUT AN INTERPRETER

If an interpreter is not available, using picture charts or flash cards can help the patient communicate some basic questions such as degree of pain or needs like water and elimination. Some patients with limited English may tend to appear agreeable and nod yes even though they do not understand. Be sure to determine that the patient understands by asking questions that require more than a "yes" or "no" answer.

If the patient understands a little English, you may be able to gather useful information without an interpreter by following these suggestions:

- Greet the patient respectfully. Be polite and formal, especially with older patients.
- Identify the patient's primary language. If you can pronounce any words in the language, use them to show you are trying to communicate. A simple "buenos dias" or "bonjour" may help to reduce the patient's anxiety.
- Speak slowly, clearly, and quietly in English if this is your only option. Do not shout. Make an effort not to appear frustrated, irritated, or hurried.
- Ask one question; talk about one symptom at a time. Use simple sentences.
- Try to avoid medical terminology. For example use "bleeding, pus, or liquid" rather than "discharge."
- Use picture cards or a phrase chart if they are available to verify patient information.
- Be aware that some patients may act as if they have understood all your questions to avoid looking ignorant or rude (Luckmann, 1999).

7 Problems with Anxiety

The Anxious Patient

Learning Objectives

- Differentiate among the cognitive, affective, behavioral, and physical symptoms of anxiety.
- Use the different manifestations of anxiety to assess the anxious patient.
- Select the most appropriate interventions for dealing with the patient with anxiety.
- Identify possible nurses' reactions to an anxious patient.

Glossary

Acute stress disorder – *A disorder characterized by a high level of anxiety immediately after a traumatic event.*

Agoraphobia – *Fear, anxiety, or avoidance of places or situations from which escape may be difficult or where help may not be available.*

Anxiety – *An unpleasant feeling of tension, apprehension, and uneasiness or a diffuse feeling of dread or unexplained discomfort; accompanied by physiological, psychological, and behavioral symptoms; may serve as an early warning that alerts the individual to impending real or symbolic threat to self, significant others, or way of life; motivates the individual to take corrective action to relieve the unpleasant feelings. The source of the anxiety is often nonspecific or unknown to the individual.*

Anxiety disorder due to a General Medical Condition – *Anxiety characterized by prominent symptoms directly related to the physiological consequences of a general medical condition (e.g., hyperthyroidism or hypothyroidism, hypoglycemia, chronic obstructive pulmonary disease).*

Fear – *A reaction to a specific danger.*

Generalized anxiety disorder – *A disorder characterized by at least 6 months of persistent and excessive anxiety and worry.*

Obsessive-compulsive disorder (OCD) – *Recurrent thoughts or ideas (obsessions) that an individual is unable to put out of his or her mind and actions that an individual is unable to refrain from performing (compulsions).*

Panic attack – *A discrete, sudden, unpredictable, intense episode of severe anxiety characterized by personality disorganization; a fear of losing one's mind, going crazy, being unable to control one's behavior; a sense of impending doom, helplessness, and being trapped.*

Post-traumatic stress disorder (PTSD) – *Anxiety and stress symptoms that occur after a massive traumatic event; often includes the feeling that the event is reoccurring, lasting for weeks, months, or years.*

Post-traumatic stress response – *A persistent, disorganizing, and distressing reaction to a catastrophic event that affects a person's emotional, cognitive, and behavioral dimensions and relationships and extends beyond the time of the immediate crisis.*

Social anxiety disorder – *Intense, persistent fear of social situations.*

Specific phobias – *Irrational fears characterized by clinically significant anxiety provoked by exposure to a specific feared object or situation, often leading to avoidance behavior.*

Substance-induced anxiety disorder – *A disorder characterized by prominent anxiety symptoms directly related to physiological consequences of drug abuse, medication use, or toxin exposure.*

Anxiety is the primary emotion from which many other emotions or responses, such as anger, guilt, shame, and grief, are generated. The term anxiety brings up images of someone pacing and wringing his or her hands with pounding heart and rapid breathing, perhaps before taking an important test in school or while waiting to hear from the doctor about results of a biopsy. Words such as worry, concern, fear, and uncertainty are often associated with the term anxiety.

Anxiety can also have a positive meaning, implying eagerness and readiness to face a challenge or perform some skill. Being mildly anxious can enhance experiences such as performing in a piano recital or completing a term paper. Anxiety is a healthy response to novel and unique experiences. In fact, being mildly anxious helps us to perform our best because perceptual, emotional, and physiological arousal can enhance learning, problem-solving, satisfaction, and pleasure during and after an event. Just as pain serves as a cue and a response to potential or actual physical danger, anxiety can serve as a cue and response to emotional, social, or spiritual danger.

Anxiety is a universal emotion; everyone has experienced some level of anxiety associated with life events. Anxiety disorders are the most common psychiatric disorder in America (Merikangus, 2006; Hollander & Simeon, 2003). Anxiety disorders affect 25% of the U.S. population (Merikangus, 2006). Social anxiety disorders are the most frequent form of anxiety disorders. It is triggered by certain types of performance situations (Bernardo, 2007). People vary significantly in their ability to manage feelings of anxiety and in their styles and patterns of coping with anxiety-producing situations. Knowing the meaning of the subjective experience to a particular individual is essential in understanding how to intervene with that individual. Fears are more specific, but the body reacts similarly to both fear and anxiety.

The DSM-IV-TR (2000) divides anxiety into these diagnostic categories: Panic Disorder with or without Agoraphobia, Social Phobia (also called social anxiety disorder), Specific Phobias, Obsessive-Compulsive Disorder, Post-Traumatic Stress Disorder, Acute Stress Disorder, Anxiety Disorder due to a General Medical Condition, Generalized Anxiety Disorder, and Substance-Induced Anxiety Disorder. Panic attacks and Agoraphobia may occur alone or in the context of several of these disorders. For treatment purposes, anxiety is often categorized into four levels: mild, moderate, severe, and panic (Table 7–1).

TABLE 7–1

Characteristics of Anxiety Levels

Level	Characteristics
Mild	• Enhanced ability to deal with stressors • Heightened awareness, problem-solving abilities; increased attention to details • Curiosity increased, asks questions • Alert, confident • Logical thinking intact
Moderate	• Hesitation and procrastination, blocking loss of train of thought • Narrowing of perceptual field • Change in voice pitch; speech rate accelerates • Selective inattention • Frequent change in topics • Repetitive questioning, joking • Increased respiratory rate, heart rate, muscle tension • Dry mouth • Palpitations • Changing body positions frequently, restlessness • Purposeless activity (wringing hands, pacing)

Continued

TABLE 7–1

Characteristics of Anxiety Levels—*cont'd*

Level	Characteristics
Severe	• Highly distorted perceptual and cognitive function • Focus on small or scattered detail, inability to see connections between events • Selective inattention, inability to concentrate • Fear of losing control • Purposeless activity (pacing, wringing hands) • Difficult and inappropriate verbalizations, inability to learn • Sense of impending doom • Sweating • Hyperventilation, tachycardia, frequency and urgency • Nausea, headache, dizziness • Gross motor tremors, trembling, shaking • Numbness or tingling sensations • Dilated pupils
Panic	• Dyspnea, choking feeling, chest pain • Extreme discomfort, emotional pain • Unrealistic, distorted perception of situation • Disruption of visual field, distortion and enlargement of detail • Inability to speak, unintelligible communication, incoherent speech • Vomiting, incontinence • Feeling of personality disintegration • Fear of losing mind, fear of dying

Mild or moderate anxiety usually speeds up physiological operations, whereas severe anxiety may slow them down. Prolonged panic can cause complete paralysis of functioning and occasionally result in death. Anxiety can also be classified as normal or abnormal. The same feelings and behaviors (uncertainties, helplessness, and an intense sense of personal discomfort) characterize both, and the level of anxiety may be equally intense.

Normal anxiety results from a realistic perception of the danger and prepares the person for defense or change in face of the threat. Normal anxiety can be motivating and useful (e.g., to motivate a student to study harder and therefore to do better on a test). Abnormal anxiety arises when the perception of danger is distorted, unrealistic, and out of proportion, resulting in maladaptive, defensive coping and inappropriate behavior.

ETIOLOGY

Theoretical approaches to anxiety are wide ranging. In the *biological* perspective, anxiety is the uneasy feeling aroused by a threat or danger and is accompanied by a physiological response. This response prepares the person for "fight or flight." The fight response (sympathetic stimulation) causes changes primarily in the cardiovascular and neuroendocrine systems. During the flight response (parasympathetic stimulation), which occurs in acute fear states, an effort is made to conserve body resources. Other evidence suggests a biological basis for anxiety. Research on the metabolism of monoamines and the function of the limbic system are central to the expression of emotions such as anxiety; the discovery of the benefits of benzodiazepines for chronic anxiety; and studies on sodium lactate in persons with panic attacks.

In *psychoanalytical* theory, anxiety represents a person's struggle with the demands and prohibitions in his or her environment, including the internal struggle among the person's instinctual drives (id), the realistic assessment of the possibility for need fulfillment (ego), and the conscience (superego). Anxiety is a signal from the ego that an unacceptable drive is pressing for conscious discharge. A conflict results between the drive, usually of a sexual or aggressive nature, and fear of punishment or disapproval. Phobias are fears that are disproportionate to the situation and cannot be explained or reasoned away. The significance and meaning of anxiety depend on the nature of the underlying conflict.

Interpersonal theorists believe that anxiety arises from experiences in relationships with significant others (SOs) throughout a person's development. If a child is treated malevolently, the foundation is laid for the child to become insecure and feel inferior and anxious in future situations. The child is forced to use coping strategies to allay anxiety; these become part of the personality when the child becomes an adult.

Learning and behavioral theorists explain anxiety as the result of a conditioning process in which a neutral stimulus has come to represent punishment, pain, or fear. The individual learns to reduce anxiety by avoiding a negative stimulus or by approaching a positive reinforcer. Extinction of behavior is a process of reducing response strength by nonreinforcement.

An eclectic understanding of anxiety, incorporating components of all these theories, is most helpful. Anxiety can be understood as experienced at conscious, unconscious, or preconscious levels. Sources of anxiety fall into two major categories:

1. *Threats to biologic integrity:* Actual or impending interference with basic human needs such as food, drink, shelter, warmth, safety and health
2. *Threats to self-security or self-esteem which can include:*
   - Unmet expectations important to self-integrity
   - Unmet needs for status and prestige

- Anticipated disapproval by SOs
- Inability to gain or reinforce self-respect or to gain recognition from others
- A severe, sudden, unexpected threat to sense of security, self-esteem, or well-being
- Guilt or discrepancies between self-perception and actual behavior

Experiences with anxiety in early life lead to the development of coping behaviors, personality traits, and defense mechanisms intended to reduce anxiety and increase a sense of security. Over time, the individual develops characteristic patterns of relief behaviors intended to provide comfort and protection in the face of anxiety. When these behaviors, traits, or mechanisms fail to relieve anxiety, the patient experiences intense emotional or physical discomfort.

Behavioral responses to anxiety can be constructive (problem-solving, task-oriented) or destructive (defensive, aggressive, violent). When anxiety levels exceed a person's adaptive coping abilities, maladaptive behaviors may develop. Disturbed coping mechanisms are characterized by the inability to make choices, conflict, repetition and rigidity, and alienation. Frustration and anxiety can lead to anger, hostility, and violence.

Anxiety often increases when a person expects one thing and is suddenly confronted with something very different. The same stressor may not always lead to anxiety or the same level of anxiety in everyone or even in the same person at different times. Generally, the patient experiences anxiety as very painful and unbearable if it continues for any length of time. Behavior patterns used to cope with anxiety include the following:

Acting out: Converting anxiety into anger, which is either overtly or covertly expressed

Paralysis or retreating: Withdrawing or being immobilized by anxiety

Somatizing: Converting anxiety into physical symptoms such as stomachache or headache

Avoidance: Evasive behaviors performed unconsciously to ward off or relieve anxiety before it is directly experienced (alcohol, sleeping, keeping busy)

Constructive action: Using anxiety to learn and problem solve (goal setting, learning new skills, seeking information)

Syndromes of abnormal anxiety frequently observed in patients include the following:

Panic attacks: Acute, intense attacks of anxiety associated with extreme changes in physical and emotional behavior that can last from minutes to hours, are severely debilitating, and are characterized by sudden, intense, and discrete periods of anxiety and fear that may occur without warning in previously calm and untroubled individuals. Recent research points to physical or organic causes for some patients.

Post-traumatic stress disorder (PTSD): Re-experience of the trauma of a previous traumatic event (e.g., rape, assault, military combat, flood, earthquake, major car accident, airplane crash, bombing, torture). The symptoms are usually more severe and last longer when the cause is a manmade rather than a natural disaster. Three subtypes of PTSD are recognized:

- Acute: Symptoms begin within 6 months of the event and do not last longer than 6 months.
- Chronic: Symptoms last for 6 months or more.
- Delayed: Symptoms begin after a latency period of 6 months or more.

Re-experiencing the trauma in PTSD may include recurrent and intrusive recollections of the event, recurrent dreams or nightmares of the event, or sudden acting or feeling as if the event were recurring because of an association with an environmental or mental stimulus. Other behaviors and affect associated with the syndrome include decreased interest in usually significant activities, feelings of detachment or estrangement from others, and constricted affect. Symptoms not present before the trauma include hyperalertness or exaggerated startle response, sleep disturbance, guilt about surviving while others died or about behavior required for survival, memory impairment, difficulty concentrating, avoidance of activities that arouse recollection of the event, or intensification of symptoms by exposure to events that symbolize or resemble the traumatic event.

Phobia: An intense, irrational fear response to a specific external object or situation. Unlike an anxiety reaction, in which the anxiety is free floating and the person cannot easily identify the cause or source, a phobia is a persistent fear of specific places, things, or situations. The major dynamic mechanism of phobic behavior is the displacement of the original anxiety from its real source and the symbolization of the stressor in the phobia (e.g., fear of sex becomes a fear of snakes).

The hallmark of phobias is that they are irrational and persist even though the person recognizes that they are irrational. The unconscious operations involved in the phobia help the person to control anxiety by providing a specific object to attach it to. The phobic person can then control the intensity of the anxiety by avoiding the object or situation to which the anxiety has become attached. Some of the more common phobias include claustrophobia (fear of closed places), agoraphobia (fear of leaving home and of open spaces), acrophobia (fear of heights), xenophobia (fear of strangers), and zoophobia (fear of animals).

Obsessive-compulsive disorder (OCD): A paralyzing anxiety disorder associated with repetitive, compulsive thoughts (obsessions) and behaviors (compulsions). These patterns of thoughts and behaviors are senseless and distressing but help achieve the goal of avoiding anxiety. This disorder has been treated very effectively with some of the newer antidepressants, leading some investigators to think this disorder is related to serotonin reuptake.

RELATED CLINICAL CONCERNS

Anxiety is the most common complaint in medical practice (Epstein & Hicks, 2005). It presents in many ways and with great variation in intensity and duration; therefore, treatment must be individualized and monitored very closely. Anxiety may be caused by many other medical and psychiatric problems such as cardiac and vascular disorders, sleep disorders, hyperthyroidism, anemia, depression with agitation, dementia, delirium, hypochondriasis, schizophrenia, mania, and personality disorders. Some medications, caffeine intoxication, and withdrawal from alcohol or sedatives may cause anxiety. Anxiety can also contribute to medical illness such as arrhythmias and labile hypertension (Epstein & Hicks, 2005). Physical illness or underlying major psychiatric syndromes must be considered and ruled out before treatment for anxiety is undertaken. Because many patients with anxiety disorders do not present to mental health providers, general medical practitioners may be the first to identify anxiety disorders.

LIFE SPAN ISSUES

Children

The anxiety most frequently experienced by children is separation anxiety. When a child is separated from those to whom he or she is attached, excessive anxiety to the point of panic may occur. Onset may be as early as preschool age. The child may refuse to go to sleep or go to school. Complaints of physical symptoms, such as headache, stomachache, and nausea and vomiting are also common. The most common sign of anxiety in children is increased motor activity (Wong, 2003).

Older Adults

Anxiety in elderly people has not been systematically investigated. It is the consensus of clinical gerontologists that anxiety is a common response to the stresses of late life, including fear of dependency, illness, dying, and multiple losses of friends, home, or lifestyle. A long-standing tendency toward excessive anxiety can persist into late life and usually is not dysfunctional in the patient who has adapted to it. Anxiety in elderly persons may be the presenting symptom of a new illness, especially depression with agitation; of early dementia; or of low-grade or chronic toxic states caused by drugs or alcohol.

POSSIBLE NURSES' REACTIONS

- May be apprehensive and even fearful about caring for patients experiencing severe anxiety or a panic attack. Intense anxiety can be very contagious, not only to staff members but also to other patients.
- May try to determine the cause of patient's anxiety and do what is possible to reassure and assist patient to decrease it, then become frustrated when patient's anxiety continues.
- May find it too strenuous to work with patient for more than a day at a time if patient's anxiety does not subside as the nurse thinks it should.
- May interpret the anxiety as a weakness in the patient, who is seen as unable or unwilling to control it or may judge the anxiety as part of a more serious psychological problem and feel very uncomfortable caring for these patients.
- May prefer to keep patient sedated.
- May feel resentment and even hostility toward anxious patients who require more attention and time than their physical conditions alone warrant.
- May want to avoid family members or SOs who are also quite anxious and make unreasonable requests in a demanding or complaining manner. Most of these behaviors may be caused by the families' own frustration or apprehension in dealing with the patient's anxiety, and they are often unaware that their behavior is affecting the staff.

ASSESSMENT

Behavior and Appearance

See Table 7–1 for Characteristics of Anxiety Levels.

Mood and Emotions

- Dread, fear, apprehension
- Lack of control or self-confidence
- Guilt
- Anger
- Grief
- Sense of imminent catastrophe

Thoughts, Beliefs, and Perceptions

- Narrowed focus of attention
- Perceptual focus scattered or fixed
- Inability to focus on reality

- Inability to learn or remember, forgetfulness
- Inability to reason or problem solve
- Difficulty concentrating, lack of awareness of environment
- Distorted perceptions

Relationships and Interactions

- Withdrawal and isolation, avoidance behaviors
- Demanding, complaining, quarreling, attention-seeking behavior
- Defensive, uses denial
- Tense, strained relationships; others frustrated over dealing with patient's anxiety and maladaptive coping

Physical Responses

See Table 7–1 for physical responses to various anxiety levels.

Pertinent History

- Medical conditions that present with anxiety as a symptom

  - Thyroid, pituitary, and adrenocortical disorders
  - Low hemoglobin
  - Hypoglycemia
  - Impending heart attack

- Use if stimulants including crystal meth, cocaine, amphetamines
- Synergistic or idiosyncratic drug reactions
- Alcohol or sedative withdrawal
- Cerebrovascular disorders
- Sequelae to head injury
- Chronic anxiety
- Recent loss of loved one, significant object, work, finances, or self-esteem
- Phobic behavior
- Recent re-exposure to anxiety-causing situation
- Traumatic experience

COLLABORATIVE MANAGEMENT

Anxiety disorders are usually treated with some form of counseling or psychotherapy or pharmacotherapy, either alone or in combination. The milder forms may be effectively treated with cognitive or behavior therapy alone, but more severe and persistent symptoms may require pharmacotherapy.

Pharmacological

The medications typically used to treat patients with anxiety are benzodiazepines and antidepressants. Benzodiazepines, such as diazepam, lorazepam, clonazepam, and alprazolam, are the medications commonly prescribed for treating most types of anxiety, including short-term (situational) anxiety and long-term (generalized) anxiety. Unfortunately, because they are so efficacious and safe, these medications are often prescribed without full appreciation of the potential problem of physical dependency. OCD and PTSD are more effectively treated by antidepressants. Several drugs in the selective serotonin reuptake inhibitors (SSRIs) class of antidepressants including fluoxetine, sertraline, paroxetine, and fluvoxamine have emerged as the preferred type of antidepressant for treatment of OCD. Clonidine and beta blockers such as propranolol and atenolol are also used. Herbal products include kava kava and valerian. Another nonbenzodiazepine used for more long-term treatment is buspirone.

Psychological

During the past decade, there has been increasing enthusiasm and demand for focused, time-limited therapies that address ways of coping with anxiety symptoms directly rather than exploring unconscious conflicts or other personal vulnerabilities. These therapies emphasize cognitive and behavioral assessments and interventions, such as relaxation training, biofeedback, systematic desensitization, reframing, thought stopping, aversion therapy, and social skills training.

The hallmarks of cognitive-behavioral therapies are evaluating cause-and-effect relationships among thoughts, feelings, and behaviors, as well as using straightforward strategies to lessen symptoms and reduce avoidant behaviors. Therapeutic modalities such as guided imagery and muscle relaxation, exercise and rest programs, aromatherapy, and music and art therapy may be used as adjuncts to medication or alone. All mental health disciplines, including psychiatric mental health nurses, psychiatric social workers, psychologists, and psychiatrists, may use these anxiety reduction approaches in their collaborative treatment of clients with anxiety.

NURSING MANAGEMENT

ANXIETY manifested by tension, distress, uncertainty related to threat to health, self-concept and lifestyle.

Patient Outcomes

- Demonstrates decreased level of anxiety
- Will report feeling less anxious after using coping strategies
- Will use coping strategies effectively when anxiety is recognized
- Demonstrates increased ability to prevent episodes of anxiety by problem-solving

Interventions

- Speak in a calm, quiet voice; convey a sense of confidence and control and a tolerant, understanding attitude.
- Place patient in quiet environment; reduce distracting stimuli (e.g., noise, activity, light).
- Use discretion in conversations with patient and near patient's room.
- Recognize factors that may stimulate more anxiety.
- Reduce demands placed on patient until anxiety is reduced. Provide rest periods between tests, activities, and visitors.
- Provide diversional activity and exercise. Monitor changes in level of activity.
- Allow supportive others (clergy, social workers, volunteers) to visit patient. Explain tests and equipment to them so they can in turn be more relaxed around patient.
- Provide realistic feedback about patient's situation; do not give false reassurances. Help patient understand the anxiety by having him or her name the feeling.
- Encourage patient to express feelings (some crying and anger are appropriate).
- Have patient identify what happened just before the anxiety started and try to identify the causative event. Discuss the possible connection between the precipitating event and the meaning it has for the patient.
- Determine patient's usual coping mechanism in similar situations.
- Encourage patient to recall and think through similar instances of anxiety, what alternative behaviors could be used to cope more adaptively.
- Attempt to discuss what patient understands as cause of anxiety or panic once the anxiety level is reduced.
- Stay with patient but do not require explanations for the distress; individuals with severe or panic-level anxiety may become more agitated by attempts to communicate with them.
- Provide measures to relieve anxiety (e.g., warm bath, back rub, walk). Discuss other techniques for reducing anxiety (relaxation exercises, stress-reduction techniques) when patient is calmer and more rested. Encourage slow, deep breathing if patient is hyperventilating; breathing with patient to set pattern may be helpful.
- Assist patient in learning and problem solving when anxiety is diminished enough to allow concentration.
- Evaluate need for antianxiety medications; anxiolytics can be very effective in relieving panic; if none have been ordered, consult with physician for pharmacologic therapy.
- Assess for potential injury or violence to self or others.

- Give feedback about patient's current coping ability; reinforce any attempts to cope adaptively.
- Refer patients with recurrent anxiety and maladaptive coping mechanisms for further psychiatric/psychological evaluation and treatment.
- For patients with panic-level anxiety:
  - Take patient to a quiet area with minimal stimuli.
  - Administer anxiolytics as needed (ask what medications patient has used in past)
  - Remain with patient through the attack.
  - Give patient clear, honest feedback ("You are having a panic attack; I will stay with you").

INEFFECTIVE COPING. Individual evidenced by anxiety/fear/avoidance of objects or events, as well as irrational thoughts related to phobias, extreme guilt.

Patient Outcomes

- Demonstrate increased ability to think rationally and without undue guilt
- Identify thoughts and situations that evoke anxiety
- Show decreased anxiety related to improved thought processes and problem solving
- Demonstrate appropriate coping strategy for reducing anxiety related to phobia

Interventions

- Realize that phobic reactions are irrational and are not changed by rational, logical explanations; work around phobias (e.g., do not require a claustrophobic patient to use an elevator).
- Promote communication that reinforces rational thinking and decreases guilt.
- Verify your interpretation of what patient is experiencing (e.g., "I understand that you are afraid to go to the radiology department.")
- Use words familiar to patient when describing new events or expectations.
- Help patient to clarify thoughts and avoid misinterpretation; ask meaning of anything that you do not understand.
- Do not talk around or whisper near patient; include patient in conversation and check that he or she heard what you actually said by asking him or her to repeat it.
- Set limits on discussing irrational material; focus on topics based in reality that you can verify.
- Avoid belittling or derogating when patient misinterprets stimuli or is irrational; do not laugh or make fun of the individual.

- Assist patient to set limits on own behavior; suggest alternative ways to cope with anxiety (e.g., take a walk instead of crying).
- Be aware of potential for violence; observe for changes in behavior indicating increased anxiety, irrational thoughts, or any destructive behavior that requires attention.
- Anticipate difficulties in adjusting to return or transfer to home or other facility; discuss concerns with family or SO.
- Let patient have some control in anxiety-provoking situation; do not force patient to do anything that seems to be extremely frightening.
- Provide time to discuss anxiety or fear while continuing supportive verbal and behavioral interventions.
- Refer patients with phobias for more specific treatment (e.g., desensitization, behavioral modification) to a psychiatrist, psychologist, advanced practice nurse, or social worker if anxiety is not managed by previous interventions.

ALTERNATE NURSING DIAGNOSES

Comfort, Impaired
Fear
Gas Exchange, Impaired
Perception, Disturbed

WHEN TO CALL FOR HELP

- Increased anxiety leading to refusal of treatment or noncompliance
- Onset of paranoid, psychotic thinking
- Onset of panic attack
- Staff conflict over management of patient behavior
- Increased staff anxiety over caring for patient.

WHO TO CALL FOR HELP

- Psychiatric Team
- Social Worker
- Chaplain
- Colleagues who know patient
- Patient's family/friends
- Coworkers

Post-Trauma Syndrome
Sleep Deprivation
Spiritual Distress
Thought Processes, Disturbed
Violence, Risk for

PATIENT AND FAMILY EDUCATION

- Teach patient and family or SO anxiety-reducing exercises such as muscle relaxation, guided imagery, music, or other activities for distraction.
- Discuss with patient and family or SO the causes and treatment of patient's anxiety.
- Review possible negative short-term and long-term effects of anxiety on physical and mental health.
- If patient is using antianxiety medications, review the need to monitor their use and potential problems when overused or discontinued without weaning.
- Educate on the use of appropriate medications to treat paralyzing symptoms such as OCD.

CHARTING TIPS

- Use objective assessment and nonjudgmental terms to describe behavior.
- Use patient's own words to describe amount and type of anxiety experienced.
- Note which interventions are most helpful in decreasing patient's anxiety and specific treatments that patient successfully learned to control own anxiety.
- Document family or SO responses to education about anxiety reduction methods.
- Document use of antianxiety medications and patient's response to them.

COMMUNITY-BASED CARE

- Discharge can be a particularly anxiety-provoking time for many patients. Begin discharge planning early and include all caretakers in planning for future care needs.
- Allow enough time to discuss alternatives and provide as much emotional support as possible during the transition time.
- Discuss available community resources: their functions, services, capabilities, and limitations.
- If transferring patient to another facility or agency for follow-up care, provide information about patient's progress in and successful interventions for dealing with anxiety.

- Refer to a psychiatrist or internist specializing in psychotropics if patient has frequent panic attacks or chronic, moderate to severe anxiety.
- Refer family for counseling early in patient's hospitalization so that therapeutic behaviors that will minimize patient's anxious behavior can be learned before patient returns home.
- To ensure consistency, record and communicate to family or others responsible for patient after discharge, those interventions that worked well.

8 Problems with Anger

The Angry Patient

Learning Objectives

- Identify three positive functions of anger.
- Identify possible nurses' reactions to an angry patient.
- Differentiate among assertive, passive, and hostile expressions of anger.
- Select the most appropriate interventions for dealing with an angry patient.

Glossary

Anger – *A state of emotional excitement and tension induced by intense displeasure, frustration, and/or anxiety in response to a perceived threat.*

Assertiveness – *Behavior directed toward claiming one's rights without denying the rights of others.*

Assertiveness training – *Learning behavioral techniques that allow an individual to stand up for his or her own rights without infringing on the rights of others.*

Frustration – *Feelings generated from the inability to meet a goal.*

Hostility – *Feelings of anger and resentment that are destructive.*

Passive-aggressive behavior – *Behavior characterized by angry, hostile feelings that are expressed indirectly, leading to impaired communication and inappropriate expression. This behavior masks anger in such a way as to obstruct honesty in relationships. It may also be associated with obsessive-compulsive personality, borderline personality, and depression.*

Rational anger – *Anger expressed in a direct, socially acceptable manner.*

Anger is a normal human emotion. It can result from frustration, fear, or rejection. When handled appropriately, anger can help people resolve conflicts and make decisions. It can energize us into action. It can also contribute to physical and emotional distress if handled in a destructive manner. Expressing anger directly can be uncomfortable. However, denying it, suppressing it, or expressing it inappropriately tends to lead to more negative outcomes. The inappropriate expression of anger may be threatening to oneself and others (Harper-Jaques & Reimer, 2005). Learning to deal with anger is an ongoing process, and when we learn how to deal with our anger and others' anger appropriately, we can gain a positive feeling of control, a sense of power and energy, and increased self-esteem. Some people fear anger because they think it could get out of control. Generally, though, anger tends to be of short duration and low intensity for most people. It does not necessarily lead to violence and aggression. Thomas (2001) asserts that expression of anger may prevent aggression and help resolve a situation.

Anger can be viewed along a continuum. At one extreme is passive-aggressive behavior, in which a person avoids direct, open expression of anger but finds hidden ways to express it. At the other extreme is aggressive expression, in which a person inflicts pain on others when he or she expresses anger. Rational anger falls in the middle. When anger is rational, feelings are expressed in a direct, socially acceptable manner that allows the person to gain some control over the threat without causing harm to others.

ETIOLOGY

No single theory can explain the complex emotion of anger. Most likely, an intertwining of biological, psychological, and sociocultural factors create each individual's unique response. Box 8–1 lists positive and negative functions of anger.

Biological theories of anger focus mainly on neurotransmitters, such as dopamine, norepinephrine, and serotonin. The balance of these and other brain chemicals seem to influence or even aggravate response to anger and stress. Actual physical changes in the brain have been noted in aggressive behavior (Watson, 2006).

BOX 8–1
Positive and Negative Functions of Anger

Positive Functions	Negative Functions
Energizes body for self-defense	Can lead to impulsive behavior
Can promote conflict resolution	Can lead to hostility and rage
Can increase self-esteem and sense of control	Can hurt others emotionally or physically

Psychological theories look at the various dynamics and learned responses that cause anger. Anger occurs as a result of a buildup of frustration. Pacquette (1998) points out that frustration and feelings of powerlessness precede expression of anger. Children often use inappropriate anger responses, such as temper tantrums, to deal with frustration and feelings of powerlessness. Positive reinforcement for this behavior can cause inappropriate anger responses to continue into adulthood. When the child's caregivers are demanding, hypercritical, and punitive, the child may develop coping mechanisms aimed at avoiding expressing anger directly for fear of displeasing the caregiver and risking emotional abandonment or retaliation. These coping mechanisms often lead to a passive-aggressive anger response and resentment, which eventually erupt into inappropriate or destructive behavior. Anger can sometimes be a normal response to fear and help the person gain control of a perceived threat, or it can be part of the adaptive process in adjusting to a loss. In addition, suppressed anger can contribute to depression and low self-esteem (Townsend, 2006). Anger can also be a motivating factor to stimulate action that in turn can raise self-esteem.

Sociocultural factors also play an important role in the way an individual expresses anger. Social groups, including families, often display common patterns in the degree of acceptance of expressed anger. For example, in some families yelling and aggressive confrontation are acceptable means of dealing with anger and conflict, whereas in others, any overt display of anger is not tolerated. Although both of these styles may work within individual families, they may not be the healthiest ways of dealing with anger. Expressions of anger are also seen in major depression, especially when the depressed person feels trapped (Fava & Rosenbaum, 1999).

Women are often socialized to deal with anger differently from men. They may tend to displace or suppress angry feelings and attempt to give in and compromise rather than deal with the conflict directly (Hollinworth, Clark, Harland, Johnson, & Partington, 2005). This behavior can lead to passive-aggressive responses or resentment that may eventually become destructive. Such repression can also be detrimental and lead to misunderstanding when dealing with male colleagues.

CLINICAL CONCERNS

Medical conditions, such as chronic illness or loss of body function, may strain one's coping abilities and lead to an uncharacteristic display of anger. Adjusting to the loss of body function includes anger as part of the grieving process. Illness often means facing feelings of powerlessness and frustration in meeting one's goals and contributes to angry responses such as irritability. Some conditions, including some brain tumors and different forms of dementia, may also directly contribute to inappropriate expressions of anger because of their influence on brain function. Emerson-Rose (2005) has found evidence that negative emotional states contribute to cardiovascular disease.

Abuse of mind-altering substances may reduce inhibitions and contribute to inappropriate expression of anger.

LIFE SPAN ISSUES

Children

Children normally respond with anger when faced with frustration. If they are raised in an environment where intense anger and violence are accepted, they can develop overly aggressive anger responses, including cruelty to others, animal abuse, and intolerance for frustration. Conversely, children who are taught that anger is unacceptable may tend to suppress or deny angry feelings and can develop extreme distress and guilt when faced with conflict. Children who learn appropriate ways to relieve tensions are more able to express anger rationally. Because children are vulnerable, they may be at increased risk of injury caused by inappropriate expressions of anger by caregivers.

Adolescents

Anger in adolescents is often seen as part of their developmental process of separation from parents and asserting their individuality. Hostility can also come from overstimulation from all they are dealing with. They may also have fears of being unable to control their impulses, leading to anxiety about anger.

Adults

Adults who must deal with difficult life experiences, such as a chronic illness or the onset of an acute illness compounding stressful life events, can become very angry. This anger can further complicate the disease by depleting coping skills and interfering with the recommended medical treatment.

Older Adults

Uncharacteristic displays of anger in elderly people may be the result of frustration caused by a variety of physical, mental, and lifestyle changes such as dementia, altered sensory function (particularly hearing loss), altered mobility, changes in sleep-rest patterns, effects of medications, depression, loss of loved ones, and fear of dying. Inappropriate behavior may cause elderly persons to be alienated, further increasing their sense of fear, frustration, and possible confusion. Additionally, vulnerable elderly people are at risk of being victims of someone else's anger.

POSSIBLE NURSES' REACTIONS

- May take patient's anger personally, causing an unhealthy emotional response.
- May respond defensively by using an aggressive response or avoidance. This can accelerate the anger cycle.
- May attribute the patient's anger to a specific event, such as the quality of care provided, and respond by feeling unappreciated and resentful.
- May feel uncomfortable or fearful and respond by suppressing or denying the anger.
- May avoid the patient for fear of emotional or physical retaliation.

ASSESSMENT

Behavior and Appearance

- Loud voice, change in pitch, or very soft voice, forcing other to strain to hear (Table 8–1)
- Intense eye contact or avoidance of eye contact
- Rapid, pacing movement
- Ruminating about an issue
- Passive-aggressive behavior, possibly including sarcastic humor; chronic complaining; socially annoying habits; pseudocompliance (agreeing to do something but not doing it)
- Possible physical violence

TABLE 8–1

Comparing Behavioral Responses to Anger

Traits	Passive	Assertive	Aggressive
Speech content	Negative: "Can I", "Should I", Puts self down	Positive: "I can", "I will", "I" messages	Hostile: "You never ...", "You always ...", Derogatory
Voice	Whispers Whiny, weak	Firm, clear	Loud
Posture Eye contact Gestures	Drooping Looks down Fidgets	Erect, relaxed Appropriate Appropriate	Tense Invasive Threatening

Mood and Emotions

- Annoyance, discomfort, frustration, continuous state of tension
- May be quick to anger, then let it go or take time to "stew" before expressing anger
- Guilt
- Powerlessness
- Vulnerability, easily offended
- Defensive response to criticism
- Passive-aggressive emotional response, possibly including being sullen, yet denying any concerns, or inappropriate cheerfulness for the situation

Thoughts, Beliefs, and Perceptions

- May believe that anger is normal and can be expressed without hurting others
- May take responsibility appropriately without blaming others
- May be angry at others but still care for them
- May lack ability to express true feelings
- May fear loss of love if anger is expressed directly
- May fear emotional or physical abandonment if anger is expressed
- May feel a sense of power when angry

Relationships and Interactions

- May communicate concerns clearly to avoid additional misunderstanding
- May avoid other hostile or angry persons
- May be catered to by others who fear patient's anger

Physical Responses

- Fight-or-flight response during confrontations, possibly including rapid pulse, increased blood pressure, rapid breathing, muscle tension, sweating, or intense feelings of wanting to attack or run
- Episodes of headaches, depression, sleep alterations, pain, or gastrointestinal symptoms associated with repressed anger

COLLABORATIVE MANAGEMENT

Pharmacological

Antianxiety medications, including benzodiazepines, are sometimes used for short-term relief of feelings of tension and anger. However, they should not be used as a substitute for acknowledging and dealing with anger, and they should not interfere with pharmacological actions of medications being taken for the underlying medical condition. In addition, antidepressants may be effective in controlling impulsive and aggressive behavior associated with mood swings. Beta blockers have also been used occasionally to control aggressive behaviors.

Common herbal products used for tension include St. John's wort, kava kava, and valerian.

NURSING MANAGEMENT

ANXIETY evidenced by tension, distress, uncertainty, restlessness, or displeasure related to threat to self-concept, frustration, or unconscious conflict.

Patient Outcomes

- Verbalizes concerns and frustrations directly at an appropriate time
- Demonstrates reduced tension including lowered voice and more appropriate anger response
- Demonstrates problem-solving skills when faced with frustration
- Demonstrates behaviors to calm self when faced with frustration

Interventions

- Use therapeutic communication techniques including open-ended questions, appropriate eye contact, and supportive gestures to encourage patient to vent feelings and concerns. Avoid providing solutions before the patient has a chance to relieve tension.
- Listen with concern without being patronizing or condescending. Phrases such as "Tell me what happened next" or "That really sounds frustrating" allow the patient to feel accepted and understood. Avoid phrases that escalate feelings of powerlessness, such as "Calm down" or "It can't be that bad."
- If needed, direct the patient to a more private setting to express his or her feelings. Having others view the demonstration of anger can make it more difficult to back down and contribute to escalation of hostility or aggression.
- When the tension of the situation is reduced, focus on identifying the source of anger and validating the problem. Explore options on how to deal with the problem more constructively. Ask the patient which methods he or she has used successfully in the past when dealing with frustration. Teach problem-solving skills. Assist the patient to identify and use more effective coping mechanisms.
- Teach tension-reducing techniques, such as deep breathing, counting to 10, walking away, and talking to self about remaining in control.
- Encourage the patient to express angry feelings toward the appropriate person. Role-playing before the confrontation may help the patient choose effective strategies.

- Recognize that an angry outburst may result from an accumulation of multiple stressors that causes the patient to overreact.
- If the patient is justifiably angry because of something you have done or not done, accept appropriate responsibility. Work with the patient or colleagues to resolve the problem. Accepting and validating the patient's feelings sends the message that you value his or her viewpoint.
- Encourage children to vent frustration by redirecting their activity, such as hitting a pillow or engaging in exercise.

INEFFECTIVE COPING evidenced by inappropriate expression of anger, distress, destructive behavior to self or others, and related to threat to self-esteem or unconscious conflict.

Patient Outcomes

- Able to identify personal strength that may help to reduce stress
- Accepts personal limits in dealing with inappropriate demands
- Demonstrates effective skills for dealing with frustration

Interventions

- Identify ways to increase the person's self-esteem as part of expressing anger by treating him or her respectfully and acknowledging his or her skills or attributes. For example, when dealing with an angry daughter's confrontation about her parent's care, state, "Your father is lucky to have you as his advocate." Avoid a defensive response or ignoring complaints.
- Focus on the patient's strengths to deal with frustration. Help him or her identify which coping skills have been successful in the past.
- Teach the patient that anger is a normal response to loss. Some individuals are unable to accept this anger as normal and experience unneeded guilt.
- Encourage the patient to state the cause of the problem clearly to avoid erroneous assumptions.
- If the patient rejects or finds fault with all of your suggestions, place the responsibility for choosing the appropriate response on the patient. You might say, "We've discussed many options. Now it is up to you to consider which one is best for you."
- Set clear limits on the patient's expressions of anger toward the staff. Refuse to listen to extensive complaining if the patient is not willing to participate in determining an acceptable solution.
- Be assertive when explaining which types of behavior are not appropriate.
- Be consistent with the demands the patient can set on the staff.
- Promote effective problem-solving.

- Encourage self-evaluation of behavior to give patient sense of control (e.g., what did you learn from that?)
- Be a role model for expressing negative emotions in a positive manner. Use "I messages," such as "I feel angry" rather than accusing the other person, which can lead to a defensive response. Speak firmly without yelling and avoid threatening gestures when confronting issues.

DEFENSIVE COPING evidenced by blaming others for his/her problems; hypersentive to criticism and related to feeling powerless.

Patient Outcomes

- Demonstrates reduced defensive behaviors
- Able to verbalize realistic causes for distress

Interventions

- Avoid challenging or criticizing the patients' responses
- Listen to his/her concerns
- Help patient identify ways to evaluate progress in changing behavior.
- Provide consistent staff so patient can establish a relationship to reduce the threat of different to his/her behavior. This will help develop trust.
- Avoid getting into power struggles with patient. Work to identify positives outcomes.

ALTERNATE NURSING DIAGNOSES

Noncompliance
Powerlessness
Self-Concept, Disturbed
Social Interaction, Impaired
Violence, Risk for

WHEN TO CALL FOR HELP

- Increased aggressiveness; violent behavior, including damaging property; increasing use of abusive language, threats made to patients or staff
- Onset of paranoid thinking or psychotic behavior
- Onset of extreme obsessive-compulsive behavior
- Increased staff conflict over management of patient behavior
- Increased staff anxiety over caring for patient

WHO TO CALL FOR HELP

- Psychiatric Team
- Social Worker
- Security if concern for potential violence
- Manager to address any conflict between staff members
- Work colleagues if you need assistance

PATIENT AND FAMILY EDUCATION

- Teach assertiveness skills by role-modeling appropriate responses and helping the patient practice these skills.
- Review with the patient frequently encountered frustrations, and explain that giving up control of the outcome may be the most effective strategy for dealing with them.
- Review potential negative health effects of inappropriate anger expression.
- If the patient is using antianxiety medications, review the need to monitor their use and avoid using them in place of trying to resolve the cause of anger.
- Review with patient/family what has helped in the past.

CHARTING TIPS

- Use objective, nonjudgmental terms to describe behavior.
- Document patient's response to frustration.
- Document the limits set on care plan or treatment plan for consistency.
- Document use of medications (including herbal products) and patient's response to them.

COMMUNITY-BASED CARE

- Communicate plan of care to all involved in discharge planning.
- Inform any appropriate agencies of patient behaviors to avoid miscommunication.
- Refer patient to counseling services or assertiveness training, if needed.
- Encourage patient's active participation in treatment plan.
- Encourage family/caregivers to take the time to understand some of the dynamics of the patient's behavior
- Inform caregivers/family of effective coping mechanisms to reduce the risk of anger escalating to violence.

The Aggressive and Potentially Violent Patient

Learning Objectives

- Identify factors that precipitate aggressive behavior.
- Describe effective techniques for verbal de-escalation of aggressive behavior.
- List possible nursing staff reactions to violent behavior in patients.
- List interventions a nurse could use in working with a violent patient.

Glossary

Aggression – *Any verbal or nonverbal, actual or attempted, forceful abuse of the self or another person or object.*

Assaultive behavior – *An intentional act that is designed to make another person fearful and produces harm.*

Chemical Restraints – *Use of medication as a restriction to manage the patient's behavior or restrict the patient's freedom of movement and is not a standard treatment or dosage for the patient's condition*

Hostility – *Anger that is destructive in nature and purpose as opposed to rational anger that is appropriate to the situation and is not destructive in intent.*

Intimidation – *The use of threats to frighten and control.*

Physical restraint – *Any physical method of restricting an individual's freedom of movement, activity, or normal access to his or her body and cannot be easily removed.*

Rage – *Engulfing emotional experience of extreme anger.*

Seclusion – *Involuntary confinement of the patient alone in a room or an area where the patient is prevented from leaving as a means of controlling impulses that might lead to the immediate harm of the patient, staff, or others*

Violent behavior – *Exertion of extreme force or destructive acts with intent to hurt another and that can cause injury.*

Workplace violence – *Violent acts including physical assaults and threats of assaults directed toward any persons at work or on duty. Four categories include violence by strangers, clients, coworkers, and personal relations.*

The presence of violence in our society has unfortunately become increasingly common. This increased violence is also reflected in the health-care setting (Winstanley & Whittington, 2004). U.S. Labor Department statistics report that hospital-related violence is higher than in other private service businesses. Health-care and social service workers have the highest rate of nonfatal assault injuries in the workplace with nurses being 3 times more likely to experience violence than other professionals. Psychiatric and emergency room nurses are at highest risk (Catlette, 2005; Emergency Nurses Association, 2006). The American Nurses Association (2002) also reports that more than 80% of assaults on nurses go unreported. NIOSH (National Institute for Occupation Safety and Health) has identified times when violent behavior may be more likely in patient care settings. These include visiting hours, meal times, when service is denied, when limits are set, and involuntary admissions.

Historically, nurses working with psychiatric patients have been taught to be alert to and manage violent, assaultive behavior; however, now all health-care workers need to be alert to this problem. Health-care facilities must institute security measures and policies to ensure the safety of staff and patients, and to reduce the fear of impending violence among staff and visitors. Consistently being confronted with aggressive and potentially violent patients, families, and visitors can cause excessive fear, stress, job dissatisfaction, lost work time, poor morale, turnover, increased errors and possible injury (Anderson, 2002; Gates, 2004). The Occupational Health and Safety Administration (OSHA) has developed voluntary guidelines for employers to address this problem. They created "Universal Precautions for Violence," which acknowledges that violence should be expected but can be avoided or mitigated by proper training, policies, and security measures.

Past history of violence is the greatest predictor of this behavior (Blair & New, 1991). In addition, a history of psychiatric illness, particularly schizophrenia, paranoia, borderline personality disorder, other personality disorders, posttraumatic stress disorder, and dementia is frequently associated with predicting an aggressive outburst. Other major risk factors include drug and alcohol use but predicting when or if a patient will become violent remains difficult (Domrose, 2007).

The causes of the increased violence in our society and, consequently, in health care are varied and complex. Some of these causes include the following:

- Attitudinal changes in society with increased acceptance of violent response to authority figures
- Increased prevalence of handguns among patients, families, and visitors
- Increased use of mind-altering drugs and alcohol
- Court decisions that give psychiatric patients the right to refuse treatment and medication
- Health care staff members who are inadequately prepared to respond to aggression or who deny the risk of violence and fail to report it
- Increasing frustrations in health-care settings, including inadequate staffing and long waits

- Health-care workers in isolated environments (e.g., examining rooms, in patient's home) with no backup, communication devices, or alarms
- Impersonal care, which may stress already frustrated patients
- Legal and ethical concerns about using chemical and physical restraints
- Media coverage of violence, which triggers additional crimes

Using restraints to manage potentially violent patients can create ethical dilemmas for the nurse concerning patient autonomy, human dignity, and informed consent. In 1993, the Joint Commission on Accreditation of Health Care Organizations (JCAHO) created standards for physical restraints, requiring each agency to provide clear policies and education on appropriate restraint use. They have continued to refine these because of ongoing problems (JCAHO, 2005, 2006, 2007). The aim is to reduce the incidence of injuries that can result from restraint use, such as loss of mobility, skin breakdown, and, possibly, death from strangulation. The least restrictive to maintain patient safety should be used when other alternatives to this restraint have been ineffective. In 1999, Medicare and Medicaid developed new federal standards for the use of restraints that included the following: the emphasis must be on prevention; health-care institutions must continually work to reduce the use of restrictive measures of restraints and seclusion; restraints can be applied only with a physician's order for each occurrence; continuous assessment of the patient while he or she is being restrained must be done; and alternatives to restraints must be tried. In 2006, The Centers for Medicare and Medicaid revised restraint and seclusion standards to include that health-care providers who use physical restraints and seclusions when treating violent or self-destructive patients must undergo rigorous training on the use of these approaches. In the medical setting, new alternatives to traditional physical restraints called freedom splints have been developed. They allow more movement but reduce the risk of interference with medical procedures like pulling out IVs or nasogastric tubes (Markwell, 2005).

ETIOLOGY

Aggressive, violent behavior has many causes. Most studies of the causes of aggression have been done on subjects with mental illness or prison populations, which may skew the results.

Biological theories include genetics, which links chromosomal abnormalities to aggressive behavior, hormone imbalances, and neurotransmitter irregularities, specifically the abnormal secretions of dopamine and serotonin.

Psychological theories on aggression are related to a person's view of the world as a source of anxiety. Individuals prone to violence often have low self-esteem and need to maintain control to enhance their own feelings of power and self-worth. Fear and anxiety can distort an individual's perception of the stimulus. The presence of alcohol or other drugs can further distort these perceptions and reduce inhibitions. Aggressive behavior temporarily reduces the anxiety and creates a temporary sense of power. In addition, individuals with poor impulse control or a personality disorder may use violence to intimidate others. Aggressive individuals may have limited ability to tolerate frustration and demand to have their needs met immediately. Individuals who have experienced emotional deprivation in childhood may be particularly vulnerable and respond with violent outbursts when they sense an attack on their self-esteem.

Social learning theory views aggression as a learned behavior. Individuals with a tendency toward aggressive, violent behavior may be more likely to respond to stressors such as illness, school or work pressures, or relationship problems with anger and hostility because they have learned that such behavior temporarily reduces their anxiety.

Sociocultural theories look at an aggressive individual's poor interpersonal skills. Exposure to aggression and violence as part of family life may also be a significantly influential factor. Children who are treated with violence may view violence as a normal way to deal with others. The cycle of family violence continues when children learn to use violence as their only coping mechanism instead of more socially acceptable ones. Poverty, deprivation, and hopelessness can also increase the risk of violent behavior.

RELATED CLINICAL CONCERNS

A wide variety of organic disorders may be associated with aggressive and violent behavior. These include the following:

Intracranial Disorders

Brain tumors

Head injury

Seizure disorders

Cerebrovascular accident

Dementia

Systemic Disorders

Endocrine disorders such as thyroid storm or Cushing's syndrome

Electrolyte imbalance

Oxygen deficiency

Septicemia

Hepatic encephalopathy

Exposure to Substances

Alcohol use or withdrawal

Use of mind-altering substances such as phencyclidine and amphetamines and crystal methamphetamine

Withdrawal from barbiturates and sedatives

Use of aromatic hydrocarbons (glue, paint)

Use of medications such as steroids, central nervous system stimulants, and antiparkinsonian agents

Exposure to toxic chemicals, pesticides, lead

LIFE SPAN ISSUES

Children

Constant exposure to violence in childhood is a major factor contributing to the cycle of child abuse and family violence. Children who learn to use violent behavior to cope with frustrations and problems are likely to carry these behaviors into adulthood and may need to learn effective coping skills. Early signs of problems may include cruelty to animals and other children, as well as difficulty controlling responses to frustration. The alarming presence of violence in schools and neighborhoods and in the media has increased the number of children who are exposed to seeing aggressive behavior and weapons used to resolve frustration in what may appear to them to be socially acceptable, normal behavior. Autism, mental retardation, learning disabilities, and attention deficit/hyperactivity disorders (ADHD) may also cause aggressive and violent behavior in children. The American Academy of Pediatrics Clinical Practice Guidelines (2000) recommend that children 6 to 12 years who present with hyperactivity, impulsivity, or behavior problems be evaluated for ADHD.

Adolescents

Adolescents may act out aggressive feelings by participating in self-destructive behavior such as drug or alcohol use, smoking, or crime. Using mind-altering substances increases the risk of violent behavior. Homicide is the leading cause of death in the 15- to 24-year-old age group (Dowd, 1998).

Adults

Aggressive behavior in adults often reflects lifelong learned patterns. For instance, persons who abuse their spouses have often witnessed abuse in their parents' relationship or been abused themselves as children.

Older Adults

Like anger, violent behavior can be a lifelong pattern or be caused by physical illness or adverse reactions to medications. Aggressive behavior may also be a self-protective response related to confusion, fear, or sensory loss (particularly hearing loss). Most frequently, aggressive behavior in elderly persons is associated with Alzheimer's disease, senile dementia, cerebrovascular accidents, metabolic disorders, and hypoxia. Management of aggressive and violent behavior in nursing homes may be impacted by policies and federal requirements to reduce use of physical and chemical restraints.

POSSIBLE NURSES' REACTIONS

- May fear being hurt by the violent or aggressive patient or one who uses intimidation with the threat of violence. This fear can cause the nurse to use poor judgment or totally deny feeling fearful. Other common fear responses include avoiding the patient or bending the rules in an attempt to appease the patient. All of these responses can affect continuity of patient care.
- May feel abused and unappreciated, leading to defensive responses such as attempting to punish the patient. Defensive responses and treating patient with less respect can escalate anger.
- May feel guilty for not being able to control the behavior or feel uncomfortable for participating in applying restraints.
- May feel offended or frustrated because the patient does not respond to care positively.
- A nurse who has been assaulted in the past may experience self-blame and question his or her competence, depression, anxiety, and hyperalertness to any situation that could lead to aggressiveness.

ASSESSMENT

Behavior and Appearance

- Pacing, restlessness
- Tense facial expression and body language
- Unpredictable behavior
- Loud voice, shouting, use of obscenities, argumentative
- Overreacting to stimuli such as noise
- Exhibiting poor impulse control evidenced by acting quickly before considering consequences of actions
- Grasping potential weapons and attempting to use them

Mood and Emotions

- Anger, resentment, rage, hostility
- Anxiety; fear of loss of control leading to panic
- Inappropriate affect for situation, labile emotions

Thoughts, Beliefs, and Perceptions

- Low self-esteem
- Low frustration tolerance

- Thoughts or plans to harm someone
- Inability to trust others to follow through without strong intimidation and suspiciousness
- Hallucinations, paranoid delusions
- Views others as out to hurt him or her
- Sense of being out of control

Relationships and Interactions

- Difficulty with close relationships; lack of trust, which causes person to fear closeness
- Others fearful of and avoid aggressive person, believing that they might be hurt or manipulated
- Family and friends have learned to meet person's demands to avoid aggressive response or exhibiting passive-aggressive behaviors in response to the person's demands

Physical Responses

- Increased muscle tension
- Increased heart rate and blood pressure
- Altered level of consciousness, confusion, lethargy
- Possible abnormal laboratory values including blood sugar, blood alcohol, drug screening
- Increased use of medications

Pertinent History

- History of violent behavior, particularly assault
- Psychiatric diagnosis
- Substance and/or alcohol abuse
- Physical, emotional, or sexual abuse in childhood or by intimate partner

COLLABORATIVE MANAGEMENT

Pharmacological

It is important to use appropriate medications in adequate doses as an alternative or adjunct to physical restraints to manage aggressive behavior. Just as physical restraints and seclusion must be closely regulated, so is the use of psychotropic medication when it functions as a chemical restraint.

Pharmacological management of acute aggressive or violent behavior may require rapid tranquilization, which involves regular, frequent administration of antipsychotic medications such as haloperidol (Videbeck, 2004). Parenteral administration may be required if oral route is not feasible. If the patient is in physical restraints, parenteral administration reduces the risk of aspiration. For example, haloperidol, 5 mg, may be administered every 30 to 60 minutes until symptoms are under control. Dosage should be reduced in elderly people. When using this drug, monitor the patient closely for hypotension and signs of extrapyramidal symptoms including akathisias and dystonia (see Chapter 21).

Antianxiety medications and sedatives may also be useful. Anticonvulsants, such as carbamazepine (Tegretol), have been used with some success. Lithium and beta blockers, such as propranolol, are other alternatives. Antidepressants have also been used to treat impulsive, aggressive behavior. When using these drugs, evaluate how they may interfere with the medications ordered to treat the patient's underlying medical condition.

Convincing an aggressive, agitated patient to accept medication can be difficult and may lead the nurse to face an ethical dilemma of giving medication against a patient's will. Be aware of hospital or agency policies and state laws regarding patient rights (Box 8–2).

Herbal products, such as valerian, have been shown to be helpful in some cases to calm the person.

BOX 8–2
Encouraging an Uncooperative Patient to Take Medication

- Have the nurse who has the best relationship with patient offer the medication. Avoid power struggles and confrontations, which would most likely escalate the situation.

- Have the medication in hand so that it can be given quickly when the patient gives consent. The patient may change his or her mind suddenly.

- Be prepared for the patient to spit out the medication. This is especially common in elderly, aggressive patients.

- Use liquid oral medication if available. It is absorbed more quickly and is less likely to be "cheeked." If medication needs to be given by injection, work quickly. Have adequate staff available in case violence erupts.

- Review with the patient the benefits of medication and that it will help him or her gain control of his or her feelings.

NURSING MANAGEMENT

RISK FOR VIOLENCE, DIRECTED TO OTHERS evidenced by overt hostility and/or aggression to others, threatening others, possession of potential weapon, assaulting others related to impaired judgment, feelings of powerlessness, impulsive behavior, inability to evaluate reality secondary to neurologic problems, psychotic thoughts, and/or drug/alcohol use.

Patient Outcomes

- Demonstrates increased self-control while in nurse's care
- Does not harm others or self while in nurse's care
- Demonstrates alternative coping mechanisms to reduce tension while in nurse's care
- Behavior does not escalate while in nurse's care

Interventions

- Help patient to verbalize angry feelings by reflecting and by clarifying your understanding of these feelings. Communicate your interest by appropriate eye contact, restating what patient has said, and asking questions. Help patient identify source of anger. Recognize that response to illness may make the person feel helpless with the need to strike out to gain a sense of control.
- Early recognition of problem behavior is essential so that staff members can develop a plan.
- If needed, allow patient to release tension physically on inanimate objects such as pillows or in prescribed exercise, as appropriate.
- Do not take patient's behavior personally. For example, if a patient calls you derogatory names, refrain from reacting emotionally. Rather, remind yourself that you represent an authority figure to the patient, and that he or she is reacting to you as such. Remember that patient may use derogatory remarks as a way to bolster his or her own self-esteem and seem to zero in on your sensitive, vulnerable points, such as weight or speech patterns. Avoid responding with sarcasm or ridicule.
- Do not ignore aggressive behavior in the hope that it will go away. It needs to be addressed. Minimization of behavior and ineffective limit setting are the most frequent factors contributing to escalation to violence.
- Set clear, consistent limits in a timely manner on what will and will not be tolerated. Clarify any specific consequences of patient behavior. For example, "If you attempt to hurt anyone, we will be compelled to control your behavior, which may mean using restraints" (Box 8–3).
- Identify one or two staff members who are comfortable with the patient to handle most of the care if possible to help provide consistent interventions. Evaluate whether a male or female staff member has a more

---

BOX 8–3
Setting Limits

1. Explain exactly which behavior is inappropriate. Don't assume the individual knows which behavior is inappropriate.
2. Explain why the behavior is inappropriate. Don't assume the individual knows why the behavior is inappropriate.
3. Give the individual reasonable choices or consequences. Present them as choices, and always present the positive first.
4. Allow time—if you don't allow time to comply, it may be perceived as an ultimatum.
5. Enforce consequences—limits don't work unless you follow through with the consequences.

Source: Reprinted from the Art of Setting Limits Participant Manual, p. 8, with permission of the National Crisis Prevention Institute, Inc., © 1991.

calming influence. Sometimes a man's presence is too threatening and powerful. Other times, it is reassuring to the patient that a male staff member is available. A male patient may be less likely to hurt a woman and may see her as nurturing and supportive. Conversely, male patients may view the female staff as less able to provide control or have other conflicted feelings toward women.

- Free patient's environment of extra stimulation, such as noise or an agitated roommate. Extra stimulation may reduce impulse control. Remove objects around patients that could be used as potential weapons such as portable IV poles or food trays and utensils. Consider providing plastic food dishes and utensils. Avoid startling the patient. Call patient by name before walking into room. Avoid sudden movements that the patient may interpret as threatening.

- Remain calm and communicate that you are in control and can handle the situation. Use a moderate, firm voice and calming hand gestures. Avoid touching patient. Table 8–2 lists a summary of staff interventions.

- Place yourself between the door and the patient. Always have a quick exit available. Never turn your back on this type of patient. Keep door of room open. Let other staff members know you are going in patient's room. Protect other patients who may get in the way of the violent individual.

- Never force an agitated patient to have a test or treatment. Power struggles will escalate aggression. Rather, prioritize care that must be given and focus only on that. Explain all procedures and ask patient's permission before beginning. Give patient choices as often as possible.

- If the patient is psychotic, he or she may be hearing voices. If so, ask what the voices are telling him or her to do. This gives you more information on

TABLE 8–2

Summary of Staff Interventions to Avoid Escalation to Aggression

Patient	Staff
Anxiety	Verbal intervention: • Assess. • Use verbal calming techniques. • Attempt to calm patient. • Do not invade patient's personal space; avoid antagonizing.
Threatening	Set limits: • Continue verbal calming techniques. • Set clear and definite limits. • Be directive and matter of fact. • Be prepared to enforce limits.
Acting out aggression	Physical management: • Recognize mounting tension. • Have a plan. • Designate team leader. • Use only after other measures fail.
Tension reduction	Emotional support: • Allow patient to express feelings. • Listen nonjudgmentally. • Show concern for patient, not anger. • Discuss events with colleagues. • Avoid blaming.

Source: Adapted from Haven, E. & Piscitello, V. (1989). The patient with violent behavior. In S. Lewis, R.D. Grainger, W.A. McDowell, R.J. Gregory, & R.L. Messner (Eds.), *Manual of psychosocial nursing interventions* (pp. 187–204). Philadelphia: WB Saunders; Lewis, S. (1993). Verbal intervention. In P.E. Blumenreich, & S. Lewis (Eds.), *Managing the violent patient* (pp. 41–52). New York: Brunner/Mazel.

what to expect. Hallucinations that command the patient to initiate aggression can be an extremely powerful force for the patient to overcome.

• A nurse who has been assaulted in the past and is now faced with a potentially violent patient may bring fears from this past experience, which could inhibit his or her response. Sharing these fears with colleagues may provide much needed support. Use agency resources for support including employee assistance or critical incident debriefing to help colleagues.

• If a patient makes threats to harm specific people, the nurse needs to notify his or her supervisor and follow protocol for notifying potential victims.

- A visitor who becomes aggressive or violent needs to be reported to the agency security staff immediately and removed from the patient care area.
- Ensure that measures and policies are in place to prevent workplace violence. For areas more prone to violence such as emergency department, work with other departments like security and other support resources to have an action plan in place if behavior escalates (Box 8–4).
- In the patient's home setting, be aware of exits in case a problem develops. Never stay alone in a home with a patient or family who is threatening violence, drinking, or displaying firearms. Consider making home visits with a colleague when there is a known risk of violence. Leave the home immediately if there is any sign of out-of-control behavior. Have access to a cellular phone in case of emergency.

RISK FOR INJURY evidenced by falls, pain, trauma, skin breakdown related to restraining patient to control violent behavior.

Patient Outcomes

- Remains free of injury and complications during restraint application
- Demonstrates control of behavior once restraints are removed

Interventions

- The decision to use restraints should be made only after other efforts to reduce tension have been tried and proven ineffective. A physician's order must be obtained each time restraints are to be used. Standing orders are not acceptable.

BOX 8–4
Preventing Workplace Violence

- Be particularly vigilant during change of shifts and on night shift. Events often occur between 8:30 p.m. and 10:30 a.m.
- Minimize stress factors such as long waits, crowded, confined spaces, and inflexible policies for patients where possible.
- Avoid wearing jewelry or neckties that can be grabbed or tugged.
- Recognize and report any signs of inappropriate angry responses in coworkers, patients and families
- Encourage coworkers to report incidents
- Immediately report all assaults to your supervisor and security.
- Be aware that many agency security staffs have minimal training.
- Receive education on local gangs and gang violence.
- Participate in agency safety committees to ensure that adequate security measures are in place.

- Once the decision is made to restrain patient, act quickly and decisively. Determine what appropriate type of restraint is to be applied before approaching patient. Restraints include cloth chest and limb restraints or leather (hard) locked restraints. (Note: When using hard restraints, make sure you have the key, and double-check that they are locked after applying them to patient.) Have equipment ready before approaching patient.

- Never attempt to restrain a patient by yourself. Have adequate staff members available (usually three to five persons) and a plan of action before attempting to physically control a patient. Recruit reliable help from all possible sources, such as security. Assess their experience in managing a violent patient and review the plan. Decide in advance who will grab which arm or leg if patient must be restrained. The presence of a number of staff members (show of force) alone may subdue a patient. Identify a leader before taking any action.

- Designate one person to talk with the patient and another to direct the other staff. Only one staff member should talk with patient, preferably someone who knows him or her. It is important to communicate in a firm manner, speaking slowly. Lack of leadership can cause confusing and contradictory messages and result in someone being hurt or the patient escaping. Remove other patients from the area.

- Maintain a firm base of support for balance if you are suddenly pushed. Remove name badge, eyeglasses, jewelry, and so on to avoid injury.

- If patient is resisting, he or she may need to be distracted. Each staff member should grab one of the patient's limbs when given the command by the coordinating person and take the patient down to the floor or bed quickly. Attempt to cradle patient's head to prevent injury.

- Once restraints are applied to bed frame, take the time to talk with the patient in a calm, concerned manner to try to humanize situation. Call patient by his or her name.

- Make sure patient has no potential weapons within reach. Patient needs to be searched for sharp objects, matches, and so on.

- Administer medications as ordered.

- Be aware of agency policy regarding application of restraints. Requirements for monitoring patients while in restraints, reasons for restraints, doctor's orders, and the length of time each order remains valid should be clearly spelled out in agency policies. If you are not sure about using restraints on someone, discuss with your supervisor to weigh your obligations to protect the patient versus going against the patient's wishes.

- Monitor the patient closely and document findings according to agency policy including vital signs, circulation extremities, and intake/output.

- Remove restraints and observe patient closely when the situation is under control. Consider removing restraints from one limb at a time so that the patient has time to adjust. For the high-risk patient, keep one arm and one leg in restraints at all times until it is clear that patient can be released. Inform other staff members that patient has been released. Establish clear criteria for reapplying restraints with patient and staff. Prepare family for patient's condition, as appropriate.

- Once the patient has regained control, discuss with him or her why that intervention was used, and allow opportunity to express feelings. This increases his or her sense of control and decreases dehumanization.
- If the patient has a gun or other weapon, never attempt to disarm him or her. Contact security and/or law enforcement agency as soon as possible. Focus on getting assistance and protecting patients and staff. Patients and staff should remain in a safe area until help arrives.
- Consider taking a specialized class on use of defensive techniques such as management of assaultive behavior. Proper training is essential to prevent injury to patients and staff. Staff members can practice with each other to demonstrate how they would handle a violent patient.
- Identify jobs at higher risk of exposure to violence and ensure that employees in these jobs have adequate training. Agency management should be providing adequate support and possibly critical incident debriefing to assist staff recovery after a violent event.

ALTERNATE NURSING DIAGNOSIS

Anxiety
Coping, Ineffective
Self-Esteem, Disturbed
Thought Processes, Disturbed

WHEN TO CALL FOR HELP

- Escalation of behavior from aggressive to violent
- Patient in possession of a weapon
- Inadequate staff members available to control behavior
- Increased staff anxiety over caring for the patient
- Staff members at risk for violence without adequate training/security
- Staff potential for injury or emotional trauma

WHO TO CALL FOR HELP

- Other colleagues in area of incident
- Security/law enforcement
- Psychiatric Team

PATIENT AND FAMILY EDUCATION

- Review early warning signs of escalation of aggressive behavior with patient and his or her family.
- Instruct patient on role of alcohol and drugs in contributing to aggressive behavior.
- Instruct on use of prescribed medications to control tension. Instruct on when to ask for PRN medications.
- If patient is in restraints, review with him or her criteria for removal and reinstatement.

CHARTING TIPS

- Document all actions taken to prevent violent behavior.
- Document application of restraints including type, length of time in restraints, reasons for application, patient response, release of limbs, and care given while in restraints. Document vital sign monitoring.
- Document need for and response to medication given.
- Document any threats made by patient
- Document alternatives tried to avoid restraints
- Document all interventions and responses to them.

COMMUNITY-BASED CARE

- Provide information to patient's family and/or caregivers about emergency psychiatric services, if needed. Discuss potential for violence with family to share possible strategies from nursing care plan.
- Provide information on shelters and/or domestic violence services, if appropriate.
- If patient is being transferred to another facility, share concerns about patient's behavior and interventions and share any history of violent behavior.
- Provide information to family and caregivers on what to do if behavior is out of control. Encourage them to call for help immediately.
- Provide information and referrals on drug treatment if appropriate.
- Provide family/caregivers with information on resources for support, how to get emergency assistance

9 Problems with Affect and Mood

The Depressed Patient

Learning Objectives

- Differentiate feeling depressed from a depressive disorder.
- Describe common physical symptoms seen in depressive disorders.
- Describe interventions for the patient with low self-esteem.
- Describe possible nurses' reactions to the depressed patient

Glossary

Anhedonia – *Loss of pleasure in activities or interests that were previously enjoyed.*

Dysthymic disorder – *Mild to moderate chronic depression lasting at least 2 years.*

Major Depressive Disorder – *Primary psychiatric illness manifested by characteristic symptom clusters such as depressed mood, lowered self-esteem, pessimistic thoughts, and loss of pleasure or interest in former activities.*

Masked depression – *Concealed depression in which patient is not aware of depressed mood or does not display obvious sadness. The depression is expressed through other means, such as physical complaints or diverse psychiatric symptoms such as phobias or compulsions.*

Psychomotor agitation – *Classic symptom cluster of depression including restlessness with rapid, agitated, purposeless movements like pacing or wringing hands .*

Psychomotor retardation – *Classic symptom cluster of depression including slow movements and speech.*

Seasonal affective disorder (SAD) – *Depression associated with shortened daylight in winter and fall. It disappears during spring and summer.*

Feeling down, discouraged, and depressed is something all people experience at different times in their lives. Periods of emotional highs and lows are normal. Depressive illness, also known as major depressive disorder, however, is very different from simply feeling depressed. Major depressive disorder is a psychiatric illness characterized by a cluster of symptoms including prolonged depressed mood, lowered self-esteem, pessimistic thoughts, and loss of pleasure or interest in former activities for at least 2 weeks. It is a painful, debilitating illness. It needs to be differentiated from short-term depressed moods or grief reactions, which are normal. Although grief displays many of the signs and symptoms of depression, it is a time-limited condition in response to an obvious loss and does not cause lowered self-esteem. The Diagnostic and Statistical Manual of Mental Disorders, 4th edition text revision, 2000, also known as DSM-IV-TR, describes dysthymic disorder as a chronic depressed mood most of the day for more days than not during a period of 2 years. Seasonal affective disorder is another form of depression. Adjustment disorders with depressed mood can also occur in response to situations like illness and loss. This disorder is of shorter duration but may progress to major depressive disorder in some cases.

Depression is the most common reason for seeking out mental health professionals. A major source of diagnosis is primary care providers who diagnose one-third to one-half of people identified as having depression (Agency for Healthcare Quality and Research, 2000). It is the leading cause of disability in the United States (Montano, 2003). About 5% to 8% of the population suffers from some form of depression at any one time (NAMI, 2007). There is a 16.6% chance of developing a major depressive disorder in one's lifetime (Kessler et al., 2005). Because the symptoms of depression can be hidden and vague, and may present as physical symptoms instead of a mood disturbance, primary care physicians may be the first to see the patient. However, the symptoms of depression can often go unrecognized and are often misdiagnosed. Undiagnosed and untreated depression is considered a major national health concern, contributing to poor work performance, family disruption, substance abuse, and premature death as a result of suicide or lack of self-care. Family history, stressful life events, and a previous history of depression are major predictors. Women are twice as likely to suffer from depression as men. Although men have a greater tendency to suffer a masked depression that can be concealed with drug use, alcohol abuse, and long work hours. Without treatment, these episodes can increase over time. It crosses all ethnic lines. In addition, depression can be part of a bipolar disorder psychosis, eating disorders, or dementia. Depression can also be secondary to a primary problem such as substance abuse or schizophrenia.

Once a person experiences a depressive episode, there is a high risk for recurrence. After one depressive episode, an individual has a 50% chance of another; after two episodes, there is a 70% to 80% risk of another; and after three episodes, the individual is at very high risk for chronic disability from depression (DSM-IV-TR, 2000).

ETIOLOGY

No single theory of depression is accepted by all theorists and clinicians. Different theories may apply to the divergent pathways that patients travel to arrive at the various types of depression.

Biological theories have focused on an insufficiency of neurotransmitters, especially norepinephrine and serotonin. These insufficiencies may be the result of inherited or environmental factors. The effectiveness of antidepressants may result from enhanced levels of these neurotransmitters. The most severe depressions are predominantly biologically determined. Hormonal factors, including abnormal melatonin metabolism, are associated with seasonal affective disorder (also called major depression with seasonal pattern).

Genetics may be a factor in more severe depressions. Relatives of people with depression have a higher incidence of this illness than those in the general population.

Psychological theories about a predisposition to depression have focused on a personal history of deprivation, trauma, or significant loss during childhood. These patients may be more susceptible to depression because current losses revive memories of former losses. They are more likely to experience low self-esteem and powerlessness.

Depression can be viewed as forbidden anger that has been turned inward. Classic psychoanalytic theory identified depression as the reaction to the loss of a significant person who has been both hated and loved. The patient handles this ambivalence by turning the hatred inward, resulting in depression and low self-esteem, whereas the memory of the departed person remains beloved and idealized.

Certain predominant issues of low self-esteem and helplessness are major contributors. For instance, low self-esteem may be based on the faulty development of an adequate, competent sense of self during childhood. As a child, the patient may have received attention and approval only when meeting parental needs and expectations. In adulthood, the absence of external support and praise and especially the loss of a supportive person may make the patient vulnerable to loss of self-esteem, which triggers depression.

Learned helplessness is displayed by a lack of adequate effort based on the belief that a person cannot be effective in getting needs met or making an impact. This person grew up in an environment that did not respond to any actions or initiative that he or she took (Seligman, 1975).

Distorted thinking can generate depression. Typically, the patient has negative expectations about himself or herself, the world, and the future. If he or she consistently overgeneralizes any mistake into the conclusion "I can't do anything right" and judges himself or herself as deficient, these negative beliefs can build toward depression. Negative expectations of the world, such as receiving no help from others or expecting only criticism, reinforce helplessness and lead to hopelessness (Beck, 1979).

RELATED CLINICAL CONCERNS

Clinically significant depressive symptoms are detectable in about 12% to 36% of the medically ill population (DHHS, 1993). The risk for depression greatly increases among people with a medical disorder (Varcarolis, 2006). Valente and Saunders (1997) reported that 20% to 25% of people with cancer experience depression that often goes untreated. Untreated depression in the medically ill can contribute to longer hospital stays, poor compliance, poorer quality of life, and increased doctor visits. It may also impact morbidity and mortality (Rouchell, Pounds, & Tierney, 2002). Major depressive disorder associated with a myocardial infarction has been shown to contribute to a higher mortality rate. This may be caused by changes in the endocrine and immune systems as well as reduced motivation and compliance (Rouchell et al., 2002). Stewart, Janicki, Muldoon, Slatton-Tyrell, & Kamarck (2007) reported that physical symptoms of depression may play an important role in the earlier stages of the development of cardiovascular disease. The patient's response to a medical illness could cause depression, and in some cases might precede it as can been seen in hypo- or hyperthyroidism, Addison's disease, and Huntington's disease. Symptoms of some illnesses such as fatigue or changes in appetite or bowel habits, can also mask depressive symptoms, making it difficult to diagnose. See Box 9–1 for a list of medical disorders associated with depression.

In addition, some medications can trigger depression (Box 9–2).

BOX 9–1
Medical Conditions Associated with Depression

- Stroke (especially frontal lesions)
- Myocardial infarction
- Adrenal disorders
- Dementia
- Diabetes
- Cancer
- Hypothyroidism
- Brain tumors
- Parkinson's disease
- Multiple sclerosis
- Chronic pain
- End stage renal disease

BOX 9–2
Drugs That Cause Depression

- Antihypertensive agents
  - Reserpine
  - Beta blockers
  - Methyldopa
  - Oral contraceptives
- Steroids
- Benzodiazepines
- Anabolic steroids
- Amphotericin-B
- Cancer chemotherapeutic agents
  - Vincristine
  - Vinblastine
  - Interferon
  - Procarbazine
  - L-asparaginase
- Psychoactive agents
  - Alcohol
  - Amphetamine or cocaine withdrawal
  - Opioids

Source: Rouchell, A. M., Pounds R., & Tierney, J. G. (2002). Depression. In J. R. Rundell & M. G. Wise (Eds.), *Textbook of consultation-liaison psychiatry* (pp. 307–338). Washington DC: American Psychiatric Press; Dubovsky, S. L., Davies, R., & Doboxsky, A. N. (2003). Mood disorders. In R. E. Hales & S. C. Yodofsky (Eds.), *Textbook of clinical psychiatry* (4th ed) (pp. 439–542). Washington, DC: American Psychiatric Press.

LIFE SPAN ISSUES

Children

Experts do not agree on the prevalence of depression in children; however, there is consensus that it does occur, even in young children. Children as young as 3 years of age have been diagnosed with depression (Varcarolis, 2006). Depression could be the aftermath of emotional deprivation, abuse, or separation. Children who were abused or neglected are known to be at a higher risk for major depressive disorder in childhood and adulthood (Widom, Dumong, & Czaja, 2007).

Because the child may be unable to express feelings or worries, other signs need to be analyzed, including acting-out behaviors, conduct disorders, inappropriate aggression, refusal to go to school, negativity, irritability, not meeting developmental tasks, sleep disorders, inability to experience joy (anhedonia), and self-destructive behaviors. There is a higher risk of depression in children when one or both parents suffer from major depression. Depression can also be a secondary reaction to other problems such as learning disorders and substance abuse. Children have been treated successfully with antidepressants in conjunction with psychotherapeutic interventions. However, precautions must be taken because of the potential increased suicide risk for children and adolescents. The Food and Drug Administration label on anti-depressants recommends close monitoring for increased suicide risk (Fochtmann & Gelenberg, 2005) leading to a dramatic reduction in prescriptions for SSRIs for young people (Leckman & King, 2007). Maternal depression while a child is young puts him or her at particularly high risk. Because the recurrence rate of depression is so high in children and adolescents, treatment is essential to prevent a lifetime of disability from it (NIMH, 2007a).

Adolescents

National Institute of Mental Health (NIMH) (2007b) estimates that 5% of adolescents suffer from major depressive disorder. Adolescents often do not express feelings of depression verbally because they may fear exhibiting feelings of vulnerability and dependency. Rather, their feelings of depression are often expressed in self-destructive or antisocial behaviors including sexual promiscuity, school truancy, threats, or petty crime. Some experts believe that substance abuse, antisocial behavior, and eating disorders in adolescence may be masking or related to depression. A depression-prone adolescent with low self-esteem will have greater difficulty achieving a positive sense of self as an adult. Adolescent victims of abuse and a history of parental depression contribute to a particular vulnerability to depression.

Postpartum

Debate continues as to whether the cause of postpartum depression is solely hormonal or represents an intermingling of psychological and physiological stressors. Although postpartum "blues" (a few days of labile mood after the birth of a baby) are extremely common, more severe reactions are relatively rare. Postpartum depression can include psychotic symptoms including delusions that often concern the newborn infant. Bonding with the infant is disrupted. Women with a history of prenatal depression and bipolar disorder are at higher risk. Once a woman experiences a major postpartum depression with psychotic features, the risk of recurrence in subsequent deliveries is between 30% and 50% (DSM-IV-TR, 2000).

Older Adults

Depression is the most common emotional disorder of later life. Elderly people are at higher risk because they experience multiple losses and more medical illnesses than the rest of the population. However, in geriatric patients, depression is more likely to be masked rather than exhibited by typical depression symptoms such as sadness, so it is often not diagnosed. Using the Geriatric Depression Scale is a useful way to capture this diagnosis. Even though these individuals may see a doctor more frequently than younger adults, it remains undertreated (Varcarolis, 2006). Symptoms are often more physical or expressed as personality changes, including irritability. Depression can also be superimposed on dementia or confused with pseudodementia because common depressive symptoms in elderly persons include confusion, distractibility, and memory loss. In addition, some of the physical symptoms of depression such as fatigue, anorexia, constipation, and psychomotor retardation can be confused with physical illness, medication interactions, substance abuse, or "signs of old age." Treatment with antidepressants must be very closely supervised because of the possibility of severe side effects, but it can be very helpful. Electroshock treatments may also be tried in an elderly patient who is unresponsive to antidepressants. Risk factors for depression in older adults include alcohol and substance abuse, dementia, cancer, stroke, myocardial infarction, functional disability, being widowed or a caregiver, and social isolation (Kurlowicz, 2003).

POSSIBLE NURSES' REACTIONS

- May feel depressed when working with these patients. A patient's despair and unhappiness can be very painful to be around and could lead to the nurse's avoidance of the patient.
- May reject the patient because of own perception of the patient's dependency. Or may become over-involved because of patient's needs and inadvertently create more dependency.
- May resent patient because of the longer time it takes to provide care.
- May feel angry or frustrated with depressed patient who isn't "helping himself or herself" or can't just "snap out of it."
- May feel inadequate when unable to make a quick impact on a patient's depression. Nurse may create unrealistic expectations of patient's recovery.
- Staff members may have inaccurate beliefs about the cause of depression, which may lead to their minimizing the degree of the patient's suffering.
- Because of the high prevalence of depression in our society, the nurse may have personally experienced it or may have witnessed a family member's struggle with depression. This can cause the nurse to identify with the depressed patient and reexperience these feelings.
- Reaction may depend on whether the nurse believes that the expression of sadness is an acceptable behavior; for example, the nurse may believe sadness is acceptable in women but not in men.

ASSESSMENT

Behavior and Appearance

- Persistently sad, anguished, or apathetic facial expression
- Dejected appearance: Head down, poor eye contact, posture slumped as if bearing a heavy weight
- Psychomotor agitation and/or retardation
- Decreased interest in grooming and self-care
- Decreased sexual interest
- Makes statements like "I don't care any more"
- May have difficulty with even simple tasks
- Anhedonia

Mood and Emotions

- Dysphoric mood: Verbalizes feelings of sadness and depression
- Inability to enjoy activities that were enjoyed previously
- Low self-esteem with feelings of worthlessness and inadequacy
- Feeling ineffective, powerless, and helpless
- Pessimistic: May appear brooding and express feelings of futility and despair
- Feelings of great heaviness
- Mild to high levels of anxiety, possibly including panic attacks and irritability
- Unexpressed anger, turned inward against self
- May express generalized anger
- Ambivalence: may feel two opposing ways at the same time

Thoughts, Beliefs, and Perceptions

- Thoughts slowed
- Poor concentration with possible temporary impairment of recent memory
- Self-doubt with relentless rumination and obsessions
- Lack of self-worth: Believes self undeserving of good experiences
- Indecisiveness
- Preoccupation with body changes
- Loss of perspective: May reject positive comments from others; gives self no credit for achievements
- Excessive guilt: condemns self; feels deserving of punishment
- Narrowing of interest to self
- Possible suicidal thoughts
- Confusion

- In severe depression: delusions; hallucinations that express feelings of worthlessness; guilt
- Believes life has no meaning and that there is no future

Relationships and Interactions

- Withdrawal from social interactions
- Deterioration of relationships because of preoccupation with self, anger, and anxiety
- Increasing dependence on others because of inability to make decisions or care for self

Physical Responses

- Slowed physiologic functioning evidenced by:
  - Lethargy and fatigue, especially in the morning
  - Constipation
  - Decreased appetite with weight loss or increased appetite with weight gain
  - Sleep problems including early morning awakening, frequent awakenings, waking up feeling tired, sleeping all the time
  - Body aches; pains such as headaches; indigestion; dizziness
- Thyroid function tests may be ordered to rule out hypothyroidism

Pertinent History

- Past history of depression, bipolar disorder, panic attacks, suicide attempts
- Family history of depression
- History of substance abuse
- History of stroke or myocardial infarction (particularly high rate of depression)

See Box 9–3 for List of Commonly Used Depression Scales.

COLLABORATIVE MANAGEMENT

Pharmacological

The advent of so many new antidepressants has provided many more opportunities for successful treatment. The American Psychiatric Association Practice Guidelines for Major Depressive Disorders (Karasu, Gelengerg, Merriam, & Wang, 2000; Fochtman & Gelenberg, 2005) recommend antidepressants be prescribed for moderate to severe depression and can be used with mild depressive symptoms if the patient wishes. Components of firstline treatment today are the Selective Serotonin Reuptake Inhibitors (SSRIs) and newer atypical antidepres-

BOX 9–3
Commonly used Depression Assessment Scales

- Beck Depression Inventory
- Zung Self-rating Depression Scale
- Geriatric Depression Scale
- Hamilton Depression Scale

sants. Because there are so many on the market that have the same effectiveness but side effects differ (AHRQ, 2007). Other variables are patient profile, history of previous response, type of depression, rate of onset, concurrent medical or psychiatric illnesses, and other medications the patient is taking. See Chapter 21 for a detailed discussion of antidepressants, their side effects, and nursing implications. Most antidepressants require at least 3 to 4 weeks of use before full benefits are obtained. Often, relief of other symptoms occurs before a change in the patient's subjective sense of feeling better. Side effects must be monitored closely. The patient may need to remain on a maintenance dose of antidepressant for many years.

Monoamine oxidase inhibitors (MAOIs) are used less today but may be a second- or third-line treatment for depressions that do not respond to the more commonly used antidepressants. If the patient is experiencing anxiety, panic attacks, hallucinations, or delusions, other medications may need to be added. A trial of stimulants such as methylphenidate hydrochloride (Ritalin) or modafinil (Provigil) may be tried in adults with severe psychomotor retardation.

Herbal products that are used for depression include stimulants such as ma huang, which contains ephedra, Gingko biloba, and SAM-e. The most common herbal product for this use is St. John's wort. As with most herbal products, there are potential side effects and drug interactions. St. John's wort is known to interact with some HIV medications and can inhibit effectiveness. However, controlled trials on St. John's wort have been inconclusive (Fochtmann & Gelenberg, 2005). An alternative, nonpharmacological approach is light therapy, particularly useful in seasonal affective disorders. Exposure to natural light is shown to reduce depression and improve alertness (Nelson, 2006).

Psychotherapy

Psychotherapy and other psychosocial treatments continue to be an important component of depression treatment. A combination of psychotherapy and pharmacotherapy is more effective than pharmacotherapy alone. Combination therapy is particularly helpful in improving treatment adherence (Fochtmann & Gelenberg, 2005). One short-term psychotherapy approach is cognitive therapy. This method is brief, structured, directive treatment designed to alter the negative thoughts so common in depression. Group therapy can also be helpful to enhance the patient's socialization.

Electroconvulsive Therapy

Electroconvulsive therapy (ECT) is a first-line treatment option only for patients with more severe or psychotic forms of depression. It may also be used for those who have failed to respond to other therapies or those with medical conditions that preclude the use of antidepressants.

NURSING MANAGEMENT

SELF-CARE DEFICIT evidenced by decreased ability to manage own hygiene, grooming, feeding, and daily activities related to loss of energy, inhibition of motivation, anxiety, and/or dependency.

Patient Outcomes

- Increased participation in self-care, daily activities
- Improved grooming and hygiene

Interventions

- Determine patient's level of self-care before onset of depressive symptoms to set realistic goals.
- Assess whether the patient is expressing certain psychological needs such as dependency or rebellion by not performing self-care. Observe whether patient acts more independently when unaware of being watched.
- Encourage as much independence as possible. Take the time to allow patient to do things for himself or herself. Assign care to staff member who may have more time or is especially patient. Make sure all staff members reinforce patient's participation. Encourage patient's participation in decisions about timing, sequence, and approaches to self-care.
- Create a positive attitude that patient can learn and progress with practice. Avoid taking over for the patient if he or she has trouble.
- If patient is not eating, encourage small meals that are high in protein and nutrition dense.
- Break down tasks into small steps so patient can experience some success. For instance, have the patient focus on washing his or her face rather than completing the whole bath. Recognize that patient's thinking processes are slowed.
- Create an environment to ease patient's participation, such as having proper utensils available at mealtime or having the walker available in room if patient is ambulating to bathroom.
- Provide reassurance and encouragement. Avoid minimizing patient's problems or infantilizing him or her.
- At times, a nurse may need to make all decisions for a very depressed patient such as when to eat. Then, as the patient begins to improve,

limited options can be presented. With further improvement, the patient should take on increasing decision making.

SELF-ESTEEM DISTURBANCE evidenced by statements of low self-esteem, misinterpreting positive or pleasurable experiences, expressions of shame and guilt related to feelings, thoughts of worthlessness, failures, and negative reinforcement.

Patient Outcomes

- Identifies positive aspects of self
- Modifies unrealistic expectations for self
- Demonstrates reduced symptoms of depression

Interventions

- Provide emotional nurturing through empathetic listening and supportive encouragement. Treating the patient as a valued individual will enhance his or her self-esteem.
- Avoid blanket reassurances like "things will get better soon." These tend to alienate the patient, who may feel that you don't understand his or her pain.
- Encourage patient to share feelings, especially negative ones. If this is too difficult, consider alternative means of expression such as writing about feelings or drawing pictures.
- Point out any specific improvement, no matter how small. Depressed people often do not see improvement because they are so focused on the negative. Consider keeping a progress chart at the bedside to record concrete accomplishments such as the number of times the patient ambulates or the percentage of food he or she eats.
- Encourage patient to speak up if he or she disagrees or feels his or her rights are being violated. Reinforce assertive response.
- Recognize and point out manifestations of self-destructive or self-undermining thinking or behavior:
  - Requiring self to be perfect or setting unattainable goals
  - Assuming responsibility for and feeling guilt about failures and events that are outside the patient's control
  - Basing entire feeling of self-worth on one achievement or attribute, a single relationship, or obtaining approval from others
  - Projecting own feelings of self-hate onto family, staff, or friends, such as "All the nurses hate me." "My family blames me for my illness."
  - Expressing self-hate directly through suicidal thoughts and behavior
  - Expressing self-hate indirectly with repeated accidents, noncompliance, provoking or being antagonistic to others, thereby unwittingly creating rejection

- Covering poor self-esteem with anger, blaming, or other maneuvers that displace responsibility onto others
- Suggest that the patient identify a few achievements from the past.
- Discuss and practice with patient alternative ways to respond to stress and to ask for what he or she wants.

POWERLESSNESS evidenced by lack of initiative, nonachievement of realistic goals, passivity; nonparticipation in decision making related to decreased motivation, decreased energy, hopelessness, perfectionistic expectations or sadness.

Patient Outcomes

- Identifies factors that he or she can control
- Participates in decisions about his or her care

Interventions

- Encourage the patient to describe feelings or the experience of powerlessness. Let the patient know that you are interested and that you understand his or her pain. For instance, you may state, "You believe there is no hope for you to ever feel better."
- Once the patient indicates that he or she feels understood, suggest alternative viewpoints. Work with patient to identify times in life when he or she felt better or felt more in control.
- Work with the patient to identify realistic goals to work toward. Encourage having patience and accepting current limitations. Break down goals into small steps and recognize progress as each is achieved.
- Allow the patient to maintain reasonable control over some of the daily routine if able.
- Have the patient list specific situations in which he or she felt powerless. Correct distorted assumptions, discuss alternative ways to handle situations, and identify helpful resources.
- Direct the patient to other topics if he or she obsesses on unrealistic goals or things that cannot be changed.

ALTERNATE NURSING DIAGNOSES

Anxiety
Coping, Ineffective
Grieving, Dysfunctional
Hopelessness
Injury, Risk for
Nutrition, Altered
Sleep Pattern, Disturbed

Social Interaction, Impaired

Thought Processes, Disturbed

WHEN TO CALL FOR HELP

- Extreme self-care deficit to point of not being able to care for basic needs
- Suicidal thoughts, threats, or attempts
- Hallucinations or delusions
- Severe side effects from antidepressants, including severe urinary retention, dramatic fluctuations in blood pressure, cardiac complications, seizures

WHO TO CALL FOR HELP

- Psychiatric Team
- Social Worker
- Attending Physician

PATIENT AND FAMILY EDUCATION

- Teach the patient that depression can generate feelings of helplessness, powerlessness, and pessimism. Encourage the patient to delay major decisions and actions based on those feelings, and reinforce the idea that the severe symptoms will abate with treatment and time.
- Reinforce the idea that depression is a treatable illness. Even though the patient may feel hopeless, the illness is not.
- For patients on antidepressants, review potential side effects and importance of taking the medication even when they start feeling better. Patient should know which side effects to report to physician. Reinforce that these medications should not be stopped abruptly.
- Inform the patient that other medications are available if the side effects from the current one are too uncomfortable.
- Encourage the patient to maintain a schedule of activity.
- Explain to the family the symptoms of depression, medication management, and interventions and what the family can do to assist and encourage the patient.
- Teach the patient and family to report signs of increasing depression or suicidal thoughts.
- Teach the patient that long-term, enduring self-esteem comes from beliefs about self as a valuable human being and is expressed through achievements, relationships, and healthful living.

- Inform the patient that the negative assumptions about himself or herself are not necessarily true.
- Direct patient to American Psychiatric Association Website for "Patient and Family Guide to Major Depressive Disorders" (healthyminds.org) and National Mental Health Association website for a confidential screening test on depression (depression-screening.org).

CHARTING TIPS

- Document patient activity, intake, sleep patterns, and bowel patterns.
- Document any expressed suicide thoughts, plans, or attempts.
- Document side effects of medication.
- Document patient response to encouragement or support.

COMMUNITY-BASED CARE

- Strongly encourage patient to seek counseling. Give appropriate referrals. If patient is too depressed to have the energy to follow through, involve family or friends in seeking help.
- If patient is unable to care for himself or herself or is potentially suicidal, work with other members of the team as well as family to determine discharge options. Patient may need psychiatric hospitalization or temporary placement in a board and care or convalescent facility.
- Refer patient for psychiatric home health care for follow-up on medication compliance and self-care activities.
- Encourage patient to maintain follow-up with physician and compliance with treatment plan.

The Suicidal Patient

Learning Objectives

- Identify risk factors for suicide.
- Differentiate between a suicide attempt and a suicide gesture.
- Describe effective interventions to protect the high risk patient in the hospital.
- Describe common nurses' reactions to the suicidal patient.

Glossary

Completed suicide – *Suicide attempt resulting in death.*

Deliberate self-harm – *Willful self-inflicting of painful, injurious acts without intent to die.*

Lethality – *The level of risk in suicide method chosen to cause death. The more lethal methods include guns, jumping, and hanging. Lower lethality methods include superficially slashing wrists, inhaling house gas, and ingesting pills because death is not immediate and there is more of a chance of being found and treated.*

Psychological autopsy – *Retrospective review of deceased person's life to establish likely diagnosis at time of death.*

Suicidal ideation – *Thoughts about harming one's self.*

Suicide – *Self-inflicted death with evidence that person intended to die.*

Suicide attempt – *Any act intended to end in suicide.*

Suicide gesture – *Any action that appears to be a suicide attempt but that is actually contrived or manipulative and that results in only minimal harm, such as superficial cuts on the wrist or a small overdose of sleeping pills.*

Suicide threat – *Verbal threat to commit suicide.*

Some nurses mistakenly believe suicidal patients are found only in psychiatric settings. However, patients with suicidal tendencies are not always easily identified, and they can be the same patients you care for in an intensive care unit, medical unit, nursing home, or in their own homes.

Many people have experienced momentary self-destructive thoughts. But obsessive preoccupation with these thoughts and acting on them is another matter. Thinking about suicide does not mean that the individual will act on those thoughts; however, anyone who talks about, threatens, or attempts suicide must be taken seriously. There are individuals who may perform deliberate self-harm when they inflict injury on themselves without intent of death. These individuals often are not suicidal, but a psychiatric evaluation would need to be done to determine this. In approximately 70% of suicides, the individual has one or more active or chronic medical illnesses at the time of death (DHHS, 1993). See Table 9–1 for key risk factors. 90% of suicide victims suffer from at least one psychiatric disorder. Major depressive disorder is most common. Others include bipolar disorder, schizophrenia, substance abuse, panic disorder, borderline and antisocial personality.

There are approximately seven suicide attempts for every completed suicide. All cultural groups are vulnerable although American Indians have a higher rate. Women make more attempts than men, but men are more likely to complete the suicide because they tend to use more lethal methods, particularly firearms (CDC/National Center for Health Statistics, 2004). Firearms are the leading form of suicide followed by suffocation and poisoning (CDC, 2004). Three factors that need to be present for a completed suicide include:

- Specific plan,
- Lethality, and
- Access to lethal method.

Suicide is the 11th leading cause of death in the United States and there are about 89 suicides per day (American Association of Suicidology, 2004). However, it may be higher because hidden suicides such as "accidental" overdoses, auto accidents, noncompliance with medical regimens, or not seeking medical care for symptoms are not reported as suicides. Most suicide attempts are expressions of extreme distress, not bids for attention (Captain, 2006).

Because suicide is basically not accepted by our culture, it generates anxiety that has led to a number of myths (Box 9–4).

BOX 9–4
Clearing up the Myths About Suicide

Myth	Truth
Asking people about their suicidal thoughts will make them more likely to act on them.	Most patients are not afraid to talk about their thoughts of committing suicide and are usually grateful that someone is available and cares. Talking can reduce the sense of isolation.
All people who attempt suicide have a psychiatric disorder.	People can become overwhelmed with life circumstances without having a psychiatric disorder.
A person who talks about suicide won't do it.	Approximately 80% of individuals who attempt or complete suicide give some definite verbal or indirect clues. As many as 50% have seen their physician within the previous month, often with vague somatic complaints.
A person who attempts suicide won't try again.	Almost 75% of those individuals who complete suicide have attempted it at least once before.
People who attempt suicide are always determined to die.	Many individuals are ambivalent and are using the suicide as a cry for help.
People who attempt suicide just want attention.	Even if the suicide attempt is manipulative, the individual may go on to complete the suicide.
As the person becomes less depressed, the risk of suicide decreases.	As the depression lifts, the individual's energy level can increase before feelings of hopelessness are relieved. Once the individual makes the decision that suicide is an effective solution to the problems, his or her mood may even elevate.

It is estimated that each person who commits suicide leaves behind at least six survivors who suffer many emotional complications. The American Association of Suicidology (2007) notes that survivors have a higher risk of suicide themselves. Surviving family and friends of the suicide victim often experience complicated grief reactions that may affect them for the rest of their lives. They are faced with the stigma of this form of death as well as many unresolved feelings of anger and guilt. Unfortunately, they may receive less support from others because of the discomfort surrounding the cause of death. In addition, many life insurance policies do not cover self-inflicted death, so the surviving family may be economically devastated.

ETIOLOGY

Suicide is not a disease in itself but a symptom of some underlying problem. *Biological and genetic* theories are closely tied to those causing depression. It is believed that low levels of the neurotransmitters, serotonin and norepinephrine, are a factor in the decision to commit suicide. There is also a strong link to alcohol and substance abuse. Suicidal behavior also runs in families. This may be related to genetics or to psychological factors in which suicide is viewed as an acceptable way to cope. The risk of suicide in family members of individuals who have committed suicide is 15 times greater than in the general population. Captain (2006) reports that psychological autopsies reveal that in 90% of completed suicides, the person had one or more mental disorders with the most common being major depression and substance abuse.

Psychological theory focuses on a number of motivating forces. Suicide can be a way to escape deep psychological pain or atone for past sins. Intense feelings of hopelessness and helplessness are key factors. It can be related to unacceptable feelings of aggression, which the individual turns inward. The individual could believe that he or she is reuniting with a loved one. The wish to instill guilt in a significant person who is perceived as abandoning or rejecting could motivate the suicidal person. Individuals with limited coping reserves who become overwhelmed with stress may seek self-destructive acts as a way to escape these feelings. Because the suicidal person may be severely depressed, the theories on etiology of depression and substance abuse may also relate to suicide.

Suicidal behavior can also be a symptom of psychosis as the person acts out hallucinations or delusions. Command hallucinations, in which voices tell the patient to kill himself or herself, create a very high risk. Severe anxiety and distress regarding psychotic symptoms as well as lack of judgment or reality testing may lead to suicide as a way to escape overwhelming anxiety or disturbed thoughts.

Suicidal gestures with nonlethal self-mutilation may occur in individuals who have poor impulse control or a high need for the attention or control of others. An individual with a history of multiple threats and gestures may have a borderline or other personality disorder.

BOX 9–5
Risk and Protective Factors

Risk Factors for Increased Risk of Suicide	Factors Associated with Protective Effects for Suicide
Psychiatric diagnosis	Children at home
Physical illness	Sense of responsibility to family
Psychosocial factors including recent lack of social support, unemployment, recent stressful event	Pregnancy
Childhood traumas such as sexual abuse	Religiosity
Family history of suicide, mental illness	Life Satisfaction
Psychological characteristics including hopelessness, anxiety, impulsiveness, aggression	Positive coping skills
Demographics including male, widowed/divorced/single, elderly	Positive social support
	Positive problem solving skills

Source: Jacobs, D. G., Baldessarini, R. J., Conwell, Y., Fawcett, J. A., Horton, L., Meltzer, H., et al. (2003). *Practice guideline for the assessment and treatment of patients with suicidal behaviors.* Washington, DC: American Psychiatric Association.

Sociological views look at a person who may feel alienated from others. A susceptible individual who no longer feels part of his or her culture or social group could be at an increased risk, especially if cultural or religious taboos against suicide are not very strong. For some, suicide is a way of expressing political beliefs. Economic losses or unemployment could also play a role as a person feels trapped and powerless to change. Suicide is an increasing problem in minority and economically deprived groups. It can also be associated with substance abuse. A psychological autopsy can be used by the psychiatry team and survivors after a completed suicide to try to understand the etiology. See Box 9–5 for Risk Factors and Protective Factors that may help to estimate suicide risk.

RELATED CLINICAL CONCERNS

Physical illness is a frequent contributor to suicidal behavior. Illnesses associated with suffering and dependency, such as advanced cancer and AIDS, are more apt to be associated with higher suicide rates. Uncontrolled pain and delirium are the key variables with these illnesses. The terminally ill patient's "right" to commit suicide has been debated for many years. Right-to-die groups have supported initiatives in several states seeking physician-assisted suicide for terminal patients. The patient's ability to remain in control until death is a key motivation for this action. Other illnesses, such as multiple sclerosis and Huntington's disease, that may not be terminal but are chronic and debilitating may also be associated with increased suicide risk. Suicidal patients with physical illnesses should be carefully evaluated and treated for depression. In addition, every effort to identify and control any uncomfortable symptoms will enhance quality of life.

Medications that contribute to depressive or psychotic symptoms could also precipitate a suicide attempt. See Box 9–2 and Box 11–4 for lists of medications that contribute to these symptoms. Patients with suicidal tendencies who are taking prescribed analgesics, tranquilizers, or sleeping pills may be at risk for saving up medications to use later for a possible suicide attempt.

LIFE SPAN ISSUES

Children

Although the rate of suicide in children is low, it is rising and is cause for great concern and analysis. Young children have tried to kill themselves by jumping out of windows, hanging themselves, or running in front of moving cars. Firearms and suffocation are also common methods in the 10- to 14-year-old age group. These actions are generally impulsive and in response to intense emotion. A suicidal act may be an attempt to gain power, punish a parent, or escape stressful situations. It could also be a response to parental neglect, rejection, or abuse. A young child who does not understand the finality of death may not understand the consequences of his or her action. Children could also be imitating parental behaviors. Suicidal behavior can also be related to substance abuse and school problems. Suicide is the 3rd leading cause of death in 10- to 19-year-olds (CDC, 2004).

Adolescents

Suicidal behavior in adolescents is considered a serious health problem. It is the second leading cause of death in teens, accidents being the first. And some accidents could be concealed suicide attempts. Teens who are depressed, socially isolated, or using drugs and alcohol are at highest risk. Low self-esteem, history of abuse, not fitting in with peers, and school pressures may be other risk factors. As with adults, girls make more attempts but boys are more likely to use more lethal methods such as firearms. The availability of firearms in our society is believed to contribute to the increase in teenage suicides. Carbon monoxide poisoning and ingestion of pills are other common methods used by adolescents. High-risk behaviors like drug use, drag racing, and gang activity could be masking suicidal thoughts. Substance abuse, psychiatric disorders, and conduct disorders are risk factors in this age group. Suicide assessment should be performed on any high-risk teen.

"Cluster" or copycat suicides, in which adolescents copy an episode of suicide of an acquaintance or celebrity, is a recent and alarming trend. To some teens the suicide of an idol can be romanticized.

Older Adults

Elderly people commit suicide more often than any other age group in the United States (Jacobs et al., 2003). Elderly white men older than 80 years of age are at highest risk (Moscicki, 1999). Guns remain the most frequent method. Suicide statistics in elderly persons are probably even higher because of the prevalence of passive suicides. Elderly people are more likely to use noncompliance with medical regimens or refusal to eat as a way to hasten their death. Risk factors include living alone, widowhood, lack of financial resources, poor health, and social isolation. In addition, misuse of alcohol and antianxiety medications may contribute.

POSSIBLE NURSES' REACTIONS

- May see a suicidal patient as weak or bad because of personal religious or moral beliefs.
- May experience feelings of anxiety with these patients, which prevent recognition of warning signs.
- May avoid dealing with suicidal patients for fear of saying the wrong thing or contributing to their suicide because of lack of adequate training. May believe talking to patient about suicide would increase risk.
- May believe he or she is rescuing patient and then experience intense guilt if patient does attempt or complete suicide. May take patient's behavior as a personal rejection.
- May feel angry with patient for creating chaos, especially if the nurse perceives that the patient has much to live for, such as children and a good job. The nurse's anger may conflict with his or her mission of promoting health and saving lives.
- May deny or minimize suicidal behavior as a defense against anxiety and helplessness.
- Patient's behavior could stir up personal feelings of depression. Nurses have six times the suicide rate of the general population and much higher lethality because of their knowledge and access to drugs.

ASSESSMENT

See Boxes 9–6 and 9–7 for suicide assessment of lethality and assessing a suicide attempt.

BOX 9–6
Assessing Current Suicide Lethality

1. Do you think about hurting or killing yourself? If yes:
2. Do you have a plan? How have you considered doing it? If yes:
3. Do you think you may or will do something to act on your thoughts? If yes, where and when? Do you feel you have control over your own behavior?
4. Do you have the means available (such as rope, rolled-up sheet, gun, saved-up pills [note lethality of plan])?
5. Have you ever tried to harm yourself in the past? If yes, how? Did you expect to survive?
6. Are you willing to contract or notify staff whenever you feel you may act on these thoughts? Our side of the contract is to be available and actively help you during these times.

If patient denies having a suicide plan, ask about other plans for the future and support systems.

1. What do you see yourself doing in a week, in a month, and in a year from now?
2. Do you feel optimistic or pessimistic about the future?
3. Do you have family members or friends with whom you can freely discuss your problems?

BOX 9–7
Assessing the Suicide Attempt

1. Did the patient expect to die? (yes, no, uncertain). Did the patient think his or her chance of dying was high, medium, or low? Did he or she underestimate?
2. How does the patient feel about surviving? If the patient regrets surviving, question him or her about any current plan to attempt suicide.
3. If the patient's objective in suicide attempt or gesture was to manipulate a significant other to behave differently, have the sought-after changes occurred? Does the patient have alternative, more adaptive methods for coping?
4. Is the support system present (helpful, unhelpful)?
5. Does the patient have any hope for the future? How optimistic or pessimistic is he or she?
6. Is the patient willing to make a no-suicide contract?

Behavior and Appearance

- Direct verbal statements (e.g., "I wish I were dead")
- Indirect verbal statements (e.g., "You won't see me when you come back to work" or asking about specific suicide methods)
- Giving away possessions
- Agitation
- Sudden changes in eating, sleeping, or usual activities
- Neglecting appearance or hygiene
- Drawing up a will
- Refusing medications

Mood and Emotions

- Depression or despair
- Sudden lifting of depression, sudden elevation in mood
- Apathy
- Hopelessness
- Helplessness
- Anxiety
- Bitter anger

Thoughts, Beliefs, and Perceptions

- Disorganized, chaotic, irrational thinking
- Tunnel vision—unable to see options other than death
- Poor judgment
- Persecutory delusions and hallucinations, especially commands
- Excessive guilt or self-blame
- Low self-esteem

Relationships and Interactions

- Social isolation; withdrawn; feels alone and abandoned
- Recent loss of significant person through death or separation
- Recent tumultuous termination or interruption of psychiatric treatment

Physical Responses

- Chronic debilitating illness
- Unrelieved pain
- Terminal illness
- Recent, catastrophic loss of physical abilities

Pertinent History

- History of suicide attempts
- Self-destructive behavior, such as drug abuse, reckless acts, or self-mutilation
- Family history of suicide attempts or depression
- Psychiatric illness
- Recent significant loss

COLLABORATIVE MANAGEMENT

Pharmacological

Suicidal patients may benefit from taking antianxiety medication, such as lorazepam, to reduce feelings of intense anxiety or distress. In addition, antipsychotic and antimanic medication may be prescribed as needed. If antidepressants are being started, it is important to remember that it will take a number of weeks to lift depression, so other interventions must be used in the interim to prevent suicide. Antidepressants could actually increase suicide risk if the patient gets a sudden burst of energy to act out the plan before the depression lifts. Overdosing on antidepressants is an increasingly frequent method of suicide. However, untreated depression puts the patient at greater risk so antidepressants are seen as protection against suicidality (APA, 2006).

Adequate symptom management for pain and other distressing symptoms must be provided to the patient with a serious or terminal illness. A patient's belief that his or her symptoms cannot be controlled could be a contributing factor in hopelessness and suicide.

Patients at high risk for suicide may need to have medications administered in liquid or parenteral form to avoid "cheeking" and hoarding pills. Outpatients should be given only a few days' supply of any medication that could potentially be used in a suicide attempt.

NURSING MANAGEMENT

RISK FOR VIOLENCE TO SELF evidenced by suicide attempts. self-mutilation, suicide plan related to suicide ideation, poor impulse control, depression.

Patient Outcomes

- Remains free from injury
- Verbalizes intent not to harm self
- Expresses more optimistic view of future in specific terms

Interventions

- Determine if patient has a plan and how potentially lethal and available that plan is (see Box 9–3). A patient in the hospital who talks about using a gun to kill himself or herself would be at lower risk (until discharge) as long as he or she does not have a gun available. A patient who has a stash of medication would be at higher risk. Seek input from other professionals to participate in this assessment. If your agency has mental health professionals on staff, it is essential to involve them in the assessment. See high risk interventions in subsequent text.

- Make a thorough assessment of patient's risk of suicide (see Table 9–1). Note: research is being conducted to develop assessment rating scales to better predict suicide potential.

TABLE 9–1
Suicide: Intensity of Risk

Behaviors or Symptoms	Intensity of Risk		
	Low	Moderate	High
Anxiety	Mild	Moderate	High or panic state
Depression	Mild	Moderate	Severe
Isolation or withdrawal	Some feelings of isolation; no withdrawal	Some feelings of helplessness, hopelessness, or withdrawal	Hopeless, helpless, withdrawn, self-deprecating
Daily functioning	Fairly good in most activities	Moderately good in some activities	Not good in any activities
Resources	Several	Some	Few or none
Coping strategies being used	Generally constructive	Some are constructive	Predominantly destructive
Significant others	Several available	Few or only one available	Only one or none available
Previous psychiatric help	None, or positive attitude toward	Yes, and moderately satisfied with the help	Negative view of help received
Life-style	Stable	Moderately stable	Unstable
Alcohol or drug use	Infrequently to excess	Frequently to excess	Continual use

Continued

TABLE 9–1

Suicide: Intensity of Risk—*cont'd*

Behaviors or Symptoms	Intensity of Risk		
	Low	Moderate	High
Previous suicide attempts	None or low lethality	One or more; moderate lethality	Multiple attempts; high lethality
Disorientation or disorganization	None	Some	Marked
Depression	Some feelings	Some feelings	Negative view of self
Hostility	Little or none	Some	Marked
Suicide plan	Vague fleeting thoughts but no plan	Frequent thoughts; occasional ideas about a plan	Frequent or constant thought with a specific plan

Source: Adapted with permission from Hatton C. & Valente S. (1984). *Suicide: assessment and interventions.* Norwalk, CT: Appleton-Century-Crofts.

- Talk openly with patient about your concern that he or she is suicidal. Let the patient know you are concerned and available to help and that confidentiality is shared among the entire health-care team for optimum care. Encouraging the patient to talk about this does not increase risk for suicide. Do not promise to keep secrets from the team. Notify all members of the health-care team of the patient's risk of suicide. Staff members must be supportive, empathetic, and familiar with treatment plan.
- If the patient has attempted suicide, see Box 9–7.
- Talk to patient about making a no-suicide contract with you. Ask him or her to wait or postpone action so that you and other professionals have time to help. Point out that depression is not permanent (with time, medication, and therapy there is hope for a change) but that death is permanent and cuts off other options. Renew the contract each shift and as needed between patient and main caregiver.
- Never attempt to work with a suicidal patient by yourself. Involve all members of the team. Seek additional resources such as social workers; notify supervisory staff.

For patients assessed to be at high risk for suicide:

- Follow agency policy for need for continuous supervision. Discourage use of family for this purpose.
- If patient is in the hospital, arrange for a room close to the nurses' station or in an ICU for closer monitoring.
- Avoid checking on patient at predictable intervals; check more frequently during danger times (changes of shift) when patient may think staff will be preoccupied.
- Remove objects with self-harm potential (such as glasses, razors, belts, or lighters) from the room. Be aware of agency policy regarding need to search personal belongings or do a body search.
- Make sure windows cannot be opened.
- If all other interventions have been ineffective, use physical restraints for brief periods to prevent patient self-harm.
- Make sure family and friends are not bringing in potentially dangerous items such as medications, alcohol, or razors.
- When patient is sleeping, ensure both hands in view.
- Meal trays should have no glass or metal silverware
- Obtain Recommendations from American Association of Suicidology for Inpatient and Residential Patients Known to be at Elevated Risk for Suicide for inpatient settings.
- Arrange (per physician) to transfer the suicidal patient to a psychiatric unit as soon as medically stable.
- If patient is not hospitalized, make sure family and friends are aware of the possible suicide risk. The patient probably should not be left alone. Give him or her a list of resources such as hotlines, therapists' phone numbers, or support people he or she can call. Call MD/Psychiatric Assessment Team if you believe the patient is still at risk of suicide.

HOPELESSNESS evidenced by expectations that there will be no improvement in situation related to depression: overwhelmed by life circumstances.

Patient Outcomes

- Verbalizes more optimistic expectations for the future
- Initiates realistic plans for the immediate future
- Demonstrates initiative in decision making

Interventions

- Recognize that extreme hopelessness is a strong indicator of suicide; assess thoroughly.
- Listen to patient's concerns and issues. Convey empathy to promote verbalizing about doubts and fears. Reflect back patient's despair without

agreeing with it. For instance, you might say "You describe a world that seems empty to you."

- Encourage patient to discuss recent events or stresses that have contributed to the hopeless view. Offer alternative analysis viewing the event without arguing or minimizing patient's concerns. Minimizing or joking about the patient's feelings will increase the patient's sense of isolation and lack of trust.
- Emphasize the patient's strengths and problem-solving abilities. Describe a recent situation in which you observed the patient being successful. Have him or her describe a past success. Point out obstacles or negative thinking that get in the way of effective problem solving.
- Provide a balanced point of view to counteract patient's tendency to judge himself or herself harshly. Point out unrealistic, perfectionistic thinking. Offer more constructive interpretations to open real options for the future.
- Acknowledge that you understand that the patient feels that everything is useless and nothing will help, but also that you believe something helpful can be done.

INEFFECTIVE COPING evidenced by repeated suicide threats/gestures, related to stunted areas of personality development with intermittent self-destructive impulses.

Patient Outcomes

- Decrease in self-destructive behaviors
- Demonstrates more adaptive means of communicating thoughts, feelings, and needs

Interventions

- Determine if self-destructive behavior is a pattern.
- Remain calm and neutral; treat patient's suicide threats and gestures in matter-of-fact manner. Treat any physical injury without excessive emotion. Avoid creating a sense of alarm about the patient's behavior. *Caution:* Do not dismiss any threat or gesture as manipulative or not serious. Any self-destructive threat or gesture should be taken seriously and not ignored.
- Ask the patient to identify any disturbing thoughts or feelings that occurred just before the threat or action. Encourage him or her to put thoughts and feelings into words rather than acting them out impulsively and destructively. Teach that anger can hide more painful feelings such as sadness and rejection.
- Teach alternate coping: talking, relaxation, distraction, exercise, music, and so forth.
- Confront the patient who wants to commit suicide for revenge and retaliation. These patients may state, "They'll be sorry when I'm dead."

Remind patient this is not a solution because he or she won't be there to see the results.

- Encourage the patient to alert staff members if feeling out of control or when having thoughts of self-harm. Consider discussing a no-suicide contract and including guidelines for behavior.
- Establish limits with patient on amount of time staff will spend listening to patient's concerns. Set limits on the patient's use of verbal abuse and demands.
- Review with the patient possible causes for self-destructive behavior that could include an attempt to get others to assume responsibility for patient's life. The patient needs to be encouraged to take more self-responsibility. See Chapter 12, The Manipulative Patient, for additional interventions.

ALTERNATE NURSING DIAGNOSES

Anxiety
Grieving, Dysfunctional
Self-Concept, Disturbed
Self-Mutilation, Risk for
Spiritual Distress (Distress of the Human Spirit)
Thought Processes, Disturbed

WHEN TO CALL FOR HELP

- Self-mutilation
- Suicide threats or attempts
- Access to highly lethal methods such as firearms, car in an enclosed space, or sleeping pills in a high-risk patient
- Hallucinations or delusions
- Lack of staff members available to manage suicidal patient
- Increasing staff anxiety and fear over patient's behavior

WHO TO CALL FOR HELP

- Security
- Psychiatric Team
- Law Enforcement
- Manager
- Critical Incident Team

PATIENT AND FAMILY EDUCATION

- Teach patient that his or her view of the options available becomes narrowed when he or she is depressed or suicidal. Review alternative ways of viewing problems. Incorporate family into this education.
- Encourage patient and family to obtain educational material including Understanding and Helping Suicidal Persons and Surviving after Suicide (suicidology.org).
- Review with the patient the idea that he or she needs to reach out to others for support and assistance. Teach the patient to reach out immediately when feeling the urge for self-harm.
- Encourage the patient to report and seek out adequate treatment for uncomfortable symptoms of physical illness, possibly including analgesics, to reduce suffering.
- Teach alternative outlets for anger rather than self-destructive ones. (See Coping Interventions.)
- Make sure that patient and family understand the purpose of close observation by staff members if patient is actively suicidal.
- Make sure that the family knows signs of increasing suicide risk and interventions.
- If a patient does commit suicide, prepare the family for the complex grief reaction that may follow (Box 9–8).

CHARTING TIPS

- Document all behaviors that could be considered a suicide thought, threat, or action, and who was notified about them.
- Note patient's response to suicide assessment.
- Document all measures in place to prevent suicide.

BOX 9–8
Information for Survivors of Suicide

- Recognize that their grief may have an added burden of guilt, shame, and anger.
- Sharing their grief with others about the cause of death will put the tragedy out in the open and provide added support.
- Recognize that factors contributing to the suicide may be out of the family's control.
- Provide information on dynamics of suicide.
- Encourage attendance at bereavement support groups specific for survivors of suicide.

- Document patient's response to a no-suicide contract and teaching.
- Document any information from others on availability of potential methods for suicide available to the patient and interventions to protect patient.

COMMUNITY-BASED CARE

- Make sure that patient and family have information on referrals for follow-up counseling. They should also have emergency numbers such as suicide hotlines. Provide written information and education.
- Determine if psychiatric evaluation needs to be made before the patient leaves the agency/institution.
- Determine the appropriate quantities of prescribed medications to send home with the patient.
- Refer for home health follow-up and make sure that the agency is aware of the patient's suicide risk. Refer for psychiatric home care if available.
- If patient is a high suicide risk, transfer to a psychiatric hospital as soon as possible.

The Grieving Patient

Learning Objectives

- Describe the variables that contribute to the intensity of the grief response.
- Describe some common behavioral responses to grief in children.
- Identify dysfunctional grief reactions.
- Describe effective nursing interventions to assist the grieving family.
- Describe common nursing staff reactions to the grieving patient.

Glossary

Absent grief – *In an effort to avoid aspects of the loss and avoid relinquishing the lost object, no grief is experienced.*

Anticipatory grief – *Grief response before and in preparation for a significant actual or potential loss.*

Bereavement – *State of having suffered a loss.*

Delayed grief – *The absence of grief behavior when it would be normally expected.*

Disenfranchised grief – *Loss that cannot be acknowledged or publicly shared.*
Distorted grief – *Abnormal extension or overelaboration of grief behavior.*
Dysfunctional or complicated grief – *Grief reaction that does not follow the usual pattern and may include delayed and/or distorted grief.*
Grief – *Subjective, emotional response to a loss.*
Loss – *Situation, real or potential, in which a valued object is rendered inaccessible or is altered in such a way that it no longer has the valued qualities.*
Mourning – *The process by which grief is resolved.*
Prolonged grief – *Continued grief behavior lasting much longer than would be expected.*

Experiencing loss is a normal part of life. Friends moving away, loss of a job, loss of functional abilities or physical health, or the death of a loved one are something we all experience.

Grief is the normal human response that usually follows these experiences. As things change in our lives, we must adapt. This process of adaptation is called grieving. The purpose of grief is to begin to face the loss, work through the emotions, and eventually let go or adapt with renewed energy to focus on new relationships and goals. Because all individuals respond to loss differently, the process of adapting varies widely and can take days, months, or years depending on many variables. Grief does not decline in a linear, predictable fashion over time. Rather, it can fluctuate over time and be affected by many factors. Variables that can influence the sense of loss include:

- The meaning of the lost object to the person (Generally, the more important the loss is to the person, the more intense the reaction.)
- The degree of preparation and past unresolved losses
- Physical health
- The degree of conflict or dependency in the relationship
- Support system
- Concurrent stressors

Culture also influences the way an individual responds to loss. Most cultures have specific rituals and traditions that provide support and reassurance during the grieving process. Grief caused by a death can be influenced by the cause of death. Unexpected deaths, deaths viewed as preventable, and the death of a child all create additional distress. Death resulting from a cause with a social stigma, such as suicide or AIDS, can be particularly difficult. With suicide, death is unexpected, violent, and possibly preventable. Survivors may experience intense anger, guilt, and self-blame. Those who lose a loved one from AIDS may have had time to prepare for the death, but many complicated feelings may still need to be resolved before grieving can be accomplished. Society's reactions to deaths caused by problems such as these may affect the type of support the mourners receive.

ETIOLOGY

There is no one comprehensive theory that explains normal grief. Research has shown that grief occurs in a sequence of phases or stages with predictable symptoms that change over time, and that these stages do not necessarily progress in an orderly, set fashion.

Acute grief symptoms were first described in Lindemann's classic study of 1944 after the Coconut Grove Night Club fire in Boston. Symptoms include sighing, sobbing, hyperventilating, and a sense of unreality or shock as the first reactions to facing a major loss. Elisabeth Kübler-Ross (1969) and Theresa Rando (1993) both describe stages through which individuals advance in their progression toward resolution (Table 9–2). These stages give us guides for expected behaviors, but each individual goes through the process in his or her own way and time.

During the initial period of shock, the mourner may experience denial or avoidance as a protective mechanism from the overwhelming stress to block out the pain. As denial and shock fade, the mourner begins to face the sadness of the loss. In addition to depression, there may be periods of anger and guilt. Anger can be directed at the lost person for leaving or the person responsible for the situation (if applicable), or it can be displaced onto others. Guilt feelings, possibly evidenced by self-reproach for real or imagined acts of negligence or omissions, can be especially painful. All of these behaviors force the individual to confront the pain over and over again. However, not all reactions cause the individual to feel discomfort. Some can provide comfort, such as a sense of being watched over by the lost person. Maciejewski, Zhang, Block, & Prigerson's (2007) research has validated the model of stages of grief and noted that depression peaked at six months post loss.

The ability to tolerate intense emotions, increasing periods of stability, taking on new roles and relationships, having the energy to invest oneself in new endeavors and ability to bring meaning to one's life (Niemeyer, 1997) are signs that the individual is recovering. Remembering both the positives and negatives of the lost person or object can also indicate successful completion of grieving. However, brief periods of intense feelings may still occur at significant times, such as anniversaries and holidays. Because each individual is unique, the extent of a grief reaction may vary. People may grieve as deeply over the loss of a pet or a longed-for goal as over the death of a family member. Disenfranchised grief can prevent outward expression of grief. This may be seen after an abortion or when the depth of relationship of deceased person is not known publicly. In addition, the length of time to resolution is individual, not necessarily fitting the 1-year tradition. How long grief should go on is less related to the calendar and more to the depth of the loss and the individual's reaction. Also, grief may be delayed because of extreme situations, such as multiple losses, and the mourner must deal with many responsibilities before taking time to experience the loss. Grief can take a more complicated or maladaptive form that interferes with the adaptation to the loss. Examples of these include absent, delayed and distorted grief. These forms of complicated grief often require professional intervention (Ott, 2003). These complicated forms of grief may be related to the circumstances that do not allow the person to

TABLE 9–2

Adapting to Loss

Stage	Purpose	Behavior
Rando's Stages of Adapting to Loss		
Avoidance phase	• Recognize the loss	• Acknowledge loss (intellectually first, then emotionally)
Confirmation phase	• React to separation • Recollect and re-experience the deceased • Relinquish old attachments to deceased and old assumptive world	• Experience pain of loss—it will impact all areas of functioning • Make changes in one's life to adapt to life without person • Change old habits, find new support systems
Accommodation phase	• Readjust to move adaptively into new world without forgetting old • Reinvest	• New relationship with deceased • Form new identity • Emotional energy into new things
Kübler-Ross's Stages: Adapting to a Loss of Self		
Denial	• Unconscious avoidance to protect self from painful reality	• "No, not me."
Anger	• Attempt to take control when feeling out of control by attacking, blaming other	• Lack of expected reaction; using unproved treatment methods; doctor shopping to avoid confronting diagnosis
Bargaining	• Attempting to change reality by making agreement, bargains for more time • Indicates beginning acceptance	• "Why me?" • Irrational demands; criticizing staff; hostile behavior

Stage	Purpose	Behavior
Depression	• Work of grief as realization hits • Involves despair, the pain of experiencing loss	• "It's me, but …" • "I want to live til my son's wedding, then I'll accept death."
Acceptance	• Resolution of feelings about death • Neither happy nor sad • Acceptance of reality, sense of peace and letting go	• Making bargains with God to change if can have more time, change reality • "It's me." • Sad, tearful, life review • Comforting others to accept impending death; remembering the past with fondness but without fighting to hang on to life

Source: Adapted from Rando T. (1993). *Treatment of complicated mourning.* Champaign, IL: Research Press; and Kübler-Ross, E. (1969). *On death and dying.* New York: MacMillan.

complete the grieving process for some reason. With a long illness, anticipatory (or preventative) grief may prepare the person for the future loss (Rando, 2000).

RELATED CLINICAL CONCERNS

The physical stress of grief can place the mourner at risk for health problems (Stroehe & Schut, 2001). Lack of sleep, poor eating, and changes in routine can predispose the individual to illness. Loss of a spouse in elderly people is associated with higher morbidity and mortality rates. Two months after a death, bereaved elderly persons report more illness, greater use of medications, and poor health ratings. Major depressive disorder associated with complicated grief can contribute to higher mortality rate, poor wound healing and immune system dysfunction (Duffy, 2005).

LIFE SPAN ISSUES

Children

Often adults try to protect children by not including them in the crisis or expressions of grief for other family members. However, they need to be included in the process, based on their level of development, so that they do not feel abandoned and left to face their fear and loss alone. Children generally display grief differently from adults, and it is important not to misinterpret their behaviors to mean that they are not grieving or that they are unaware of what is happening. Children often use symbolic or nonverbal language to communicate their awareness of loss and may even feel ashamed of their loss because they feel differently from their peers. Because they may also need more time to really assimilate what has happened, grief reactions may be delayed (Table 9–3).

Children's initial reaction to death is often shock and sadness but can quickly return to seemingly inappropriate laughter or activity. But their suffering may continue under a different guise (Brown-Saltzman, 2006).

TABLE 9–3
Children's Understanding of Death

Age	Understanding of Death	Common Behaviors in Response to Death
Infant to toddler	• Unable to comprehend death • Fears separation and abandonment	• Frightened, difficulty separating
3–5 years	• Views illness as punishment for real or imagined wrong-doings • May view death as sleep; cannot comprehend death • Magical thinking; may think they caused the event by their thoughts or actions	• Sadness • Clinging to parent • Nightmares, sleep disruption • Regression in toilet habits • Complaints of stomachache and headaches • Temper tantrums
School age	• Associates death with punishment multilation, violence • May feel responsible for event • By age 9, understands that death is final	• School phobia, diminished school performance • Aggressive behavior • Preoccupation with parent's health • Loss of appetite • Change in relationship with friends
Adolescence	• Understands own mortality • May seem to have adult view of death but not emotional view	• Acting out; substance abuse • Increased time with peers • Withdrawal from family • Depression

Adolescents

As they struggle with dependency issues, the adolescent may feel vulnerable to express feelings of grief. They may appear to deny or avoid the dying patient, act out their frustration in such ways as school truancy, substance abuse. This may be very distressing to other family members who may view the teen as uncaring.

Older Adults

Elderly people face multiple changes, often including the loss of a spouse, friends, job, financial status, health, and mobility. In spite of the extent of these losses, most elderly persons seem able to adapt, probably because of their past experience. However, the death of a spouse or partner still remains one of the major losses in life. This loss requires multiple life changes that become more difficult with increasing age. Grief can be masked by symptoms of dementia, depression, suicidal ideation, and substance abuse. Brown-Saltzman (2006) notes that the older adults may suffer disenfranchised grief as they experience multiple losses which others may consider normal for this age.

POSSIBLE NURSES' REACTIONS

- May feel helpless and uncomfortable, not knowing what to say. This could lead to avoidance or inappropriate hopefulness.
- May fear saying the wrong thing that will cause the patient or family to feel more pain.
- May fear losing control of emotions, crying.
- May make judgments regarding the degree of intensity of grief behavior, such as thinking that a family is "not upset enough" or too upset for a dying 95-year-old parent.
- May feel guilty for "causing" client to cry when discussing the loss.
- May become detached from the situation and attempt to minimize the loss to the patient with phrases like "This was for the best" or "At least you can have more children."
- May expect all people to experience the stages of grief in the same way.
- May relive past and unresolved personal losses, causing intense emotions.

ASSESSMENT

Behavior and Appearance

- Crying, agitation
- Extreme change from usual behavior patterns
- Unable to concentrate, distractible
- Taking on behavior traits of lost person
- No apparent reaction when one would be expected
- Unkempt, not caring for self

Mood and Emotions

- Shock, numbness
- Depression (Table 9–4)
- Anxiety, panic

TABLE 9–4

Differentiating Grief From Depression

	Uncomplicated Grief	Major Depression
Reaction	• Labile • Heightened when thinking of loss	• Mood consistently low • Prolonged, severe symptoms lasting more than 2 months
Behavior	• Variable, shifts from sharing pain to being alone • Variable restriction of pleasure	• Completely withdrawn or fear of being alone • Persistent restriction of pleasure
Sleep patterns	• Periodic episodes of inability to sleep	• Wakes early morning
Anger	• Often expressed	• Turned inward
Sadness	• Varying periods	• Consistently sad
Cognition	• Preoccupied with loss • Self-esteem not as affected	• Focused on self • Feels worthless; has negative self-image
History	• Generally no history of depression	• History of depression or other psychiatric illness
Responsiveness	• Responds to warmth and support	• Hopelessness • Limited response to support • Avoids socializing
Loss	• Recognizable, current	• Often not related to an identified loss

Source: Adapted from Ferszt, G. G. (2006). How to distinguish between grief and depression? *Nursing, 36,* 60–61; Brown-Saltzman, K. (2006). Transforming the grief experience. In R. M. Carroll-Johnson, L. M. Gorman, N. J. Bush (Eds.), *Psychosocial nursing care along the cancer continuum* (2nd ed) (pp. 293–314). Pittsburgh, PA: Oncology Nursing Press.

- Mood swings
- No obvious emotional reaction or one that is inappropriate to situation
- Anger
- Guilt, remorse
- Relief that ordeal is over

Thoughts, Beliefs, and Perceptions

- Self-blame
- Idealizing lost person
- Remembering only positive aspects of lost person
- Ruminating over events leading to the loss
- Obsession with lost person
- Illusory phenomena in which mourner thinks lost person is present
- Preoccupied with thoughts that can bring only pain
- Imagining that lost person is watching over mourner
- Difficulty making decisions

Relationships and Interactions

- Seeking support from others, may become more dependent
- Fear of being alone
- Unable to participate in conversation because of preoccupation with loss
- Feeling that others do not understand the pain ("How can they have a good time when I hurt so much?")
- Projection of anger onto others

Physical Responses

- Initial symptoms that may include hyperventilating, sighing, sobbing, muscle tension, chest pain, fainting
- Gastrointestinal distress
- Loss of appetite
- Change in bowel habits
- Insomnia, constant fatigue
- Dehydration

Pertinent History

- Unresolved or multiple past losses
- Ambivalent relationship with lost person
- History of psychiatric disorder or substance abuse
- Tendency to isolate self

COLLABORATIVE MANAGEMENT

Pharmacological

Sedatives and tranquilizers are often used in the early stages of grief to reduce the impact of the intense emotions and promote rest and sleep. However, these medications suppress the intense emotions and interfere with the purpose of the grief process. Antidepressants may be useful, along with psychotherapy, when depressive symptoms are prolonged.

Spiritual

As people face loss and grief, they may be more likely to reach out for spiritual support. They may question their beliefs, talk about an afterlife, and face past wrongdoing. Allow the patient to express feelings and, as needed, seek out clergy available within the agency or ask the patient's or family's own clergy to assist. Churches and temples may also offer special support programs. If the patient requests, provide information on important religious rituals such as the Sacrament of the Sick and prayer, and provide religious articles such as Bibles, prayer books, medals, rosaries, candles, and special clothing. Clergy may also provide important support for staff members who may be struggling with helping patient or family with spiritual issues.

NURSING MANAGEMENT

GRIEVING evidenced by denial, anger, depression, sorrow related to significant personal loss (actual or potential) including change in relationship, unexpected outcome, illness, death.

Patient Outcomes

- Acknowledges loss
- Expresses concerns, feelings of grief
- Verbalizes feeling of being supported in the grieving process
- Identifies potential coping mechanisms, support systems

Interventions

- Accept all grieving behavior. Recognize that responses to grief are highly individual.
- Provide private environment for person to acknowledge loss and express grief.
- Recognize your role as listener. Providing an accepting, supportive environment to share feelings is extremely important. Recognize that words are often less important than just being present at these times.

- Support grief rituals used by individual from his or her culture. These can provide reassurance and comfort to the bereaved.
- Accept feelings, tolerate mourner's expressions of extreme emotions such as sobbing, wailing.
- Provide privacy for the mourner.
- Recognize that it is not only acceptable but preferable to talk about the loss and express feelings. Not talking or not expressing feelings is a greater concern.
- If you are helping someone who just heard about the death or other loss, provide needed information such as mortuary, support groups in small amounts. Information may need to be repeated several times. Focus assistant on helping to get other family members or friends to assist so that mourner will not be alone. Assist with making phone calls. Provide concrete written information whenever possible.
- Seek assistance from colleagues if possible. Dealing with acute grief can be very draining.
- Use touch; holding the mourner can be very supportive. Recognize that waves of emotions will come and go. Be prepared for more intensity as the person relives events leading to the death or other loss.

GRIEVING, DYSFUNCTIONAL evidenced by inhibition, suppression, absence, prolongation, or distorted grief reactions related to significant loss, multiple losses, unresolved guilt, lack of support system, difficulty expressing feelings.

Patient Outcomes

- Acknowledges the loss
- Demonstrates absence of abnormal, prolonged, excessive reactions to loss
- Resumes or develops social relationship.
- Expresses feelings expected with the loss

Interventions

- Recognize that the individual needs to confront the loss slowly and accept it into his or her reality at the individual's own pace. Part of this process will include talking about the loss, reliving memories, talking about events leading to the loss, and expressing feelings.
- Use supportive phrases such as "It must be hard for you now" or "I'm so sorry to hear of your loss." These phrases acknowledge the loss and encourage the person to tell his or her story. Avoid phrases such as "At least you had him for 20 years." These statements diminish the loss to the mourner and can lead to feeling isolated and misunderstood.

- Monitor for signs of dysfunctional grieving, including prolonged denial, lack of emotional response, living in the past, or self-destructive behavior. If the mourner exhibits these behaviors, monitor closely and talk with him or her about your concerns. Point out feelings or reactions that the individual might be experiencing, for example, "You might be feeling like you're in a dream right now" to encourage expressing feelings.
- Encourage involvement in new activities and meeting new people. Help the person to set small goals to begin these activities very slowly, and identify realistic expectations.
- Assist the mourner to redefine the relationship with the lost person or object. This includes remembering the positives and negatives and acknowledging possible angry feelings.
- If the mourner does not acknowledge the loss, bring up the subject. You might say "I notice you never mention your deceased husband. How has it been for you?"
- Provide spiritual support as requested. Encourage involvement of clergy.
- Recognize that patients with histories of psychiatric disorders or substance abuse may need additional support to maintain their past improvements during these times.

ALTERNATE NURSING DIAGNOSES

Anxiety
Coping, Family: Compromised
Coping, Ineffective
Knowledge, Deficient
Powerlessness
Self-Esteem, Disturbed
Sleep Pattern, Disturbed
Social Isolation
Spiritual Distress (Distress of the Human Spirit)

PATIENT AND FAMILY EDUCATION

- Prepare patient and family for the normal stages of grieving.
- Inform them that anticipatory grief does not necessarily reduce the emotional impact of the loss. Mourners still may expect an intense reaction.
- Tell the family the signs of dysfunctional grief and encourage them to seek help if they begin to experience them.
- Tell the patient that feelings of anger and guilt may be normal. Encourage seeking professional help if he or she is having difficulty resolving these feelings.

WHEN TO CALL FOR HELP

- Disturbing behavior including hallucinating, delusions, obsessions
- Evidence of intense prolonged preoccupation with the loss
- Recurrence of psychiatric symptoms, substance abuse
- Dwelling on detailed events leading to loss or death long after the event
- Long periods of depression, possibly including suicidal thoughts or gestures
- Living in the past many months or years after loss occurred
- No emotional reaction to loss for a prolonged period of time
- Or if the staff exhibits: Intense emotional reaction to death of patient; Difficulty in dealing with personal grief to the extent that it impacts on patient care

WHO TO CALL FOR HELP

- Social Worker
- Chaplain
- Psychiatric Support
- Bereavement Counselor
- Critical Incident Team/Employee Assistance

- Encourage mourner to be very patient through this process. Time is needed to slowly face the grief. Discourage making major decisions early on in grieving.
- Discourage use of tranquilizers as a way to avoid intense emotions.
- Let the mourner know that his or her feelings may be intensified at key times such as holidays and anniversaries and that they may last for a few days.
- Encourage good nutrition and good health habits, especially for elderly people. Encourage seeking medical attention, as needed, during the bereavement period because the mourner is at an increased risk of illness.
- Prepare mourner and family for delayed grief reaction when intense feelings may occur in response to future loss.
- Provide written information on grief for family members.

CHARTING TIPS

- Document grieving behaviors.
- Document use of medications such as tranquilizers and analgesics.

- Avoid documenting judgments about patient behavior.
- Document available resources identified to support grieving individual.

COMMUNITY-BASED CARE

- Provide information on bereavement counseling and support groups. Provide the information in writing because mourners may be unable to concentrate.
- Inform referring agencies and home health agencies about patients' recent losses and grief reactions.
- Identify opportunities for socialization. Encourage involvement in activities when appropriate.
- Encourage involvement of family and friends to expand mourner's support system.
- Provide follow-up phone calls to mourner to reinforce information given.

The Hyperactive or Manic Patient

Learning Objectives

- List the outstanding characteristics of mania.
- List possible contributing factors to manic episodes.
- Describe effective nursing interventions for a manic episode.
- Describe possible nurses' reactions to manic behavior.

Glossary

Bipolar Disorder – *Psychiatric disorder marked by shifts in mood, energy and ability to function. Alternating moods are characterized by mania, hypomania, depression. There are two types: Bipolar I disorder: Characterized by the occurrence of one or more manic episodes or mixed episodes. Often, but not always, individuals with this disorder also have one or more major depressive episodes. Bipolar II disorder: Characterized by the occurrence of* one or more major depressive episodes with the presence (or history) of at least one hypomanic episode.

Cyclothymic disorder – *A chronic mood disturbance lasting at least 2 years that can be thought of as a muted version of bipolar disorder*

Hypomania – *A distinct period that is similar to a manic episode but with less severe symptoms. There is impairment of social or occupational functioning, mood is clearly different from usual nondepressed mood, but psychotic features may not be present.*

Mania – *A distinct period during which there is an abnormally and persistently elated, expansive, or irritable mood possibly accompanied by inflated self-esteem or grandiosity, decreased need for sleep, pressured speech, flight of ideas, or subjective experience that thoughts are racing, distractibility, increased involvement in goal-directed activities or psychomotor agitation, and excessive involvement in pleasurable activities with a high potential for painful consequences. Marked changes in social or occupational functioning or need for hospitalization or psychotic features must be present.*

Mixed episode – *A period during which the criteria for both a manic and a major depressive episode are met nearly every day.*

Rapid cycling – *At least four episodes of a mood disturbance in the previous 12 months that meet criteria for a major depressive episode or a manic, mixed, or hypomanic episode.*

Schizoaffective disorder – *An uninterrupted period of illness during which, at some time, there is a major depressive, manic, or mixed episode concurrent with the characteristic symptoms of schizophrenia.*

Bipolar disorder, formerly called "manic depression," is best viewed as a recurrent, life-long illness. Episodes of mania or depression can last from days, to weeks, to months. 1.2% to 1.6% of the population suffer from some form of bipolar disorder (DSM-TR-IV, 2000). There is a 3.9% lifetime risk of developing this disorder (Kessler et al., 2005). First episodes are more likely in a younger population especially if there is a family history. More than 90% of patients who experience a first manic episode go on to have future episodes. The majority of individuals with bipolar disorders eventually return to a fully functional level between episodes. Many patients with bipolar I disorder return to work when properly medicated. Manic and hypomanic episodes often precede or follow major depressive episodes in a characteristic pattern for a particular person. The frequency of manic episodes varies. Some have periodic episodes separated by years, and some have close repetition. Long-term, even life-long medication may be necessary. (Medication-free trials should be tried only under physician supervision.) Cyclothymic disorder may also require medication.

In the early phase of a manic episode an individual can become engaging, outgoing, and charming, presenting as one who is achieving and successful with excessive energy and optimism. During the hypomanic episode, the person accelerates to an "abnormally and persistently elevated, expansive or irritable mood lasting at least 4 days." (APA: DSM-IV-TR, 2000, p 365). Mania can continue to accelerate to a continuously frenzied, out-of-control pace, leading to seriously impaired decision making and potentially very hazardous activity. An increasing manic episode can be viewed as a series of stages during which the symptoms become more intense and severe. For example, an initial overestimation of abilities ("I can earn more money than any other salesman in the United States") can balloon to grandiose delusions ("I am Jesus Christ") and hallucinations. What begins as pressured, rapid, but still organized speaking can escalate to constant, loose, flitting verbalizations from topic to topic with little or no connections and, eventually, incoherence. Irritability, especially when demands are not met, can escalate into belligerent explosiveness and combativeness. Restlessness can peak into a state of continuous motion. A patient in an escalated manic phase frequently denies the seriousness or even the existence of illness, both medical and psychiatric. This individual could walk endless miles for days, expecting cars to clear a path for him or her, ignores the need for any food and sleep, and disregards any physical impairment. Without medication, a manic episode can last months. Individuals may be prone to abuse substances like tranquilizers to sleep or control some aspect of the manic episode.

Interestingly, descriptions of manic episodes reflect a mirror image of depression. Depression is characterized by an insidious slowing down of movement, thought, self-esteem, and initiative, accompanied by dejected, constricting, pessimistic, and even despairing mood. Internally focused guilt abounds, and anger is usually self-directed. In mania, everything seems to speed up, including thought, speech, decisions, activity, mood, self-esteem and a belief that all desires and dreams can be fulfilled. Externally focused anger and blame are directed outward: Guilt is noticeably absent. In the extreme forms of both depression and mania, there is a psychotic break with reality, including delusions and/or hallucinations.

During the acute manic phase, the primary goal is maintaining patient safety and hospitalization may be required in severe cases. When the manic episode has resolved, the patient may need to deal with substance abuse issues and need help to reduce the risk of relapse. Long term the goal is to try to prevent or at least reduce the severity and duration of future episodes. People often emerge from a manic episode in a confused and startled state with minimal memory of what happened. They may be shocked to see what has happened to their lives—bills, destroyed relationships, legal problems (Varcarolis, 2006).

Depressive episodes in bipolar patients tend to have a greater impact for the patient but there is less research on this phase of the illness (Hirshfeld, 2005). Schizo-affective disorder may also be present in a patient with schizophrenia.

ETIOLOGY

Bipolar disorder is a complex phenomenon in which a variety of factors converge.

Biological theory predominates. Studies indicate that this disorder is caused by an imbalance in neurotransmitters, particularly norepinephrine, dopamine, and serotonin. Increased levels are believed to be present in manic episodes and decreased in depressive ones. Impaired interrelationships of the hormonal and endocrine systems are currently being explored. Investigation of brain electrical activity is also being studied because valproate, carbamazepine, and other anticonvulsants have been successfully used with lithium-resistant manic episodes. Electroencephalographic changes have been linked to mood disturbances as well. Disruptions in circadian rhythms and exposure to light, as in light therapy for depression with seasonal pattern, can contribute to manic episodes.

A *genetic* link has also been demonstrated through family studies. Bipolar patients have a significantly greater percentage of relatives with bipolar and depressive disorders than the general population. Studies done on twins and adopted individuals provide strong evidence of a genetic influence for bipolar I disorder. When a family history is present, the first episode tends to be at a younger age.

Sociologically, there are no reports of differential incidence of bipolar I disorder based on race, ethnicity, or sex. Mania is more often the initial episode in men and depression in women. Bipolar II disorder may be somewhat more common in women.

Psychological theory views mania as a defensive flight from an underlying extreme depression with its attendant painful feelings of hopelessness, worthlessness, and emptiness. It is suggested that the individual uses denial as a defense mechanism. Hypotheses requiring further investigation are that the patient uses manic symptoms to covertly get dependency needs met; approval from others maintains self-esteem, whereas manic symptoms prevent others from setting limits and containing out-of-control behavior. Psychological factors may be a larger factor in precipitating relapse.

RELATED CLINICAL CONCERNS

Hyperactive symptoms caused by substance abuse, medication use, or a general medical condition are not considered to be a bipolar disease. Under these circumstances, the diagnoses would be substance-induced mood disorder or mood disorder caused by a general medical condition but not be considered bipolar disorder (Box 9–9).

Manic episodes can be induced in susceptible individuals by other somatic treatments for depression, such as ECT or light therapy for depression with sea-

---

BOX 9–9
Drugs and Physical Illnesses That can Cause Manic States

Drug Related	Infections
Steroids	Influenza
Levodopa	Q fever
Amphetamines	St. Louis encephalitis
Tricyclic antidepressants	**Other Illnesses**
Monoamine oxidase inhibitors	Hyperthyroidism
Methylphenidate	Multiple sclerosis
Cocaine	Systemic lupus erythematosus
Thyroid hormone	Brain tumors
	Stroke

Source: Dubovsky S. L., Davies, R., & Doboxsky, A. N. (2003). Mood disorders. In R. E. Hales, S. C. Yodofsky (Eds.), *Textbook of clinical psychiatry* (4th ed.) (pp. 439–542). Washington, DC: American Psychiatric Press; McDaniels J. S., & Sharma S. M. (2002). Mania. In M. G. Wise & J. R. Rundell (Eds.), *Textbook of consultation liaison psychiatry* (2nd ed.) (pp. 339–359). Washington, DC: American Psychiatric Press.

---

sonal pattern (exposure to increased amount of bright visible-spectrum light during seasons of the year with diminished daylight).

Sleep disturbance is both a symptom of manic episodes and an irritant that can exacerbate manic episodes and worsen the overall condition.

Patients with extreme manic episodes may be at risk for illness owing to physical exhaustion and immune system compromise.

LIFE SPAN ISSUES

Children

Studies indicate that frequently bipolar disorders have their onset before the age of 20. This disorder is now being diagnosed in younger people. Children may manifest bipolar disorder as an ongoing, continuous mood disturbance that includes both depression and mania rather than distinct phases (Child and Adolescent Bipolar Foundation-CABF, 2007). Children may be misdiagnosed as having a conduct disorder such as attention deficit hyperactivity disorder (ADHD). Before putting a child on a stimulant for ADHD, an evaluation for history of bipolar disorder should be done. A stimulant could precipitate a manic episode in an at-risk child. If one parent has bipolar disorder, a child has a 15% to 30% chance of having this disorder (CABF, 2007).

Adolescents

Manic episodes in adolescents are more likely to include psychotic features and can be misdiagnosed as schizophrenia. As with younger children, behavioral problems can lead to the misdiagnosis of conduct disorder. Approximately 10% to 15% of adolescents with recurrent major depressive episodes will go on to develop bipolar I disorder (DSM-IV-TR, 2000). Assessments should include a family history of mood disorders.

In adolescents, manic and hypomanic episodes may be associated with school truancy, antisocial behavior, suicide attempts, school failure, or substance abuse. A significant minority of adolescents appear to have a history of long-standing behavior problems preceding a frank manic episode. It is unclear whether these problems represent a prolonged prodrome to bipolar disorder or an independent disorder. The Child and Adolescent Bipolar Foundation has developed consensus guidelines for diagnosis and treatment for this age group (Kowatch et al, 2005). Screening for substance abuse should be done with any teen with bipolar disorder.

Antimanic medications can be used in adjusted doses along with psychotherapeutic interventions in this age group.

Adults

The majority of first manic episodes in bipolar disorder occur between 20 and 30 years of age with preponderance in the early 20s. If the onset of a first manic episode occurs in a patient 40 years of age or older who has no previous psychiatric illness, medical conditions and drug-inducing manic symptoms should be ruled out.

In the adult years, uncontrolled symptoms can result in job losses, marital and other relationship breakups, grave financial problems, or serious legal repercussions from violating laws. During manic episodes parents may be unable to care for and provide safety for a child. Child abuse, spousal abuse, or other violent behaviors may occur during severe manic episodes or during those with psychotic features.

Postpartum

"Postpartum onset" is applied to manic, depressive, or mixed episodes that occur within 4 weeks after delivery of a child. The symptoms remain the same. If delusions are present, they often concern the newborn child. If a manic episode develops in the postpartum period, risk for recurrence in subsequent postpartum periods may be increased.

Older Adults

The intervals between episodes tend to decrease in bipolar I disorder and to increase in bipolar II disorder as an individual ages. Medical conditions and drug reactions as causative factors in manic episodes need to be carefully evaluated particularly when initial episodes occur in elderly people. Managing patients with bipolar disorder in long-term care settings can create major challenges for staff members.

POSSIBLE NURSES' REACTIONS

- May be entertained or amused by the initial exuberance and acting out and not set limits
- May become irritable, anxious, or angry when patient is noncompliant with healthcare regimen or routine
- May be embarrassed or sense lowered self-esteem if the nurse believes that a "good" nurse should be able to control patients or prevent them from behaving strangely
- May feel verbally abused and unrecognized by the patient
- May feel manipulated, outsmarted, and defensive, needing to justify actions and motives
- May feel frightened if patient becomes violent

ASSESSMENT

Behavior and Appearance

- Excessive in all areas: bizarre, garish, flamboyant, eccentric
- Pressured speech (profuse, rapid, as if generated by an engine)
- Poor personal grooming and excessive and bizarre clothing or make-up changes
- Restlessness, hyperactivity with constant moving and pacing
- Flitting attempts to participate in multiple activities, unable to complete things, impulsive
- Poor judgment in decision making; undertakes risky or dangerous endeavors without awareness of consequences, including buying sprees, foolish business investments, reckless driving, hypersexuality
- Behavior inappropriate to situation
- Complaints, hostile comments, and angry tirades; may be violent

Mood and Emotions

- Elation; heightened sense of pleasure; unrealistic optimism
- Lack of shame or guilt
- Anger escalating to rage, especially when wishes are thwarted
- Labile mood swings including depression, irritability, and anger

Thoughts, Beliefs, and Perceptions

- Distracted; unable to concentrate on task at hand; overly attuned and responsive to stimulation from people and events
- Grandiose overestimation of own abilities, talents; exaggeration of past achievements; inflated self-esteem; impaired judgment

- Complicated plans to acquire unlimited fame, fortune, and/or power
- Poor insight; unaware of his or her distortion and negative effect on others
- Makes puns, plays on words, and jokes
- Flight of ideas (continuously jumps rapidly from one topic to another)
- Suspicious; escalates to delusions or hallucinations of grandiosity or persecution

Relationships and Interactions

- Excessively gregarious; can be charming; lacks true concern for others
- Forms superficial relationships quickly but becomes manipulative, demanding, intrusive, taunting
- Attempts to engage everyone into his or her plans and activities; constantly demands attention
- Manipulates self-esteem of others by flattery
- Irresponsible; gives quick, deceptively plausible excuses for own actions; puts responsibility on others
- Intimidating

Physical Responses

- Sometimes initial overeating; weight gain, even food hoarding
- As mania escalates, inadequate nutritional intake leading to weight loss and even dehydration
- Physical exhaustion with insomnia, reduced need for sleep, changes in sleep patterns
- May exhibit side effects of drug abuse and symptoms of general medical conditions that can cause mania
- Patients on lithium must have blood levels monitored for therapeutic level

Pertinent History

- Earlier episodes or family history of depressive and/or manic episodes
- Dramatic changes in personality during manic phases
- Psychiatric diagnosis and treatment of schizophrenia or schizoaffective disorder may occur; differential diagnosis is often confused because extremes of manic episodes have similar symptoms
- History of substance abuse

COLLABORATIVE MANAGEMENT

Pharmacological

Patients may need to take antimanic (mood stabilizer) medications for the rest of their lives; therefore education and compliance are very important.

Lithium carbonate remains first-line treatment for a severe manic episode (Hirschfeld et al, 2002). An antipsychotic medication may be added as well. Lower maintenance doses are often continued in the intervals between episodes. Blood levels and side effects need to be monitored because lithium can reach a toxic range, possibly causing seizures, coma, and even death. Therapeutic lithium levels are between 0.5 and 1.2 mEq/L for most patients. Blood lithium levels can be elevated when there is significant lowering of body fluids as in such conditions as limited fluid intake, dehydration, profuse sweating, or chronic diarrhea. It is essential to constantly monitor for adverse drug reactions because some individuals can become toxic at blood levels considered normal for most people. Onset of sedation, nausea, and vomiting are early warning signs of lithium toxicity. As toxicity increases, tremors and muscle twitching may occur as well as renal failure when blood levels approach 2.0 mEq/L.

Lithium can take 7 to 10 days to reach the desired effect. If psychotic symptoms are present, antipsychotics can be used on a regular or as-needed basis. The need should diminish as lithium or other antimanic medications reach therapeutic levels. The antipsychotic drug aripiprozole (Abilify) has been used to treat severe agitation in bipolar disorder.

Antimanic drugs are available only in oral forms. If the patient is unable to take oral medications, other medications may be used, such as antipsychotics or antianxiety drugs, which can be given parenterally.

Anticonvulsants, such as carbamazepine and divalproex, are also used. Carbamazepine can cause agranulocytosis with lethal implications. The incidence of this adverse effect is low; however, it is important to monitor the patient continually for changes in white blood cell and granulocyte count and any signs of infection. Agranulocytosis subsides promptly when the drug is discontinued. Antidepressants that are normally used to treat depression unrelated to bipolar disorder may be used but they need to be combined with a mood stabilizer (Hirschfeld, 2005).

Herbal products such as valerian root and chamomile may be used to calm the person. During depressive periods, the individual may use stimulants to recreate some of the feelings of the hypomanic period.

Dietary

A patient in an escalated manic phase may be too restless to sit down and eat. Patients may need "finger foods" that can be carried, such as sandwiches and milkshakes. A high-calorie diet should be provided if patient is in constant movement.

Psychotherapy

Maintaining a psychotherapeutic relationship is an important part of the total treatment program to prevent or reduce the severity of relapses and promote compliance with the lifelong medication regimen. The patient has to take the time to work through the denial and, later, anger over having an incurable condition. Medications can control the frequency and intensity of manic episodes, but exacerbations can still happen. The patient may need assistance in dealing with shame over behavior during manic episodes. He or she may also need to learn how to discriminate normal from abnormal moods and will probably need help in learning to tolerate more dysphoric feelings and moods.

As life becomes flatter and less colorful without mania, the patient may need to grieve for the losses associated with giving up mania, such as fantasies, high or euphoric states, increased level of energy and sexuality, decreased need for sleep, and possibly decreased degree of productivity and creativity.

Developmental tasks may have been overshadowed by the illness. For example, the adolescent tasks of establishing a separate identity and learning about relationships may have been disrupted. Once the patient is stabilized, these issues will need to be addressed. If the patient has an alcohol or drug abuse dependency, this needs to be acknowledged as a problem, especially because the patient usually denies the problem. Mood disorders can mask substance abuse just as substance abuse often masks mood disorders. Effective substance abuse treatment should be used concurrently with approaches for bipolar disorder (Goodwin & Jamison, 1990). In extreme depressive phases when the patient exhibits suicidal ideation or psychosis, electroshock therapy may be needed.

NURSING MANAGEMENT

ANXIETY evidenced by hyperactivity, distractibility, disorganized and unrealistic thoughts related to manic phase of bipolar disorder.

Patient Outcomes

- Slower and more controlled speech and behavior
- No evidence of delusions or hallucinations
- Demonstrates an increased ability to concentrate
- Demonstrates more realistic decision making
- Complies with medication regimen

Interventions

- Determine psychiatric care provider for treatment of mania. If none, strongly encourage immediate referral and assessment. Make sure that physician and other staff members are aware of the patient's history.
- Provide firm, clear limits. Describe exactly what is expected and what is not allowed. Be realistic. For instance, patient may need to have a designated area in which to pace without being disruptive.
- Administer ordered antimanic medications; monitor blood levels, adverse effects, and signs of possible toxicity.
- Assess for psychotic symptoms; evaluate for need to administer PRN antipsychotic medications.

- Do not reinforce patient's delusional beliefs. Present reality without arguing with the patient.
- Be consistent even if the patient produces seemingly plausible reasons and excuses. Do not participate in verbal battles—just repeat the rules. Avoid power struggles. Keep directions simple and specific.
- Use a calm, relaxed approach.
- Provide a focus to conversation if patient jumps from one topic to another. Interrupt to slow him/her down. Refocus on the chosen topic. Phrase questions so that they require a brief answer. If the patient's thoughts are speeding to the point of confusion, do not encourage continued speaking, and, if possible, arrange for someone to sit quietly with patient. Supervise other caregivers who are unfamiliar with manic patients.
- Explain to staff, patients, and visitors who complain about patient's constant need for attention that the patient will feel better in a quiet atmosphere. Encourage them to limit interactions with the patient without abandoning him or her.
- Remove patient from external stimulation. If possible, place patient in a room in a quiet area and use dim lighting. A private room is preferable. Calming music may help.
- Assess whether patient should be allowed to verbalize anger or fear. If patient becomes overly agitated, change or redirect the topic of conversation. As the mania decreases, the patient may be better able to tolerate more processing of emotion.
- Limit the patient's choices. Attempt to limit the number of objects patient has in the room. Encourage family and/or friends to take home unnecessary possessions.
- Remove hazardous objects from patient's room.
- Provide brief activities because of short attention span. Tasks can be more complex as mania decreases.
- If the patient's behavior is unacceptable, distract with more productive activities. Do not reinforce inappropriate behaviors by giving them a lot of attention.
- Assess for activities patient can do in his or her room, such as writing or drawing.
- Provide an outlet for excessive energy. Assess whether a stationary bike or other equipment can safely be placed in the patient's room. Supervise any physical activity. Consider physical and/or occupational therapy evaluation.
- Support and encourage the patient's ideas that are realistic and consistent with the healthcare regimen.
- Assess for any injuries, bruises, and signs of infection.

- Assess for substance abuse.
- Assist the family in dealing with any negative feelings they may have toward the patient so that they can interact more constructively with him or her.
- Obtain support from peers and other resources if patient's manipulations begin to erode the nurses' abilities to maintain an effective approach.

SLEEP PATTERN, DISTURBED evidenced by inability to lie down at night, sleeping only brief periods, and erratic sleep patterns related to manic/uncontrolled activity.

Patient Outcomes

- Remains alert and awake during the day without daytime fatigue
- Sleeps at least 5 hours per night
- Does not require naps during the day

Interventions

- Monitor sleep patterns and assess for signs of fatigue.
- Use calming techniques just before bedtime: warm milk, soothing music, or warm bath. Avoid stimulants such as caffeine.
- Decrease stimulation at bedtime: lights out, curtains drawn, phone unplugged. Avoid loud noises nearby and loud talking. Some patients may respond well to having someone sit quietly just outside the room until he or she is asleep. Encourage the patient to remain in bed long enough to fall asleep.
- Provide ordered sleep medication if patient is unable to sleep.
- Encourage the patient to go to bed at the same time each night.
- If naps are needed during the day, encourage taking them at the same time each day.

ALTERNATE NURSING DIAGNOSES

Coping, Ineffective
Fluid Volume, Deficient
Injury, Risk for
Noncompliance
Nutrition, Imbalanced: Less Than or More Than Body Requirements
Social Interaction, Impaired
Therapeutic Regimen Management: Ineffective
Thought Processes, Disturbed
Violence, Risk for

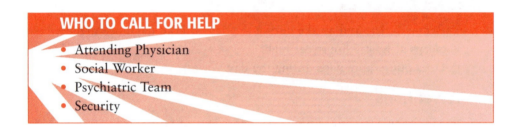

WHEN TO CALL FOR HELP

- Out-of-control verbalizations and behavior
- Psychotic symptoms
- Patient refusing health care or refusing to take medications
- Gross interference in other patients' care
- Symptoms of lithium toxicity
- Laboratory values indicating agranulocytosis in patients taking carbamazepine

WHO TO CALL FOR HELP

- Attending Physician
- Social Worker
- Psychiatric Team
- Security

PATIENT AND FAMILY EDUCATION

- Avoid health teaching until patient displays significant reduction in psychiatric symptoms and demonstrates good awareness of reality.
- Teach the family the symptoms of a manic episode so they can recognize what is occurring and not personalize the patient's interactions with them.
- Teach the patient and family the importance of continuing psychiatric medications and treatment, monitoring signs of medication adverse effects and toxicity, and noting early signs and symptoms of recurrent episodes.
- Teach patients, especially those on lithium, to maintain normal diet, fluid, and salt intake.
- Teach patients on lithium to check with their physician about withholding drug if excessive diarrhea, vomiting, or diaphoresis occurs.
- Provide educational resources such as healthymind.org for Bipolar Disorder pamphlet.
- Teach the patient to make a contract with a family member or a trusted significant other to encourage and assist the patient to make contact with psychiatrist or counselor if there is a resurgence of symptoms. Often family members are the first to notice behavioral changes.
- Help the family to make plans for hospitalization so they will be able to act quickly if an emergency situation arises.

- Teach patient about the process of realistic decision-making and the effect of one's decisions on others.
- Teach patient that life includes accepting periods of sadness, disappointment, and uncomfortable feelings.
- Teach patient about his or her effect on others.
- Explain to the patient and family that alcohol or drug abuse can undermine bipolar treatment.
- Encourage continuing in psychotherapy even when symptoms have stabilized.

CHARTING TIPS

- Note the presence or absence of adverse effects of lithium.
- Document the amount of PRN antipsychotics given and the results if used.
- Document any factors that could lead to dehydration.
- Document percentage of food eaten and weight changes.
- Note changes in patient's behavior and thoughts expressed.
- Document patient's compliance or lack of compliance with health-care regimen.

COMMUNITY-BASED CARE

- Reinforce the idea that it is essential that the patient continue in medical and psychiatric treatment and take prescribed medications after discharge.
- Make sure that patient has appointments for required blood level tests and follow-up referrals.
- Social service referrals may be helpful for patients who may have alienated friends, family, or associates before hospitalization. Financial and legal issues may be pending because of unwise actions such as excessive spending sprees.
- Recommend assessing the need for transfer to psychiatric facility if patient's behavior and thought processes are not sufficiently stabilized.
- Recommend that the patient attend community support groups for bipolar disorder such as the Manic Depressive and Depressive Association; refer for alcohol or drug problems if indicated.
- Recommend that the family attend support groups such as those sponsored by the National Alliance for the Mentally III (NAMI).

10

Problems with Confusion

The Confused Patient

Learning Objectives

- Differentiate between dementia and delirium.
- List the most common types of dementia.
- Describe common nurses' reactions to the confused patient.
- Describe effective nursing interventions for the confused patient with the following: memory deficits, unable to verbalize his or her needs, and at risk for falling.

Glossary

Agnosia – *Loss of ability to recognize objects*

Agraphia – *Difficulty writing and drawing*

Alzheimer's disease – *Progressive deterioration of memory, and intellectual functioning, often leading to complete loss of functioning and personality. Autopsy reveals brain atrophy, senile plaques, and neurofibrillary tangles.*

Apraxia – *Inability to carry out motor activities despite intact motor function*

Delirium – *Rapid fluctuations in mental status, memory deficits, disorientation, and perceptual disturbances over a short period of time.*

Dementia – *Multiple cognitive deficits: aphasia, apraxia, agnosia, or disturbance in executive function such as organizing or abstracting.*

Mild cognitive impairment – *Subtle but measurable memory disorder when memory problems are greater than what are normally expected with aging but no other dementia symptoms.*

Mixed dementia – *Vascular dementia and Alzheimer's disease simultaneously.*

Nocturnal delirium (sundowning syndrome) – *Increased confusion and agitation at dusk.*

Prompts – *Staff actions used to help dementia patient initiate self-care or other desired behaviors after loss of verbal comprehension.*

Pseudodementia – *Depression in elderly people that appears similar to dementia.*

Substance-induced persisting dementia – *Dementia caused by intoxication or withdrawal from a substance such as alcohol or drugs.*

Vascular dementia – *Dementia caused by multiple strokes that have usually occurred at different times and involve the cortex and underlying white matter.*

Confusion is not just a state of the mind seen in elderly people. It has many causes and can occur at any age. It significantly influences a patient's dignity, independence, personality, and support system, and can complicate the diagnosis and treatment of an illness. Confused patients are experiencing an alteration in higher level brain functioning such as comprehension or abstract thinking caused by delirium or dementia (Boxes 10–1 and 10–2). These patients have difficulty remembering, learning, following directions, and communicating needs and pains.

BOX 10–1
Factors That Contribute to Misdiagnosis in Dementia and Delirium

- The symptoms of dementia and delirium are similar.
- Several causes may occur simultaneously to bring about dementia.
- Delirium occurring in a patient with a dementia can exacerbate already existing symptoms.
- Health-care personnel may harbor unfounded beliefs that serious memory deficits, confusion, and other progressive intellectual deficits are a normal part of the aging process.
- Health-care personnel may harbor unfounded beliefs that confusion always indicates Alzheimer's disease in an older patient.
- Confusion and behavioral changes may be the first sign of medical illness in the elderly.
- Head injuries and other conditions causing brain tissue trauma may present with symptoms similar to those of dementia.
- Confusion is an adverse reaction to many medications.

Source: Gorman, L., Raines, M., & Sultan, D. (2002). *Psychosocial nursing for general patient care* (2nd ed). Philadelphia: FA Davis.

BOX 10–2
Characteristics of Delirium and Dementia

Delirium	Dementia
• Fluctuating levels of awareness and symptoms	• Slow, insidious onset with less fluctuation of symptoms
• Sudden onset	• Deterioration of cognitive abilities
• Clouding of consciousness	• Impaired long-and short-term memory (memory impairment always present)
• Perceptual disturbances (hallucinations, illusions)	
• Memory disturbance, more often for recent events	• Personality changes
• Highly distractible	• May focus on one thing for a long time
• Reversibility possible with treatment	• Often irreversible

Nursing care must be modified to help these patients to retain and regain the mental abilities that can be recovered and to compensate for those that cannot.

Delirium is a reaction to underlying physiologic (illness, drug reaction, or exposure to a toxin) or psychologic stress. Nurses in the intensive care unit often see delirium induced by the disorienting and confusing environment, sensory deprivation, or sensory overload. It may also occur postoperatively related to anesthetic or electrolyte changes. It is also very common in advanced cancers and in the terminally ill (Kuebler, Heidrich, Vena, & English, 2006). Delirium is caused by a temporary malfunction of the brain. When the underlying causative condition is resolved, the delirium generally resolves. It is a medical emergency. If left untreated, it could progress to dementia, coma, or death depending on the underlying cause. It is often under-recognized until the symptoms become more flagrant. Delirium can take 3 forms: hyperalert-hyperactive, hypoalert-hypoactive, and mixed (Irving, Fick, & Foreman, 2006). See Table 10-1 for Types of Delirium.

Dementia is generally a permanent condition caused by a variety of factors that lead to cellular brain changes or malformations. It is characterized by slow, insidious onset affecting memory (impaired ability to learn new information or to recall previously learned information), intellectual functioning, and the ability to problem solve. Types of dementia include Alzheimer's disease, vascular dementia, substance-induced dementia, and dementia caused by other medical conditions including HIV, Parkinson's disease, and Creutzfeldt-Jakob disease.

Alzheimer's disease is the most frequently seen type of dementia, affecting between 4 to 5 million Americans (Alzheimer's Association, 2006). The number

TABLE 10–1

Types of Delirium

Assessments	Hypoactive-Hypoalert	Hyperactive-Hyperaltert	Mixed
Level of alertness	Lethargic, falls asleep between questions, difficult to arouse	Overly attentive to cues	Alternates between hyper-alert and hypoalert states within hours or days
Motor activity	Decreased activity	Moves quickly	Alternates within one episode of delirium
Ability to follow commands	Follows a simple command, e.g., lift your foot Is passively cooperative	May be combative, pulls at tubes, tries to climb out of bed	Alternates between hypoactive and hyperactive states, may be unpredictable
Thinking Ability	Difficulty in focusing attention, disorganized	Easily distracted, rambles May mumble, swear, or yell	Alternates between hypoactive and hyperactive states in an unpredictable manner

Source: Adapted from Forrest, J., Willis, L., Holm, K., Kwan, M. S., Anderson, M. A., & Foreman, M. D. (2007). Recognizing quiet delirium. *American Journal of Nursing, 107(4),* 35–39.

affected has doubled since the 1980s because people are living longer. The current rate of dementia is expected to triple by 2050 (Davis, 2003; Hebert, Scherr, Bienias, Bennett, & Evans, 2003). It strikes at least 50% of people older than 85 years because the risk to develop it increases with age. Initial changes occur so slowly that they may not be recognized. The person may be regarded as absent minded. Changes in communication, personality, and social skills occur gradually. Because the decline is usually so slow, patients and families may deny its existence until a crisis occurs. The person with Alzheimer's disease loses the ability to relate to the environment and recognize loved ones. This contributes to families experiencing a prolonged grief process as they slowly lose who their loved one was. Because of the long trajectory, this disease has many financial impacts because the patient will require care for many years. In later stages, the individual may develop gait and motor disturbances and eventually become mute, bedridden, and incontinent. Death often occurs from severe debilitation, aspiration pneumonia, and recurrent infections. The average duration of the illness from onset of symptoms to death is 8 to 20 years.

Vascular dementia, the second most common form, is caused by multiple strokes. Symptoms are variable depending on the extent, location, and timing of the strokes. Decline tends to occur in steps rather than a gradual decline. There is usually more fluctuation in functioning. Impairment is limited and distinct depending on the area of the brain affected. This contrasts with more global intellectual impairment in Alzheimer's disease. Evidence of strokes, such as one-sided weakness, sudden onset of loss of speech, and focal neurological signs, such as hyperactive deep tendon reflexes, occur with vascular dementia. Treatment of underlying hypertension and vascular disease may prevent further progression.

In 2001, guidelines for Mild Cognitive Impairment were developed by the American Academy of Neurology. This condition may be a predictor of dementia in about 50% of patients (Gauthier et al, 2006).

ETIOLOGY

Delirium can have biological and psychological causes. *Biological* causes include a variety of medical conditions, exposure to toxins, and drugs. The onset of symptoms is related to exacerbation of a medical condition or introduction of a new medication for example, and contributes to the diagnosis. *Psychological* causes include sensory deprivation or overload, relocation or sudden changes, sleep deprivation, and immobilization.

Dementia can be caused by a variety of *biological* factors including the direct physiological effects of a medical condition, the persisting effects of a substance (drug of abuse, medication, or toxin), or multiple etiologies such as the combined effects of a stroke and Alzheimer's disease. Alzheimer's disease destroys brain cells and nerves leading to shrinkage as gaps develop in the temporal lobe and hippocampus where storing and retrieval of new information occurs. Diagnosis can now be made by magnetic resonance imaging (MRI) and positron emission tomography (PET) scan to document the brain atrophy.

The etiology of Alzheimer's disease remains the focus of much research. Current theories under investigation include decrease in the activity of the neurotransmitter acetylcholine and presence in the brain of the protein beta-amyloid. Thus far, theories of environmental toxins, poisons, or a slow-acting virus are unsupported. Genetic factors may also be present. There is a greater incidence of Alzheimer's disease in the family members of patients who acquire the disease before the age of 60 (Schutte, 2006).

RELATED CLINICAL CONCERNS

Delirium

Medical conditions that can generate delirium include systemic infections, hypoxia, hypercapnia, hypoglycemia, fluid or electrolyte imbalances, hepatic or renal disease, thiamine deficiency, sequelae of head trauma, postictal states, postoperative states, and complications of cancer. Some of the risk factors for delirium include vision impairment, cognitive impairment, restraints, malnutrition, and addition of more than three new medications (Samuels & Neugraschl, 2005). Elderly patients and cancer patients with pain are particularly vulnerable (Kuebler et al., 2006). Delirium is the most common cognitive disorder seen in palliative care and in as many as 80% of patients with advanced cancer (Elsayem, Driver, & Bruera, 2003). The presence of delirium increases the risk of complications associated with a medical illness and increases the risk of mortality.

Substance intoxication delirium can occur from ingestion of alcohol, amphetamines, cannabis, cocaine, hallucinogens, phencyclidine (PCP), opioids, hypnotics, and sedatives. Substance withdrawal delirium can occur from abruptly stopping significant abuse of alcohol (formerly called "delirium tremens"), hypnotics, antianxiety medications, and corticosteroids.

Many prescribed medications can contribute to delirium, including analgesics, anesthetics, anticonvulsants, antihistamines, antiparkinson drugs, corticosteroids, gastrointestinal medications, and psychotropic medications with anticholinergic side effects.

Dementia

Medical conditions that contribute to development of dementia include stroke, Parkinson's disease, Huntington's disease, AIDS, Creutzfeldt-Jakob disease, hypothyroidism, multiple sclerosis, traumatic brain injury, brain tumors, anoxia, lupus, and hepatic failure. Substance-induced persisting dementia can also occur with a long history of alcohol or substance abuse.

The dementia patient is at risk for many complications including unrelieved pain due to inability to express it. In addition this patient is at risk for skin breakdown, aspiration pneumonia, weight loss, and sepsis.

LIFE SPAN ISSUES

Children to Adolescents

Children may be more susceptible to delirium than adults, particularly in the presence of febrile episodes and in response to some medications such as anticholinergics. Assessment may be complicated by difficulty in eliciting the signs of problems in thinking, memory, and orientation. In fact, delirium can be mistaken for uncooperative behavior. One indication of delirium may be the inability of familiar figures to soothe the child. Children and teens may be at risk for delirium when they abuse club drugs, PCP, inhalants, or combinations of several illicit drugs.

Dementia is rare in children and adolescents but can occur as a result of medical conditions including AIDS, brain tumors, and head injury. As with delirium, dementia can be difficult to identify in young children. It may present as a deterioration in function, as in adults, or as a significant delay or deviation in normal development. Deterioration in school performance may be an early sign.

Older Adults

Delirium is extremely common in medically ill elderly people. It is a complex process that is caused by many age-related physiologic changes in the brain and other organs (Bond, Neelon, & Belyea, 2006). Ten percent to fifteen percent of hospitalized elderly persons exhibit delirium on admission (DSM-IV-TR, 2000); 15% to 30% of hospitalized medically ill older people may develop it at some time while they are in the hospital. Multiple medications, multiple chronic illnesses, use of over-the-counter medications, and impaired kidney and liver function contribute to the development of delirium. Specific conditions that put the elderly patient at greater risk include urinary tract infections, sepsis, stroke, bypass surgery, myocardial infarctions, and dehydration (Liptzen & Jacobson, 2006). A masked depression can appear as confusion (pseudodementia). Acutely confused elderly persons are often inappropriately labelled "demented," when potentially reversible conditions go undiagnosed and untreated.

Dementia in general is most common after the age of 85 and is often seen in residents of nursing homes. It occurs with increasing frequency after the age of 65 but is not a normal or expected part of the aging process. Mixed dementias are also more common as people continue to live longer.

POSSIBLE NURSES' REACTIONS

- May have a more positive attitude and take more active measures in care of patients if they believe the confusion is reversible.
- May feel very frustrated and helpless because of lack of improvement, constant need to repeat instructions or break tasks down step by step, repetition of the same question, and time requirements for care of patients with irreversible dementia.
- To avoid feeling hopeless and helpless, may become emotionally detached and give only impersonal care.
- May find themselves bored, unfocused, or confused if patients have considerable problems in communicating verbally.
- May be angry with patient's pathology; may believe patient can control own behavior.
- May become impatient with negative, hostile, impulsive patients who are very slow to respond.
- May feel repulsed by poor hygiene, messy eating behaviors, incontinence, or inappropriate behaviors.

ASSESSMENT

Behavior and Appearance

- Disheveled, inappropriate clothing; poor grooming
- Restless, agitated, impulsive, aggressive
- Wandering
  - Perseveration (involuntary repetitive movements, speech [most common] or activity)
  - Apraxia
  - Agraphia
  - Loss of coordination; stiff awkward movements; impairment of learned skilled movements
  - Unsteady, shuffling gait; stooped, leaning posture
  - Loss of ability to perform activities of daily living (ADLs)
- Types of aphasia including
  - Echolalia (repetition of word, phrase, or syllable just said by someone else)
  - Repetitive questions
  - Palilalia (repeating sounds or words over and over)
  - Anomia (difficulty finding wanted words) leading to paraphasia (using similar-sounding words) and circumlocution (using many words in place of the one word that is wanted)
  - Slurred speech
  - In late stages, may remember only a few key words used inappropriately in all situations (such as no)
  - May become mute
  - Hoarding
  - Regression
- Hypersexual behavior such as obsessive masturbation
- Hyperoral symptoms including increased appetite
- Inappropriate eating and toileting behavior
- Sleep disturbance including nocturnal delirium (sundown syndrome)
- Overreaction to neutral stimuli (catastrophic reactions)
- Inability to tolerate stress and change

Mood and Emotions

- Emotional lability
- Depression

- Suspicion, paranoia, hostility
- Anxiety

Thoughts, Beliefs, and Perceptions

- Loss of recent or remote memory or both
- Disorientation, first to time, then place, then person
- Impaired concentration
- Loss of abstract thinking ability
- Loss of ability to calculate
- Inability to learn and use new information
- Loss of ability to plan, initiate, sequence, monitor, and stop complex behavior
- Agnosia
- Ability to read words without knowing what they mean
- Loss of ability to read
- Confabulation
- Loss of awareness of spatial relationships; loss of awareness of own body parts and how they are organized in relation to each other
- Illusions
- Delusions, hallucinations
- Impaired insight and judgment

Relationships and Interactions

- Personality changes: accentuation or alteration of premorbid traits that affects previous relationships (e.g., caretaker role reversals); family unsure how to interact with patient
- Loss of social skills; social withdrawal
- Clinging, demanding
- Inability to sustain real relationships as memory gaps eliminate continuity; in later phases, may not recognize family or friends
- Negative, belligerent, briefly combative at times; hostility caused by brain damage or by misinterpreting events; not necessarily by the behavior of others

Physical Responses

- The patient may not verbalize or demonstrate common physical signs of pain or other symptoms such as bladder distention, constipation, dehydration, injuries, or urinary tract infections.
- Laboratory data, medication history, and possibly drug screening should be performed to evaluate patient at the onset of confusion.

Pertinent History

- Complex medical history
- Chronic illness
- Substance abuse
- Head trauma

COLLABORATIVE MANAGEMENT

Pharmacological

A great many medications cause confusion. Confused patients who are taking multiple medications may need to have the medications withdrawn one at a time to determine their impact on the symptoms and the underlying illness. Any medications used to treat confusion should be started at lower dosages. Drugs that commonly cause delirium include anticholinergics, benzodiazepines, steroids, antiemetics, and opioids.

Confused patients often become disruptive and may need to be controlled to protect the patient and environment. Haloperidol (Haldol) is frequently used to treat agitation and aggression. Atypical antipsychotics like resperidone are also useful. Side effects such as orthostatic hypotension must be closely monitored because the patient may not be able to verbalize how he or she is feeling. Other medications used with this population include short acting benzodiazepines like lorazepam and selective serotonin reuptake inhibitors (SSRIs).

Buspirone (Buspar) has been used successfully in patient's with Alzheimer's disease, although it may take several weeks to take effect fully. Hypnotics, antidepressants (particularly SSRIs used for irritability), and anticonvulsants (used for rage) are also useful. However, using medications to control agitation should not replace other interventions. There can be a tendency to use medications to sedate the patient rather than pursue behavioral techniques.

Medications to slow down the decline of Alzheimer's disease include cholinesterase inhibitors such as donepezil hydrochloride (Aricept), rivastignine (Exelon) and Galantamine (Rozadyne) have been used to temporarily improve cognitive function. Memantine (Namenda) is used to treat moderate to advanced Alzheimer's disease. It is a NMDA antagonist that protects brain cells against the influx of calcium into the nerve cells. It does not stop the disease but may help increase independence in activities of daily living and slow the progression.

Rehabilitation

A multidisciplinary approach for the patient with dementia is essential. Physical and occupational therapy, nutritional support, speech therapy, psychiatry, social work, nursing, and medicine all need to be part of the long-term management of this patient. It is important that families use all available resources to reduce their isolation and stress. A variety of nonpharmacological approaches have been helpful to reduce agitation. Some include pet therapy, massage, therapeutic touch, and aromatherapy.

NURSING MANAGEMENT

IMPAIRED VERBAL COMMUNICATION evidenced by inability to name objects or sensations such as pain; inability to comprehend verbal instructions; inability to communicate needs; inappropriate, dramatic reactions or accusations, catastrophic reactions related to confusion, disorientation, memory loss.

Patient Outcomes

- Demonstrates understanding of nurses and communication
- Able to communicate thoughts and needs
- Responds appropriately

Interventions

- Look directly at patient when speaking. Call patient by name frequently. Identify yourself by name before each conversation and refer to others by their names rather than "he" or "she."
- Keep interactions simple. Use short words and simple sentences that express one thought or question at a time.
- Ask specific questions such as "Does your stomach hurt?" rather than general ones like "How are you?"
- Reinforce speech with nonverbal techniques. For example, point, touch, or demonstrate an action while talking about it. For instance, if the patient is trying to tell you about his or her body, point as well as ask "Is this where it hurts?"
- Note in the chart or on the care plan the phrases, key words, and techniques that the patient responds to so that others can use them as well.
- If patient keeps repeating a question, try distraction and give reassurance that he or she will be cared for. Repetitive questions may indicate anxiety, and you want to be reassuring.
- If patient is searching for a particular word or trying to communicate something, guess at what it is, and ask if your guess is correct. If you are unable to determine what he or she is trying to say, focus on the feelings possibly being communicated. Always ask patient to confirm whether your determination is correct.
- If patient is reacting inappropriately, remain calm and reassure him or her that you are there to help. Avoid arguing or trying to convince patient that he or she is overreacting. Clarify any information or instructions. Assist patient with the next step of a task that is the source of frustration. Try to distract patient by removing him or her from disturbing situation.

- If patient makes inappropriate accusations, such as accusing the staff of stealing his or her glasses, help look for the missing item. Remember that the patient may accuse you of stealing because of memory loss. Also, routinely check wastebaskets for missing items.
- Family/caregiver support to deal with difficult behaviors. Resources for support should be provided to avoid reactions to behavior with frustration and aggression.

IMPAIRED MEMORY evidenced by confusion, decreased ability to perform activities of daily living (ADLs), or inability to follow therapeutic regimen; inappropriate emotional or behavioral responses related to delirium, dementia, or other cognitive deficits.

Patient Outcomes

- Demonstrates improved orientation to person, place, and time
- Demonstrates improved ability to perform ADLs
- Displays less emotional or behavioral agitation

Interventions

- Establish a baseline assessment of patient's mental status and functioning:
  - Observe ability to perform ADLs.
  - Use a standardized method of mental status assessment such as that found in Table 3–1.
  - Ask the patient orientation questions. For example, ask patient personal questions such as names of his or her children or home address. Make sure that you can verify the answers from the chart or family.
- Assess if patient is willing to discuss memory lapses. Determine emotional responses to these lapses. Do not push the discussion if the patient becomes agitated or defensive.
- Be aware that patient may try to disguise memory loss by confabulation, avoiding responding, or by speaking in a rambling style to hide the fact that no thought or information is being expressed.
- Be aware that when social skills and personality are still intact, patient may mistakenly appear stubborn and resistant rather than unable to remember.
- Do not argue with patient about what he or she remembers. Rather, focus on immediate and specific tasks to be completed. Give patient step-by-step instructions on what needs to be done. Be directive without being domineering.
- Do not make demands that the patient cannot handle or focus on topics that clearly cause distress. Such demands will only add to the confusion and/or agitation.

- Break down complex tasks into individual steps. The seemingly simple act of brushing one's teeth can take over 10 steps. Be aware of the steps the patient can handle himself or herself and those requiring assistance. Use prompts to cue each step of the task.

- Establish a regular and predictable routine. Try to do things at the same time and in the same order each day, such as shave, bathe, and then eat breakfast. Communicate routines to the staff to coordinate patient's care and ensure that the same techniques are used. Obtain input from the family on patient's usual routine. Use prompts such as consistent cue words or signs to remind patient of the routine.

- Attempt to arrange for consistent staff to care for patient.

- Keep surroundings simple. Reduce clutter. Do not leave equipment in the patient's room if possible.

- Personalize the patient's room. Have the family bring in photos and favorite objects. Encourage the family to create a memory box with meaningful items from the patient's past (wedding photos, special momentos).

- Place a large, visible clock and calendar in the patient's room. Cross each day off the calendar daily. Place large signs on the wall noting where patient is and special events such as when the family is coming and the next upcoming holiday.

- Write lists of daily activities or tasks patient needs to do if still able to read and comprehend. Put labels on possessions and patient's name on his or her door in large letters.

- Avoid an overstimulating environment. In the hospital, the patient's room should be close enough to nurses' station to monitor safety yet far enough away to avoid noise. Restrict the number of people visiting at one time.

- If the patient tends to wander, make sure all staff are aware of this problem and can bring him or her back to the unit. Consider using alarms, if available, for a patient at high risk of leaving the area. Monitor all exits. Draw a large red octagon-shaped stop sign and hang it by the exit. At home, make sure exits are monitored. Have the family notify neighbors of the problem and elicit their assistance to monitor for wandering. Make sure the patient always has some form of identification stating that he or she is confused, such as an identification bracelet. Maintain photos of the patient to be shown if he or she is missing.

- Provide some form of night light. If the bathroom is connected to patient's room, leave the bathroom light on. Otherwise, use reflective tape in the shape of arrows to direct the patient to the bathroom door. Encourage the use of a bedside commode.

RISK FOR INJURY evidenced by falls and bumping into objects. related to problems in gait, vision, hearing, lack of coordination, confusion, or lack of understanding of environmental hazards.

Patient Outcomes

- Remains free of injury
- Demonstrates appropriate actions to avoid injury
- Reduce use of restraints

Interventions

- Be aware of factors that increase risk for falls (Box 10–3).
- If patient is a fall risk, keep side rails up and bed in lowest position. At home consider taking the mattress off the bed frame and putting it on the floor to avoid injuries from falls. In the inpatient setting, bed alarms and hip protectors can be used to prevent injury.
- Even with side rails up, be aware that patient may get out of bed. Keep area around bed free from clutter. Make sure that there is always a clear path to the bathroom because that is the place where the patient will most often attempt to go. Make sure that patient uses the bathroom before going to bed at night. Plan administration of medications such as laxatives and diuretics so that they are not given in the evening. Recognize that the patient with dementia may have sleep pattern disturbances and become more confused at night.
- Make rounds frequently for patients at high risk for falling. Keep the patient's door open, and make sure all staff members know that this patient is at risk.
- Use restraints only after all other methods are ineffective. In some instances, restraints can increase confusion in elderly patients.
- If the patient has an unsteady gait, have him or her take your arm instead of the reverse while walking. Make sure the patient has access to any needed equipment such as walkers or wheelchairs. Provide instruction as appropriate within the patient's ability to understand. Ensure that any furniture or objects the patient leans on for support are sturdy and well balanced. Railings in hallways and bathrooms are very helpful. The patient may need prompts to perform simple actions, such as walking.
- Make sure the patient receives adequate exercise within the limitations of his or her abilities and condition.
- If the patient wears glasses or a hearing aid, make sure that these are in place before any activity. Be sure to check that the hearing aid battery is good.
- Ensure that the room is adequately lighted for any activity and that the call light is within reach when patient is in bed, in bathroom, or sitting in chair.
- Check the patient routinely for bruises, cuts, or burns.

BOX 10–3
Causes of Increased Risk of Falls and Injury

- Stiff, awkward movements caused by damage to areas of brain that control muscle movement:
  - Difficulty getting out of bed
  - Stooped or leaning posture and shuffling gait as disease progresses
  - Apraxia, with inability to make or coordinate movements
- Overmedication: Changes in drowsiness, walking, posture, stiffness, agitation, falling, increased postural hypertension
- Visual problems:
  - Cataracts
  - Increased near- or farsightedness
  - Inability to distinguish between similar color intensities (may have difficulty identifying railings that are same color as walls; may stumble into walls of color intensity similar to that of floor)
  - Poor depth perception
  - Blurred vision (may be side effect of medication, anticholinergic action)
- Hearing problems: May not hear approaching machinery or people
- Agnosia: May bump into furniture, not recognizing what it is
- Diminished or absent pain perception:
  - Inability to recognize or communicate injury (for example, patient may try to walk on broken leg)
  - Only manifestation may be change in behavior
  - May burn self while smoking
- Sundowning syndrome (increased confusion at night) with night restlessness, wandering
- Any factor, including concurrent delirium, that increases confusion and disorientation

---

Source: Gorman, L., Raines, M., & Sultan, D. (2002). *Psychosocial nursing for general patient care* (2nd ed). Philadelphia: FA Davis.

- Use colored waterproof tape along the area of the bathtub where patient is to stop filling with water. Decorative markers that stick to the bottom of the shower or tub can compensate for spatial disorientation.
- Use brightly colored materials in the room, if possible.
- Be aware that the patient may try to pull out catheters or intravenous tubing. Try to reduce risk of the patient's pulling out the tubes by reducing the discomfort associated with tubes. For instance, use the smallest-

size nasogastric tube or cover the IV site with a large bandage to avoid the patient's pulling on the tubes. Wrist restraints, freedom splints, or monitoring by a family member may be required to avoid injury.

- Be aware of medication interactions that could add to confusion and the risk for falls.

NUTRITION, IMBALANCED: LESS THAN BODY REQUIREMENTS, AND FLUID VOLUME DEFICIT evidenced by weight loss, electrolyte imbalance, increased confusion, or other signs of dehydration, related to impaired recognition of hunger and thirst, memory loss, impaired movements.

Patient Outcomes

- Receives adequate nutritional and fluid intake
- Displays ability to recognize signs of hunger and thirst
- Demonstrates ability to feed self

Interventions

- Assess the patient's ability to feed and care for self (Fig. 10–1).
- Provide assistance, as needed, for dressing, personal hygiene, and eating.
- Determine how much patient can safely do independently. Perhaps just opening containers or cutting meat is all that is needed to promote independence. Provide verbal cues to keep patient on track.
- Determine patient's food preferences and provide these foods, if possible. Encourage the family to bring familiar foods from home if appropriate.
- Make sure that dentures are in place and that they fit correctly before serving a meal.
- Allow hot foods to cool to prevent burn injury.
- Simplify the meal routine. The patient may be able to cope with only one food or one utensil at a time. Provide finger foods if utensils are difficult to use.
- Reduce distraction during mealtimes. For instance, turn off the television or radio.
- Assess regularly for signs of dehydration and aspiration (coughing after eating/drinking). Use thickened liquids or pureed diet.
- Make sure that patient can see his or her food and hear your instructions.
- Consider liquid supplements if eating solid food is too difficult.
- Assess for constipation.

Self-care Checklist

Ambulation:
Independent with steady gait _____
Uses cane _____ walker _____ wheelchair _____
Needs staff to accompany when walking _____ assist sitting/getting up _____
assist in/out of bed _____ assist up/down stairs _____
Effective techniques for assistance

Resists using necessary equipment/assistance: Yes _____ No _____
If yes, nursing approach: _____
_____

Feeding:
Independent _____ Adequate nutritional intake _____
Difficulty swallowing _____ Needs staff to locate dining area _____
Provide assistance prompts _____ Feed patient _____
Effective techniques for assistance

Requires special feeding routine: Yes _____ No _____
Requires special food/supplements: Yes _____ No _____
If yes, describe:_____
_____

Fluid intake:
Independent _____
Adequate amount _____
Needs staff to monitor daily amount of fluid intake _____
Provide prompts to drink _____ hold cup while drinking _____ drink with straw _____
Effective techniques for assistance _____
_____

Toileting:
Independent: Yes _____ No _____
If no, words/behaviors patient uses to express need to toilet: _____
Diarrhea _____ Constipation _____ Frequency _____
Uses bedpan _____ urinal _____ commode _____ adult diapers _____
Needs assessment of frequency/circumstances of urination _____ defecation _____
Needs staff to take to toilet at scheduled times (every hour _____ before going to bed _____)
Effective technique to encourage patient to use toilet _____

Bathing/Hygiene:
Independent: _____
Areas of skin breakdown _____
Areas of paralysis _____
Needs staff to provide assistance and prompts _____
Wash certain body areas (list) _____
Full bath _____
Mouth care _____
Effective means for assistance _____

Dressing/Grooming:
Independent _____
Hearing aid _____ Glasses _____
Needs staff to provide assistance and prompts _____
Change clothes _____
Provide grooming (for example, comb hair)
If yes, specify steps that require assistance or if total care is needed: _____
_____

Effective techniques for assistance _____
_____

FIGURE 10–1. Self-care checklist.

- For patient with end-stage dementia, family may face decision on whether to pursue aggressive nutrition intervention if patient refuses to eat or is unable to swallow. Provide support for the family in attempting to weigh these difficult options. Consider offering ethics consultation or palliative care/hospice assistance, if appropriate.

ALTERNATE NURSING DIAGNOSES

Confusion, Acute
Confusion, Chronic
Family Processes, Interrupted
Sensory Perception, Disturbed
Sleep Pattern, Disturbed
Therapeutic Regimen Management: Ineffective
Thought Processes, Disturbed

PATIENT AND FAMILY EDUCATION

- Provide simple instructions based on patient's current ability to comprehend.
- Teach the family techniques to control uncooperative and aggressive behavior.
- Give the family information about the disease so that they can better understand that the patient has no control over his or her behavior.
- Teach the family or caregivers about the need to avoid stress and fatigue for the patient because this can increase behavior problems.
- Encourage family to obtain material and newsletters from the Alzheimer's Association (alzheimers.org). Also encourage them to obtain a copy of *The 36-Hour Day* by Mace and Rabins.
- Alert family to signs of caregiver abuse.
- Teach the family or caregivers to build support systems to maintain a balance in their lives. Give information on obtaining caregivers.
- Encourage family to consider options for the future such as nursing homes, in-patient dementia programs.
- If the patient is in the early stages of dementia, encourage discussion of wishes for resuscitation and feeding tubes when the disease advances. Encourage completion of an advance directive.
- Review realistic expectations from Alzheimer's drugs and symptom management medications.

- For patients with delirium, help the patient/family identify possible sources of the delirium so the risk can be minimized in the future.
- Teach the family about the emotional strain created by caring for the confused patient. Educate them that, with Alzheimer's disease in particular, the family may go through a mourning process for the person who their loved one used to be. This process is complicated because the patient looks the same but no longer has the same personality. Adult children must be prepared to reverse roles and become caretakers.

CHARTING TIPS

- Document any changes in levels of confusion, memory, behavioral routines, or consciousness.
- Document which activities the patient cannot do.
- Document if patient is able to start an activity but requires a prompt to continue. Document words or physical directions that work as a prompt.
- Document stimulus that causes the patient to have catastrophic reactions, such as too much noise or too many demands at the same time.
- Document the patient's response to medications.
- Document any techniques that have been effective in calming patient.

WHEN TO CALL FOR HELP

- Sudden onset of confusion
- Episodes of patient's becoming physically combative
- Patient who becomes a danger to self or others because of poor judgment (driving, cooking, etc.)
- Severe agitation unresponsive to medication or other interventions
- Delirium that does not remit or gets worse

WHO TO CALL FOR HELP

- Social Worker
- Security
- Psychiatric Team
- Geriatrician

COMMUNITY-BASED CARE

- Be sure that the family has the needed information on financial resources and legal information for power of attorney.
- Report all indications of caregiver abuse.
- Assist the family or caregivers to set a plan to provide them with needed rest and recreation. Encourage family and caregivers to seek out support of friends or clergy. Encourage attendance at local support groups.
- If the care demands become too great, families need to consider placing the patient in a nursing home, specialized Alzheimer's program, or day care. Provide information on any specialized programs in the community and suggestions for what to look for in a facility. Provide families with support to make this difficult decision.
- Give specific information on this patient's management to home health agencies and skilled nursing facilities.
- Give information from local Alzheimer's Association chapters on treatment programs, research, and facilities.
- Patients with end-stage dementia may be appropriate for referral for palliative care or hospice care when they are bedbound, experiencing repeated infections, and are having difficulty with eating and drinking.
- Refer to home health agency if patient to be discharged home with a feeding tube or needs further instructions on prevention of aspiration, skin breakdown.

11

Problems with Psychotic Thought Processes

The Psychotic Patient

Learning Objectives

- Differentiate between schizophrenia and other psychoses.
- Describe effective interventions for the hallucinating and delusional patient.
- Describe possible nurses' reactions to the psychotic patient.
- Discuss specific interventions for the patient experiencing intensive care unit psychosis.

Glossary

Brief psychotic disorder – *Sudden onset of psychosis precipitated by severe stress with patient returning to premorbid state within 30 days.*

Delusional disorder – *Persistent suspicions, persecutory ideation, and delusions or delusional jealousies with resentment, anger, and sometimes grandiosity without other signs of psychotic thoughts or mood disorders. Patients are usually able to maintain daily functioning. (Previously known as paranoid disorder).*

Delusions – *False, fixed beliefs that cannot be corrected by feedback and are not accepted as true by others in the same culture.*

Good reality testing – *The ability to accurately identify and evaluate events. Absence of delusions, hallucinations, and other distorted perceptions.*

Hallucinations – *Sensory experiences that are very real to the patient but that do not exist in external reality, occurring while the patient is awake and when no one else has a similar experience.*

Poor reality testing – *Defects in a person's ability to accurately assess external events and interactions with others.*

Psychosis – *Severe distortion of and withdrawal from reality accompanied by severe disorganization of the personality.*

Schizoaffective disorder – *Symptoms of major depressive disorder or the manic phase of bipolar disorder as well as some of the symptoms of schizophrenia.*

Schizoid personality – *Individual who is indifferent to social relationships and with a very limited range of emotional experiences and expressions*

Schizophrenia – *A severe thought disturbance characterized by impaired reality testing, hallucinations, delusions, limited socialization; diagnosis requires the symptoms to last at least 6 months.*

Caring for a patient who is hearing voices, believes that the staff is trying to kill him or her, or exhibits other bizarre behavior can be confusing, disorienting, frightening, and disarming for the nurse. Although nurses in the psychiatric setting may frequently see psychotic patients (more than 50% of psychiatric beds are occupied by patients with schizophrenia [Berkow, 1992]), nurses in other settings may be unprepared for managing the psychotic patient. These patients are often feared and shunned by healthcare workers.

Hallucinations and delusions can be frightening for both the patient to experience and the nurse to observe. Even hallucinations that begin as fairly innocuous experiences can become frightening or accusatory to the patient (Box 11–1). Subjects of delusions vary. Common delusions are described in Box 11–2.

Hallucinations, delusions, or other psychotic thought disorders occur in patients with a primary psychiatric disorder such as schizophrenia, delusional disorder, brief psychotic disorder, or severe depressive disorder. Physiological

BOX 11–1
Recognizing Hallucinations

Affected Sense	Example
Visual	"I watch gypsies bring different babies to my apartment, each night."
Auditory (most common)	"The voices are calling me a prostitute."
Tactile	"When I touched my arm, I could tell my arm is made of stone."
Olfactory	"I don't want to stay in that room. I can smell the odors of the people who died there."
Gustatory	"I taste milk in my mouth all the time."
Kinesthetic (bodily or movement sense)	"It feels as if the rats in my head are eating up my brain."

BOX 11–2
Common Delusions

Delusion	Example
Grandeur (belief of exaggerated importance)	"I am Napoleon Bonaparte."
Paranoia (belief of deliberate harassment and persecution)	"The FBI is following me and wants to kill me."
Reference (belief that the thoughts and behavior of others is directed toward self)	"Those people on the TV show are talking to me."
Physical sensations (belief that parts of body are diseased, distorted, or missing)	"I have no blood in me."

changes or drug and alcohol use or withdrawal can also cause these thought disorders. Whether or not the etiology of the symptoms is known, the basic interventions are similar.

Psychotic thought disorders lead to severe distortion of and withdrawal from reality, accompanied by major personality disorganization. This disorganization leads to hallucinations, delusions, and bizarre behavior such as catatonia (assuming inappropriate postures or becoming completely immobile) or echolalia (repetition of words heard).

Schizophrenia, a psychiatric diagnosis characterized by changes in cognitive, perceptual, affective, motor, and social domains, is one of the most common forms of psychosis. Schizophrenics have psychotic episodes, but not all psychotic episodes are caused by schizophrenia. The word *schizophrenia* refers to splits between different components of the personality; for example, what the patient says does not match the emotion shown. The onset of schizophrenia occurs between the ages of 17 and 25 for 75% of cases (Moller and Murphy, 2001). Earlier onset is associated with poorer outcome. The lifetime prevalence of schizophrenia is 1% worldwide, with no differences related to race, social status, culture or environment (Mariani, 2004). All socioeconomic and cultural groups are affected, but schizophrenics tend to cluster in the lower socioeconomic levels because of their difficulty maintaining employment and functioning in society. Schizophrenia is a chronic, disabling condition, although symptoms can usually be controlled with appropriate medication. Schizophrenic patients can also have features of depression, manic behaviors, or both (schizoaffective disorder). Predictors for schizophrenia include social maladjustment and schizoid personality. See Box 11-3 for the various forms of schizophrenia.

Other types of psychoses include delusional disorder, brief psychotic disorder and psychosis due to general medical condition.

Patients without a psychiatric illness who experience sensory deprivation or overstimulation can become psychotic. A common example is referred to as intensive care unit (ICU) psychosis. However, the patient does not need to be physically located in the intensive care unit to experience this problem. Psychological stress, sleep deprivation, sensory overload, and immobilization all con-

BOX 11–3
Types of Schizophrenia

Type	Characteristics
Disorganized	Regressive and primitive behaviors
Catatonic	Marked abnormalities in motor function
Paranoid Schizophrenic	Delusions of persecution or grandeur
Undifferentiated	Does not meet criteria for other types

tribute to the critically ill person's developing personality changes, hallucinations, and delusions. A delirium from a medical condition or drug reaction can also contribute to psychotic behavior. Physiological changes such as hypoxia, renal failure, and response to medications also contribute.

ETIOLOGY

No single cause of schizophrenia has been identified. *Genetic* theories recognize possible hereditary tendencies because there is a higher incidence in families with one schizophrenic parent or sibling. *Biological* theories have received increasing attention. Some causes may be brain dysfunction in the limbic system and prefrontal cortex or biochemical disruption in neurotransmitters such as dopamine. Antipsychotic medications work by blocking dopamine activity. *Psychological* theory focuses on deficits caused by severely inadequate parenting throughout development, with special recognition of the devastating impact of deprivation during the first years of life. The more research validates the genetic and biologic theories, the less psychological theories appear to be causal. Clearly, though, personality is affected by psychological development and in turn affects outcomes in patients with schizophrenia. *Cognitive* theories indicate that the patient with schizophrenia has problems with attention or information processing. The person is unable to filter stimuli, leading to disorganization of mental functioning. *Family* theory has examined communication patterns that present unrealistic and unworkable expectations for the susceptible individual.

Other types of psychotic disorders may develop in individuals with fragile egos who become flooded with anxiety under severe stress.

RELATED CLINICAL CONCERNS

Certain physical conditions and medications, drug and alcohol withdrawal, and sleep and sensory deprivation cause some type of brain dysfunction that may result in psychosis. Examples of physical conditions include brain tumors, head injuries, high fever, septicemia, AIDS, encephalitis, epilepsy, and hepatic encephalopathy. Box 11–4 lists the types of psychotic reactions caused by med-

BOX 11–4
Drugs Associated with Psychotic Reactions

- Amphetamines
- Antidepressants (particularly tricyclics)
- Anticholinergics (e.g., atropine)
- Anticonvulsants (e.g., carbamazepine, valproic acid)
- Antihistimines (e.g., diphenhydramine)
- Antiparkinsonians (e.g., L-dopa)
- Antituberculosis (e.g., isoniazid)
- Antivirals (e.g., acyclovir, amantadine)
- Antiarrythmics (e.g., Lidocaine)
- Alcohol
- Beta blockers (e.g., propranalol)
- Corticosteroids
- H2-receptor blockers (e.g., cimetidine)
- Cyclosporine
- Digitalis
- Dilsulfiram (antabase)
- Anesthetics (e.g., ketamine)
- Antibiotics (e.g., cephalosporins, ciprofloxacin, sulfonamides)
- Opioids (e.g., morphine, hydromorphone)

Source: Adapted from Goff D.C., Freudenreich, O., & Henderson, D. C. (2004). Psychotic patients. In T. Stern, G. L. Friccione, N. H. Cassem, M. S. Jellinek, &. J. F. Rosenbaum (Eds.), *Massachusetts General Hospital handbook of general hospital psychiatry* (5th ed.) (pp. 155–173). St Louis: Mosby.

ications. Withdrawal from alcohol as well as effects of drugs such as LSD, PCP, stimulants and cocaine can also produce psychosis.

Disorders, medications, and environmental factors can alter cerebral perfusion and chemistry to create biological states that mimic some psychiatric disorders, including exhibiting psychosis and thought disorders. The combination of medications, sensory and sleep deprivation, fear and anxiety, and illness put the patient in an intensive care unit at risk of experiencing psychotic episodes. If this occurs, a thorough assessment is essential to accurately determine the underlying cause.

A patient with a psychotic disorder may also misuse drugs or alcohol as a way to self-medicate for uncomfortable symptoms. These medications could intensify psychotic symptoms and confuse the diagnosis and treatment. Dual or co-occurring diagnosis is the term used to describe someone with a substance dependency and a major psychiatric disorder.

LIFE SPAN ISSUES

Children

Although schizophrenia is rare in children, it has been identified. Symptoms include inappropriate affect, hallucinations, and mutism. It is often confused with autism, which is the most severe developmental disability of childhood, but it is not the same disorder. Children with psychotic disorders can be treated with antipsychotic medications, but side effects such as sedation and weight gain are a concern.

Children of parents with schizophrenia are at high risk for developing the disorder. As children of the mentally ill, they are at risk for being victims of abuse because they may be inadequately protected as a result of parental illness. They are likely to take on more responsibility to care for the household and less likely to have developmentally appropriate social skills because of the poor skills of their parents. Because so many people with schizophrenia are homeless, their children may be living on the streets.

Adolescents

The diagnosis of schizophrenia is more common in adolescence. Teens may be more likely to experiment with drugs in an effort to self-medicate to deal with distressing symptoms of anxiety and hallucinations. The move to college can trigger a psychotic episode in an at-risk teen or an exacerbation of long standing mental disorder. Being away from home, increased pressure to make independent decisions, and exposure to drugs and alcohol can all contribute to a psychiatric crisis in an adolescent at risk for psychosis.

Postpartum

Postpartum psychosis is a relatively rare disorder. Psychotic behavior tends to be evident within 4 weeks of delivery. Women with a past history of this are at higher risk for recurrence with succeeding pregnancies. If the symptoms last longer than 4 weeks, other diagnoses need to be considered. For patients at risk for this condition, precautions need to be in place to prevent child abuse and/or neglect.

Older Adults

Elderly schizophrenics often have fewer and less severe symptoms, especially hallucinations and delusions, although symptoms of emotional flattening and loss of motivation often continue. These patients often do not verbalize pain or discomfort, which leads to under-treatment of medical conditions. The first signs of physical illness in these patients may be changes in ability to perform activities of daily living. They are also more prone to the nonreversible drug side effect of tardive dyskinesia (constant involuntary movements). See Chapter 21 for further discussion. With elderly persons living longer and mentally ill people less likely to be institutionalized, it is believed that there will be an increase in the number of these patients in nursing homes and retirement settings.

A new onset of psychotic behavior in elderly people must be closely assessed to rule out physical illness, delirium, or medication toxicity. Because elderly persons may already have some sensory deprivation, illness, and use a variety of medications, the simple fact of their being hospitalized can increase anxiety and can make them at risk for confusion and psychosis. Symptoms can easily be confused with those of dementia, which could lead to inappropriate treatment.

POSSIBLE NURSES' REACTIONS

- May avoid psychotic patients because the nurse feels that he or she lacks knowledge or experience with them.
- May feel strangely uncomfortable or detached because of patient's lack of emotional connectedness.
- May feel frustrated and angry and have unrealistic expectations regarding the patient's self-care.
- May feel afraid because of patient's bizarre behavior. May fear violence and personal harm.
- May feel confused when patient responds unpredictably.
- May ignore patient's complaints because "he's crazy."
- May feel rejected if patient's extreme mistrust or fear of others is not understood.
- May feel that he or she has to control patient's bizarre behavior to be effective.
- May feel unable to intervene, leading to the nurse's giving up on the patient.

ASSESSMENT

Behavior and Appearance

- Strange or bizarre appearance, poor grooming, disheveled, eccentric clothing
- Unusual gestures, mannerisms, facial grimaces, posturing
- Neglect or difficulty performing activities of daily living
- Incoherent, repetitive speech; mumbling; talking to self
- May not answer questions or responds only partly; frequently asks that questions be repeated.
- May be watchful or withdrawn: head positioned, eyes moving, watching something that is not there.
- Socially unacceptable behavior and speech; may make up words
- Marginal functioning, such as being unable to maintain employment

Mood and Emotions

- Displays emotions inappropriate to situation such as crying when others are laughing
- Displays contradictory emotions at same time; unpredictable mood changes
- Flat affect
- Highly anxious, panic
- Difficulty controlling emotions: outbursts of rage, crying, laughing

Thoughts, Beliefs, and Perceptions

- Poor concentration
- Impaired ability for abstract and/or logical thinking
- Loose associations (ideas shift rapidly from one unrelated subject to another)
- Hallucinations; sensory distortions such as seeing objects or people change in size and shape
- Delusions
- Extreme sense of worthlessness; overwhelming, inappropriate guilt
- Decreased recognition of own body sensations, such as hunger, pain, and urge to urinate
- Depersonalization (sense of feeling separated from body)
- Suspicious; paranoid
- Extreme ambivalence; impaired decision-making ability; inability to problem solve
- Altered sense of self; uncertain where own body stops and external objects and people begin

Relationships and Interactions

- Dependent on others for basic needs
- Fear and distrust of others
- Unable to maintain close relationships
- Lack of social skills
- Interactions seem cold and detached
- Poor eye contact; withdrawn

Physical Responses

- Complaints of unusual or bizarre symptoms
- Blunting of pain

Pertinent History

- Psychiatric hospitalizations
- Ongoing or periodic outpatient psychotherapy
- Substance abuse

- Childhood behavior problems such as being isolated or described as "odd"
- Minor infractions of law
- History of suicide attempts

COLLABORATIVE MANAGEMENT

Pharmacological

Although they are not cures, antipsychotic (or neuroleptic) medications can reduce and control many of the symptoms of psychosis. See Chapter 21 for a detailed discussion of these medications. Antipsychotics are especially effective in managing agitation, combativeness, and belligerence. Newer antipsychotics, often called atypical, such as risperidone (Risperdal), quetiapine (Seroquel), and olanzapine (Zyprexa) are particularly effective in treating social withdrawal, flat affect, hallucinations, and delusions. These are now being used for patients with schizophrenia that is refractory to other antipsychotics. They have fewer extrapyramidal side effects than the older antipsychotics. One of the original atypical medications, clozapine, can cause agranulocytosis. Though more effective, these drugs are considerably more expensive than traditional antipsychotics. Patients with schizophrenia may need to remain on these medications for the rest of their lives, and symptoms can recur if they stop taking them. Approximately 25% of patients with schizophrenia do not respond adequately to traditional antipsychotics (Moller & Murphy, 2001). For patients with chronic psychotic processes, finding the right antipsychotic with minimal side effect profiles can take months or even years of trial and error. Traditional antipsychotic drugs like haloperidol are used less today due to the extrapyramidal side effects which impact functioning.

Antipsychotics can be given on an occasional basis to manage acute agitation, such as might be seen in ICU psychosis or drug reaction. They control the symptoms until the problem resolves or the cause can be treated.

NURSING MANAGEMENT

RISK FOR VIOLENCE evidenced by agitation, aggressive behavior related to delusions and hallucinations.

Patient Outcomes

- Able to maintain control of own behavior
- Demonstrates less anxiety
- Does not cause harm to self or others

Interventions

- Reassure patient that he or she is safe and that the staff will provide protection. Be aware that the psychotic patient is more timid and frightened than dangerous.

- Avoid putting patient on the defensive. Avoid ultimatums.
- Maintain nonstimulating environment. Use a calm voice with relaxed, nonthreatening body language.
- Ask if patient is hearing voices and if he or she can tell you what they are saying.
- Ask the patient if he or she is hearing "command" hallucinations, such as voices commanding him or her to act a certain way. If these commands are for dangerous behavior, monitor the patient closely.
- Reinforce the patient's ability to remain in control of his or her behavior.
- Be aware of signs that indicate tension level is increasing.
- Monitor patient's behavior closely. If having hallucinations or delusions that are very frightening, patient could inadvertently harm self or others (e.g., the patient has to protect himself or herself from a monster in the room or voices saying to kill himself or herself). Observe closely if this occurs and seek out additional assistance.
- The patient may interpret even the most innocent behavior as threatening (turning up the thermostat could be interpreted as turning on poison gas).
- Administer ordered antipsychotic medications. Consider injectable ones for faster onset of action. Patient may need these medications administered frequently (rapid tranquilization) until behavior is controlled. Monitor closely for side effects including postural hypotension and extrapyramidal symptoms.
- Determine if use of touch calms patient or adds to his or her distress. Ask the patient's permission to be touched.
- Set limits on destructive behavior. Let the patient know what behavior is and is not allowed. Reinforce to staff members that everyone must support the same approach.
- If patient is out of control, use restraints only as last resort. See Chapter 8 on managing violent behavior and restraint application. For the psychotic patient, restraints can represent a relief from the tremendous anxiety and loss of control being experienced, or they can significantly increase anxiety and persecution delusions. Have adequate, trained staff available to manage potential violence.

DISTURBED THOUGHT PROCESSES evidenced by inability to evaluate reality; hallucinations, delusions related to schizophrenia or other psychoses.

Patient Outcomes

- Demonstrates clear communication to others
- Maintains reality orientation (person, place, time, situation) and demonstrates good reality testing
- Demonstrates improved ability to participate in treatment plan

Interventions

- Determine if patient's behavior is a chronic problem or if this is a new onset. If chronic, determine baseline behavior, medications taken, psychiatric care received, and provider. If new, determine possible causes.

- Make short, frequent contacts to help build trust by helping the patient feel secure.

- Focus on the present reality rather than future or past. Speak simply. Focus on concrete subjects. Keep directions simple. Give only one step at a time. Avoid theoretic or philosophical topics.

- Provide a quiet, nonstimulating environment.

- Use one form of communication at a time; avoid using a lot of hand motions while speaking.

- Although psychotic speech is unclear, listen for unconsciously symbolic communication.

- Avoid giving choices to severely disorganized patients to avoid provoking anxiety.

- If possible, problem solve with the patient about ways to cope with anxiety.

- Provide frequent reality orientation: review location, date, and so on.

- Arrange for the same staff members to care for patient, if possible.

- Find ways to provide structure in patient's day; provide a written schedule to follow.

- Make sure patient is taking and swallowing prescribed antipsychotic medications. Recognize that hallucinations and especially delusions may take weeks to months to diminish fully once the medication is started.

- Patient can easily misinterpret what you are saying or doing. Obtain frequent feedback from patient.

- Monitor patient's decisions. Poor judgment may indicate an exacerbation.

- Ask the physician to arrange for a psychiatric consultation.

- For the patient who may be reacting psychotically to the stressful hospital environment:
  - Ensure that patient is able to get adequate rest and sleep.
  - Make sure patient is oriented to the time of day.
  - Explain equipment and noises and their significance to patient.
  - Call patient by name and personalize his or her care.
  - Encourage family to bring in personal belongings such as photographs.
  - Vary stimuli around the patient; for example, turn on music or TV at times.

- If the patient is hallucinating:
  - Ask patient directly about his or her hallucinations. For instance, you may say, "Are you hearing voices? What are they saying to you?" "Are they telling you to do anything or not to tell?"
  - Watch patient for cues that he or she is hallucinating: eyes darting to one side, muttering, or watching a vacant area of the room. Patient may deny hallucinations per imagined commands to do so.
  - Avoid reacting to hallucinations as if they are real. Do not argue back to the "voices."
  - Do not negate patient's experience, but offer your own perceptions. For instance, you may say, "I don't see the devil standing over you, but I do understand how upsetting that must be for you to be seeing that."
  - Focus on reality-based diversions and topics such as conversations or simple projects. Tell patient, "Try to not listen to the voices right now. I have to talk with you."
  - Be alert to signs of anxiety in the patient, which may indicate that hallucinations are increasing.
- If the patient is having delusions:
  - Be open, honest, and reliable in interactions to reduce suspiciousness. Respond to suspicions in a matter-of-fact and calm manner. Ask patient to describe the delusions: for example, "Who is trying to hurt you?"
  - Avoid arguing about the content of the delusions, but interject doubt where appropriate: for example, "I don't think it would be possible for that petite girl to hurt you."
  - Focus on the feelings that the delusions generate, such as "It must feel frightening to think there is a conspiracy against you."
  - Once patient describes delusion, do not dwell on it. Rather, focus conversation on more reality-based topics. If patient obsesses on delusions, set firm limits on amount of time you will devote to talking about them.
  - Observe for events that trigger delusions. If possible, discuss these with patient.
  - Validate if part of the delusion is real, for instance, "Yes, there was a man at the nurse's station, but I did not hear him talk about you."

ALTERNATE NURSING DIAGNOSES

Coping, Ineffective
Injury, Risk for
Self-Mutilation
Self-Care Deficit
Sleep Pattern, Disturbed
Social Isolation

WHEN TO CALL FOR HELP

- Self-mutilation
- Suicide threats or attempts
- Aggressive behavior escalating to violence
- Hallucinations or delusions with increasingly violent, bizarre content
- Patient's inability to care for self
- Increasing staff anxiety and fear over patient's behavior

WHO TO CALL FOR HELP

- Psychiatric Team
- Security
- Social Worker

PATIENT AND FAMILY EDUCATION

- Teach patient signs of escalating symptoms.
- Teach patient effective interventions to control anxiety and fears, such as distraction, listening to music.
- The patient needs to have strategies for coping with hallucinations. Some suggestions include reading aloud, telling voices to go away, physical acivity, calling someone for help.
- Review with patient ways to validate whether what is being experienced is real, such as asking others if they see or hear the same things.
- Make sure family or caregivers are aware of signs of escalating symptoms and provide suggestions for managing them. For chronic psychotic disorders, give the family written information on the diagnosis or suggest appropriate reading, such as *Surviving Schizophrenia: A Family Manual* by E. F. Torrey.
- Teach the importance of taking prescribed medications and ways to manage side effects.
- Teach the importance of informing the physician of new symptoms, delusions, physical symptoms, and pains.

CHARTING TIPS

- Document patient's behavior and content of delusions and hallucinations.
- Document the administration of medications, side effects, and patient's response to the medication.

- Document efforts and effectiveness in controlling patient's behavior.
- If restraints are needed, document the type used and appropriate monitoring provided.
- Document the family response to patient and the education and discharge plan.

COMMUNITY-BASED CARE

- Determine psychiatric care and provider. Reinforce the need to continue in treatment. Reinforce to the family or caregivers their responsibility for getting the patient to follow-up appointments. Give patient and family written referrals and specific appointments for psychiatric care.
- Emphasize to the family their need for emotional support. Refer to appropriate programs or support groups, such as local chapters of the National Alliance for the Mentally Ill.
- If the patient has a chronic psychiatric disorder, determine patient's functional ability. Referrals may be needed to programs to assist with employment skills and living arrangements.
- If the patient has difficulty functioning in society, he or she may need to be transferred to a psychiatric hospital or more protected living arrangements, such as a halfway house, group living home, or day treatment program.
- Reinforce need to continue follow-up medical care. Give written specific appointments.

12

Problems Relating to Others

The Manipulative Patient

Learning Objectives

- Identify types of manipulative behaviors.
- Identify some possible nurses' reactions toward manipulative patients.
- Describe "staff splitting" and characteristic manifestations.
- Define confrontation and limit setting as therapeutic responses.
- List effective nursing interventions to deal with manipulative patients.

Glossary

Adaptive manipulation – *Skillful management or use of one's self to affect or change a situation to one's best advantage. It is goal oriented, used only when appropriate, considers others' needs and welfare, and is only one of several coping mechanisms used.*

Antisocial personality disorder – *A psychiatric disorder in which there is a pervasive pattern of disregard for and violation of the rights of others. Individuals with this disorder rarely feel motivated to change.*

Borderline personality disorder – *A psychiatric disorder in which there is a chronic state of instability with changes in relationships, self-image, and mood.*

Cognitive behavior therapy – *Form of psychotherapy that focuses on challenging core beliefs that adversely affect self-perception*

Dialectical behavior therapy – *Form of cognitive behavioral therapy for the borderline client that focuses on gradual behavior change, teaching skills to regulate emotions, group social skills training, and psychotherapy.*

Maladaptive manipulation – *Similar to an addiction and not goal directed, it is the predominant, continuous controlling of others whether or not it is appropriate, effective, or attains specific goals.*

Personality disorder – *A group of psychiatric disorders in which specific, pervasive patterns of inflexible, enduring maladaptive thinking about one's self and the environment cause difficulties in interpersonal relationships and the ability to do work.*

Splitting – *An unconscious defense mechanism found in certain manipulative people that causes them to experience others only in the extremes of love or hate, or good or bad.*

Staff splitting – *An unfortunate staff response to a patient that leaves the staff members arguing and not coordinating with each other. The staff members whom the patient treats well think highly of the patient and the others do not.*

The word *manipulation* usually conjures up negative images of pushy, untrustworthy individuals who are concerned only with getting what they want with no regard for other people's feelings, priorities, or needs. However, manipulation can be viewed more accurately as a tool that is not inherently bad and that can be used in either constructive or maladaptive ways. For instance, adaptive or constructive manipulation is an effective technique for a charge nurse making assignments to ensure the best use of nursing personnel to meet patients' needs while considering the nurses' preferences and learning needs. Some people use maladaptive manipulation strategies during periods of stress to avoid uncomfortable, anxiety-arousing feelings and to gain a sense of security. The patient may use manipulation to compensate for feeling overwhelmed, out of control, and frightened by illness, hospitalization, or personal or occupational concerns.

People who consistently use maladaptive manipulation regardless of the circumstances may have a personality disorder. Personality disorders are frequent in the general population and may coexist with other psychiatric diagnoses. *Borderline personality* is the most common personality disorder seen in the clinical setting (Oldham et al, 2001). People with this disorder make up about 1% to 2% of the population and 20% of psychiatric inpatients (Gunderson, 2001). These individuals operate using ingrained behavior patterns that have been effective for them, and they may not be aware of their manipulative behavior, the cause-and-effect relationship between their actions and resulting consequences, or the possibility of alternative, effective approaches. This behavior can be very difficult to change because the person is repeatedly rewarded by achieving his or her goal when the manipulation is successful. People with borderline personality disorder manipulate to gain nurturance. They are so fearful of separation that they use manipulation to try to achieve a goal of maintaining closeness. They may exhibit both clinging and distancing behavior as they struggle with these issues (Townsend, 2006). The family of borderline patients may have a long history of frustration and exhaustion with having to deal with multiple impulsive acts. Another common disorder is *antisocial personality disorder*. Individuals with this disorder manipulate to gain power, possessions, or some other material gratification. Antisocial personality disorder is also associated with social irresponsibility and reckless or criminal behavior. Manipulative behavior stemming from personality disorders can be either blatant or insidiously covert. The manipulative person may appear superficially pleasant. However, the person being manipulated often recognizes the impact or results even if he or she is unable to describe clearly how they occurred.

Manipulative behavior can also take the form of sexually inappropriate behavior such as provocative language or inappropriate touching or threats of violence as a way to maintain control over others (Manos & Braun, 2006).

The first sign of a patient's use of maladaptive manipulative behavior may be the staff's growing frustration and anger. Manipulative patients may unconsciously project their own thoughts and feelings onto staff members and see one or some of them as a mirror image of themselves. As a result, the patient perceives the staff members as manipulative, unreliable, and even verbally abusive. When the patient feels threatened, he or she tries to control the situation by manipulating, attacking, or avoiding the staff members.

Two effective techniques for working with manipulative patients are *confrontation* and *limit setting*. Both of these techniques need to be used consistently with concern for the patient. Although the word *confrontation* is usually associated with hostile, antagonistic battles, it is used effectively as an intervention to dispassionately point out to the patient a discrepancy among words, actions, or feelings. For instance, "You said you have not seen a doctor before coming to the ER, but you have a bottle of prescription drugs dated last week. Where did you get that?" *Setting limits* is teaching and maintaining boundaries of the nurses' and the patient's roles and acceptable behaviors. This may mean telling a patient what he or she may or may not do under certain conditions or in certain situations (see Box 8–3).

Despite protests, manipulative patients feel more secure and less out of control when their behavior is contained. Using these techniques, nurses can alleviate much of the patient's insecurity and help to create the appropriate boundaries of acceptable behavior. Before being successful at using these techniques, however, you need to feel comfortable being assertive and being in the role of an authority figure. The nurse's past experiences with authority figures and individual personalities influence his or her ability to master these techniques. It is important to realize that no one can completely control another person's behavior.

Manipulative patients who unconsciously block painful feelings by *splitting* their perceptions of people into the extremes of all good or all bad can have a very disruptive, divisive effect on the staff. *Staff splitting* is a possible response to splitting when the patient idealizes certain staff members, treating them as all worthy and good while viewing others as all bad and criticizing and devaluing them. The staff may respond similarly, each one either intensely liking or disliking the patient and eventually becoming alienated from each other (Box 12–1).

BOX 12–1
Warning Signs of Staff Splitting

A manipulative patient can have a devastating effect on the staff and functioning of the unit. Staff group behavior that can indicate that staff splitting has occurred includes:

- The staff viewed as "all bad" by the patient demonstrates resentment toward the other staff members who are liked by the patient.
- Lunch hour and coffee breaks are dominated by discussion of the specific patient.
- The nucleus of an in-group believes that only they can help the patient.
- Loss of morale and confusion in the out-group.
- Criticizing each other for how they handle patient issues
- Blurring of staff-client role boundaries (for instance, patient and staff discuss another staff member, staff share personal information with patient, give personal phone number to patient, spend off time worrying about the patient).
- Split in- and out-groups make accusations: "ins" accuse "outs" of being cold and insensitive; "outs" accuse "ins" of being too permissive and gullible and of spoiling patient.
- Splits between departments in a hospital agency structure.
- Staff keeping secrets about the patient.
- Staff members use poor judgment in decisions about this patient.

Source: Adapted from Lego, S. (1990). Borderline personality disorders. In E. Varcarolis (Ed.), *Foundations in mental health nursing* (pp. 408–420). Philadelphia: WB Saunders; Groves, J. E. (2004). Difficult patients. In T. A. Stern, G. I. Friccione, N. H. Cassem, M. S. Jellinek, & J. F. Rosenbaum (Eds.), *Massachusetts General Hospital handbook of general hospital psychiatry* (5th ed.) (pp. 293–312). St. Louis: Mosby; Manos, P. J., & Braun J. (2006). *Care of the difficult patient.* New York: Routledge.

ETIOLOGY

According to *psychological* theory, manipulative patients do not trust other people to like or accept them, to be responsive to them, or to be responsible toward them. Consciously or unconsciously, they rely on manipulative behavior to demand that others supply what they need and want.

Manipulative behavior in health-care settings may reflect the patient's ongoing, habitual mode of interaction, or it may be an escalation of milder, more common control mechanisms. In the hospital setting, the patient may regress and have unrealistic expectations that his or her every need will be instantly gratified. Disappointment results in fury and an increase in manipulative behavior.

Chronic manipulative behavior may result from childhood dilemmas if parents undermined attempts toward independence and autonomy. Manipulative individuals have come to suspect that any person or institution may try to control them, rendering them powerless and vulnerable to attack. Even being cooperative can be viewed as giving in or being weak, negatively affecting self-esteem. Authority figures are seen as being stronger and having too much control over the patient's life. The patient may seek ways to equalize the power by controlling staff, not complying with medical regimen, and making excess demands. Suicidal gestures may be a frantic attempt to regain control or block painful feelings of helplessness or dependence. Fear of rejection and abandonment or expectation of increased responsibility are also triggers for self-destructive acts.

The *learning* theory of manipulative behavior focuses on the concept that the behavior may have been learned in childhood based on adult role models, peers, and even the media. The *family* theory suggests that manipulative behavior may have been developed, especially in younger years, as the only way to cope with a severely dysfunctional family.

Antisocial personality disorder frequently arises from a chaotic home environment with early parental deprivation. There may be some genetic link. Borderline disorder is associated with separation issues concerning parental figures. Brain dysfunction causing poor impulse control and mood instability have also been implicated in the etiology of borderline personality (NIMH, 2001). Personality disorders are generally associated with depression.

RELATED CLINICAL CONCERNS

These patients may rely on sedatives, analgesics, or other substances to reduce feelings of anxiety. These substances may trigger reduced inhibitions and increased aggressive responses. These patients are high users of inpatient services because of multiple crises (Shoemaker & Varcarolis, 2006). Borderline patients may use the hospital for multiple medical problems and results of self-destructive behaviors.

LIFE SPAN ISSUES

Children and Adolescents

Manipulative behavior begins in the earliest years, partly as a way to test the responses of parents and other caretakers. Toddlers have temper tantrums and quickly learn whether or not they can get their way. Children of all ages mimic the manipulative behavior of parents and siblings, such as making promises that are not kept. Or they may try getting permission from one parent after receiving a "no" from the other. They also learn from their peers. They may try to obtain privileges or possessions by saying that all their friends have these already.

Disturbed, maladaptive manipulative behaviors manifested in conduct disorders are seen in childhood and adolescence. Those who rely on deceitfulness can also display cruelty to animals or other children, destructiveness of property, and serious violations of rules. This can evolve into antisocial personality disorder in adulthood. These children may have experienced more severe deprivations such as multiple rejections, neglect, or abuse.

Adults

People who have successfully used manipulative behavior as children tend to become more proficient at this behavior as they grow older. They tend to flourish in systems where they are able to manipulate. People who are extremely manipulative and exploitative may violate laws and end up in the criminal justice system. Those who exhibit strong manipulative tendencies but are able to stay within legal confines may become successful in using people, personally and professionally, for their own goals.

POSSIBLE NURSES' REACTIONS

- May feel angry, frustrated, or resentful for being tricked; may have lowered self-esteem if unable to stop the manipulation; or may feel embarrassed or humiliated.
- May feel helpless in relieving patient's apparent distress or when attempting to get patient to conform to nurse's expectations of reasonable conduct.
- May feel vulnerable and afraid of patient's attacks.
- May take manipulations personally and react defensively, especially when challenged in authority or position.
- May reject patient because the experience of coping with personal reactions is too draining and demoralizing.
- May avoid patient, spend minimal time needed to provide physical nursing care, or assign a different nurse to the patient each day.
- May compensate by becoming overcontrolling or engage in power struggles with patient.
- May experience desire for revenge, retaliation; may become punitive, want to counterattack by insulting, hurting, or embarrassing patient. May secretly hope things go wrong for patient.
- May experience guilt about negative feelings toward patient.
- May become overinvolved or overattached and wish to rescue patient.
- May feel total responsibility for patient's improvement or lack of improvement.
- May be punitive in setting limits or confronting the patient or may be inconsistent or hesitant in enforcing rules for fear of patient's reaction.

Older Adults

As people age and become more dependent on others for assistance in activities or socialization, they may resort more frequently or aggressively to manipulative behaviors to get their needs met. If inducing guilt has been a personal trait, declarations such as "I don't want to be a burden" may be intended to stir guilt and get attention.

ASSESSMENT

Behavior and Appearance

- Frequent disregard of rules
- Argumentative
- Can be superficially charming and entertaining
- Demanding; the more staff try to cater to demands, the more they escalate
- Impulsive and unpredictable; lacks ability to tolerate frustration; can easily become out of control
- Uses threats to get demands met
- May use intimidation to control or feel superior
- Frustration causes more intense manipulative behavior
- Destructive toward self, others, property without taking responsibility
- Suicide threats and/or attempts
- Lies, cheats, steals
- Intense manipulation around medication; overuse of medication
- Noncompliant with health-care treatment
- Undermines treatment of other patients, such as encouraging them to ignore doctor's recommendations or suggesting alternate treatments

Mood and Emotions

- Anger predominates. Behavior can be cutting, sarcastic, and vicious.
- Anxiety rises rapidly to panic, which precipitates impulsive actions. May not experience anxiety unless facing a threat to self-image or self-esteem.
- Views self as very vulnerable and frightened, even when being intimidating, or as totally invulnerable to harm or negative consequences, resulting in reckless behavior.
- Has labile moods and emotions. The more patient is in crisis, the more frequently moods and emotions may fluctuate over the course of a day. May appear resistant to depression or may have periodic depressive reactions.
- May have inflated or diminished self-esteem. If inflated, denies or distorts information that would lower self-esteem.

Thoughts, Beliefs, and Perceptions

- Thinking can contain gross distortions of some specific events or people and yet maintain accurate perception and good reality of others.
- Projects own thoughts and feelings onto others, resulting in feelings of fear and manipulation by others.

Relationships and Interactions

- May seek or avoid attention
- Exploitative with little real concern for others; limited capacity for empathy; demonstrates caring only to get own needs met
- Quick to recognize vulnerable areas in others
- Limited ability to see others for who they really are; distorted perceptions of how others experience self
- Needs to feel either in control or helpless and vulnerable (Life is seen as a seesaw competition. If someone else is up, then patient feels down)
- Does not feel a sense of obligation to reciprocate favors or helpful acts
- Devalues others to feel good about self
- Sees others as attacking or dangerous
- Feels and acts as if he or she were entitled to having needs met without comparable effort or cost
- Becomes a "special patient" to the staff
- Blames others for mistakes and problems without taking personal responsibility; confuses taking responsibility with being blamed, worthless, and vulnerable to attack
- Belief of being superior; cannot admit lack of knowledge and has great difficulty asking for assistance and information; obtains information by using indirect manipulation; unable to accept suggestions or criticism

Physical Responses

- Physical complaints that cannot be substantiated with testing
- Magnifies any subjective symptoms that cannot be measured
- With documented disability, usually requires more frequent medication and higher dosages; recovery takes longer than usual

Pertinent History

- Erratic, impulsive behavior with marked instability; frequent changes in jobs, relationships, and physicians
- Drug or alcohol abuse
- Long history of many physical complaints

- Suicide threats and attempts
- Psychiatric diagnoses including major depression, borderline or antisocial personality disorder

COLLABORATIVE MANAGEMENT

Pharmacological

If the patient is given tranquilizers to reduce anxiety, there is a risk for drug dependence and power struggles (e.g., patient may try to manipulate the nurse to get extra doses). Individuals with personality disorders may benefit from antidepressants to address depression and reduce impulsive behaviors. Fluoxetine and olanzapine have been helpful in controlling rapid mood shifts. The anticonvulsant carbamezepine has been used to improve mood stability. Avoiding PRN medications can reduce power struggles with the nurse. Regular dosing schedules of analgesics if needed can be useful. Herbal products may be used as a way to self-medicate uncomfortable symptoms.

Multidisciplinary Team Communication

When staff members have extremely different experiences with the same patient, infighting among each other can occur when discussing care for the patient. These variations in experiences can occur between or among individuals in the nursing staff, different shifts, nurses and physicians, or all staff members and administrators. To overcome this staff splitting, the group needs to recognize the patient's dynamics and cooperatively share their different perceptions to gain a more complete picture of the patient. They need to identify whom the patient sees as "all good" or "all bad" and how this affects interactions.

Once the team has identified the problem behaviors, it is essential to formulate a united, consistent care plan. Each staff member should monitor the intensity of his or her individual reactions to the manipulative behavior. This will help to avoid becoming entrapped into feeling the need to be special or the only one who can help or avoid getting caught in power struggles. A supportive and coordinated multidisciplinary team approach helps neutralize the manipulative patient's ability to identify vulnerability in team members and discord in the health-care organization.

Psychotherapy

Psychotherapy represents the core treatment for borderline personality (Gunderson, 2001; Oldman, 2005). Dialectal behavior therapy (DLT) has been shown to have the best results for borderline patient with substance abuse (Oldman, 2005). Dialectal behavior therapy uses a multimodal approach of individual and group therapy as well as education. Other useful therapeutic approaches include family therapy, cognitive behavior therapy, and traditional psychotherapy.

NURSING MANAGEMENT

INEFFECTIVE COPING evidenced by noncompliance with rules and treatments related to impulsive, manipulative behavior.

Patient Outcomes

- Decreased use of maladaptive, manipulative behaviors
- Complies with treatment regimen and hospital rules
- Demonstrates use of effective coping patterns
- Demonstrates more adaptive methods of dealing with stress, such as using problem-solving skills

Interventions

- Carefully assess patient's mode of interaction and frequency over time before labeling behavior as "manipulative."
- Determine if the patient is using manipulation to indirectly express a need, anxiety, or distressful emotion. Active listening and empathetic responses to underlying issues can help diminish the patient's anxiety and need to control others.
- Approach patient in a calm and matter-of-fact manner, using a neutral tone of voice.
- Provide feedback to patient, who may not be aware that manipulative behaviors are being used. State specific observations about his or her style of interactions without arguing. If patient argues or denies, calmly repeat your observation without becoming defensive. Describe options and consequences. Follow through consistently with consequences.
- Don't state consequences that you do not have the authority to exercise.
- State which behaviors are not acceptable without personally rejecting the patient.
- Help patient identify when using manipulative behavior becomes an attempt to control anxiety. Encourage patient to identify triggers for anger and frustration.
- Encourage patient to verbalize feelings instead of acting them out. Ask the patient to identify what he or she is experiencing and what feelings and thoughts preceded the behavior.
- Evaluate whether patient's manipulative behavior increases or decreases when not reinforced by nurse's attention. Be aware that even when ignoring provocation is effective over time, there may be an initial escalation to test responses.
- Avoid power struggles and attempts to outmanipulate the patient. Point out that the patient is undermining his or her own care. State explicitly that the patient will not be forced to accept treatment and that each individual is responsible for the outcome of the treatment.

- Explain as early as possible rules and regulations and the reasons for them. If allowable limits are not stated, patient may push and test until they are clarified. If he or she attempts to break the rules, review firmly the stated expectations.
- Include the patient in decisions about limits and provide opportunities for personal decision making to enhance sense of control. When all rules are rigid, the patient may feel a greater need to rebel. Be careful not to allow patient to dictate nursing decisions.
- Written contracts defining both staff and patient expectations can be most effective. Specifically define any consequences of patient's continued manipulation and lack of cooperation. Nurse and patient can sign contracts.
- Describe in detail on the care plan the limits set and the consequences of breaking them. In periodic staff meetings and multidisciplinary case conferences, give current information and promote agreement about the patient, which will enable staff members to work more consistently and cohesively.
- Make sure all staff members are aware of limits and consequences. Confront colleagues who are observed not following the treatment plan.
- Consult with physician when patient seems to exaggerate complaints of pain or becomes preoccupied with timing of medications. The physician may decide to convert a PRN order to low doses of regularly administered medications to avoid power struggles.
- Assess for signs of substance abuse or withdrawal if patient has such a history or shows symptoms.

IMPAIRED SOCIAL INTERACTION evidenced by attempts to undermine, control and influence, and cause conflict related to splitting, distorted perceptions of others, impulsivity, and anxiety.

Patient Outcomes

- Uses acceptable methods to interact with others to communicate and obtain needs
- Positively responds to confrontation and limit setting
- Demonstrates tolerance of frustration and waiting
- Does not reject or denigrate the staff as "bad" when they are unable to respond in desired manner
- Demonstrates more trust in relationship with at least one staff member by sharing personal thoughts and feelings

Interventions

- Maintain assertive, centered, firm but fair, and even-toned stance when patient tries to manipulate or undermine you.

- Tell the patient that he or she may understand events and interactions differently than the staff does.
- Direct patient who complains about staff member to discuss the problem with implicated staff person. Do not allow yourself to be used as an intermediary; do not take sides.
- Use "I" statements indicating how patient made you feel. Avoid becoming defensive, which can escalate manipulative behavior.
- Confront the patient with your perception that he or she is trying to put you down. This can have an impact even if patient denies it.
- Take time to think about effective responses and to diminish the intensity of your reactions if patient is trying to manipulate. Use stress reduction techniques.
- Role play or discuss situation with other staff, if necessary.
- Return to original topic if patient tries to divert topic to a personal attack.
- Be aware of patient interactions that can increase staff divisiveness by blaming, accusations, or comparisons. Monitor your own responses.
- Provide praise and reinforcement when patient communicates directly and openly about needs and concerns.
- Use kind but firm approach. Clarify that setting limits is constructive and caring rather than punitive.
- Establish from the beginning that you take all of the limits very seriously. More flexibility can be introduced later as the patient takes more responsibility.
- Find neutral actions and topics for conversation. This will help to present you as a person interested in the patient and not just a rule keeper.
- Be aware that patient may need to test limits repeatedly to see whether there are repercussions and to be reassured that the staff will follow through on the consequences.
- Let patient know immediately that threats or verbal abuse is unacceptable, that you expect these will never be repeated, and state the consequences of repeated abuses.
- Confront patient when he or she attempts to undermine other patients' treatment.
- Do not allow patient to manipulate, flatter, seduce, bargain, or intimidate staff into granting him or her special status. Do not accept gifts or favors or share personal information, especially about any current difficulties.
- Never agree to keep a secret with a patient. Remind patient that the entire health team needs to be aware of patient's concerns in order to offer the best care.
- Assess interactions with family. If patient uses same approaches with them, family members may need information on changing their response.

ALTERNATE NURSING DIAGNOSES

Anxiety
Coping, Defensive
Noncompliance
Powerlessness
Self-Esteem, Disturbed

WHEN TO CALL FOR HELP

- Threats or actions of physical harm to others or self, including suicidal threats or gestures
- Undermining own or other's health care and unresponsive to nursing interventions
- Repeated violation of agency rules
- Evidence of staff splitting
- Noncompliance, which jeopardizes patient's health status, such as refusing to take medications

WHO TO CALL FOR HELP

- Psychiatric Team
- Social Worker
- Manager
- Attending Physician
- Advanced Practice Nurse
- Critical Incident Team/Employee Assistance

PATIENT AND FAMILY EDUCATION

- Teach patient to ask directly for what he or she wants and needs in words, not actions. Teach problem-solving skills.
- Help patient recognize that his or her desires may not require immediate action and that he or she may not always get desired responses.
- Explain the consequences of manipulative behavior.
- If a patient will not take responsibility for own actions, explain how his or her behavior contributed to the unwanted response or consequences and that taking responsibility is not the same as being blamed.

- Teach patient that understanding of one's own behavior and developing improved interactions are the avenues for developing stable support networks.
- Involve family in patient education. The same skills used in working with the patient may be helpful for the family.
- Provide information for family members of individuals with personality disorders. Several websites provide information including www.mental-health-matters.com/borderline.html and nimh.nih.gov for patient information on borderline personality

CHARTING TIPS

- Describe specific manipulative behaviors objectively rather than just labeling the patient as manipulative.
- Develop a detailed treatment plan with interventions so that the team can respond consistently. Chart patient's responses to interventions. Update team care plan as needed.
- Document usage of PRN medication, reason for use, and patient's response.

COMMUNITY-BASED CARE

- Begin discharge planning as early as possible to decrease last-minute impulsive and inappropriate decisions the patient might make without consideration for consequences. When last-minute disruptions to the plan occur, maintain a consistent, clear approach on the plan that has been developed.
- Inform the family and patient together of patient's healthcare needs to reduce manipulative behavior with family.
- Inform referring agencies of patient's behavior, team care plan, and short-term treatment planning goals.
- If appropriate, make referrals for individual and group psychotherapy as well as substance abuse treatment if needed.

The Noncompliant Patient

Learning Objectives

- Identify factors that contribute to a patient's noncompliance with treatment plans.
- List the principles of adult education that contribute to effective patient education.

- Identify nursing interventions to reduce noncompliance in the patient whose cultural beliefs impede compliance.
- List some nursing staff reactions to the noncompliant patient.

Glossary

Compliance – *Patient's accurately following a prescribed regimen of treatment. Sometimes referred to as adherence.*

Ineffective management of therapeutic regimen – *A pattern of regulating and integrating into daily living a program for treatment of illness and the sequelae of illness that is unsatisfactory for meeting specific health goals.*

Noncompliance – *State in which an individual desires to comply but factors are present that deter adherence to health-related advice given by healthcare professionals. Sometimes referred to as nonadherence.*

*C*ompliance and *noncompliance* are terms that are used to describe patient behaviors in response to information they are given about their health care. Compliance usually requires some form of motivation, perception of vulnerability, and the belief that the recommendation will control or prevent an illness (Carpenito-Moyet, 2006). What makes a patient follow, change, or ignore health teaching is complex and may not always be related to the amount and quality of information provided. Nurses need to be aware that noncompliance is a symptom of an underlying problem and not the actual problem, and that labeling behavior as "noncompliant" can have negative connotations, such as blaming or criticizing a patient who is not following instructions. Once you have identified that the patient is not following the medical regimen, you need to investigate what barriers prevented the patient from following the recommendations. Carpenito-Moyet (2006) describes noncompliance as occurring when the patient is prevented from compliance due to factors like overly complex instructions, lack of understanding of instructions, and lack of funds to follow through with recommendations. If the patient makes an autonomous, educated decision not to follow recommendations, that behavior is not noncompliance as long as the individual understands the risks and benefits of not following the recommendations. Some educators prefer the term adherence rather than compliance.

The cost of noncompliance is greater than can actually be documented. Besides factors such as the cost of medications purchased but not taken or taken incorrectly, poor results of diagnostic tests caused by poor preparation, and more severe illness from not following recommended treatments, both patients and health-care providers can experience a great deal of frustration. Although not the only reason for noncompliance, inadequate or inappropriate patient education is among the most common.

When teaching adults, the nurse needs to incorporate principles of adult learning (Box 12–2). Adults have different learning needs than children do. Adults are goal oriented. The goals need to be clearly identified and attainable, and adult patients need to consistently be made aware of their progress toward their goal. Adults need to understand how the education will benefit them. Adults tend to learn better when they understand the rationale for what they are learning, apply what they learn immediately, and can compare what they are learning to knowledge from past experiences. Learning is inhibited when authoritarian teaching methods are used. Interpersonal relationships with teachers are important.

ETIOLOGY

Many factors can interfere with the patient not being receptive or not be able to receive or follow health information:

- *Denial:* This may be a conscious or unconscious method of believing that he or she is not sick. For example, by not checking blood sugars, the patient can block the diagnosis of diabetes from his or her mind.
- *Power struggles:* At times, the patient who feels a lack of control over his or her body uses noncompliance as a way to maintain some control over a sense of destiny or over health-care providers.
- *Counterdependence:* The patient could be concerned that following recommendations would increase dependency on others. Because dependency can enhance feelings of loss of identity, noncompliance becomes a statement of independence and individualism.
- *Loss of coping mechanisms:* Often, health teaching involves asking the patient to give up habits that are part of the person's usual coping strategies.

BOX 12–2
Adult Learning Principles

- Adults need to participate in the learning process. Avoid directive approach. Give them some control.
- Adults need to understand the purpose behind any information they receive.
- Adults learn more effectively if past experiences are integrated into the teaching.
- Put new information to immediate use.
- Give specific feedback to learner of progress made in learning process.
- Match medication format with learning style
- Barriers to learning are addressed

Source: Knowles, M. A. (1970). *The modern practice of adult education.* Englewood Cliffs, NJ: Prentice-Hall; Russell, S. S. (2006). An overview of adult-learning processes. *Urologic Nursing, 26(5),* 349–352.

For example, smoking, diet changes, or exercise may need to be altered or avoided. If the patient has not yet developed alternative coping mechanisms, the anxiety created by the loss of these habits may be overwhelming.

- *Conflict with self-image:* Noncompliance may be a method of self-protection against the threat of an altered body image, particularly in individuals whose health and activity are a source of pride. Taking medication or imposing limitations on activity may represent a threat to the individual's self-image.
- *Fatalistic viewpoint:* A patient may believe there is no point to following instructions because of the belief that nothing will change the outcome.
- *Hidden benefits of illness:* Some people may consciously or unconsciously perceive benefits from the sick role, such as attention, avoidance of responsibility, controlling the destiny of another, or maintaining stability in a rocky relationship.
- *Self-destructive behavior:* A patient could be consciously or unconsciously participating in a wish to die or hurt himself or herself, possibly reflecting depression or suicidal tendencies. It could represent behaviors associated with a serious personality disorder.
- *Psychiatric disorder:* Psychiatric illness or altered thought processes may make consistent compliance with a health routine impossible.
- *Family influence:* Family members may discourage or undermine compliance because they are using denial, lack the understanding of the treatment, or unconsciously need to maintain the patient in the sick role.
- *Lack of economic resources:* If the patient has insufficient funds or no insurance, he or she may need to decide between eating or feeding the family and buying needed medications.
- *Lack of social resources:* Lack of funds, fear of being dependent on others, or lack of social contacts may cause the patient to miss appointments because there is no transportation.
- *Unsatisfactory relationship with health-care team:* If the patient perceives the doctors or nurses as cold, uncaring, not knowledgeable, or authoritarian, he or she may resent or ignore instructions. This may stir up in the patient such issues as resentment of authority and feeling unrecognized as an individual. This patient may minimize or distort information given because of his or her emotional response. Long waits and uncomfortable waiting areas may also contribute to the poor relationship.
- *Lack of trust in information given:* Patient may not believe health information given because it has not proved useful in the past. Also, with the increase in media reporting of conflicting reports of studies, patients may think the information is not trustworthy enough to warrant a change in life-style.
- *Cultural beliefs:* Cultural or religious beliefs may influence the way the patient views his or her illness and the treatments that are acceptable. For instance, women in some cultures may not allow a male health-care provider to examine their breasts or a Jehovah's Witness may not accept a blood transfusion.

- *Inability to read or understand instructions:* Some patients may be too embarrassed to acknowledge that they cannot read English. This may apply to those who speak another language or even to those who do speak English. Literacy rates in the United States are dropping, so some patients who function well in society may not be able to read. Also, be aware that some patients will not admit that they do not understand language that is too technical or that contains too much jargon. To be understood by the majority, patient education materials should be written at the average reading level, which for most adults is the fifth to eighth grade level. Low health literacy contributes to higher rates of hospitalization and use of emergency services (Contillo, 2007). The Joint Commission for Accreditation of Healthcare Organizations (JCAHO) has addressed the unsafe care that is provided because patients do not understand medical jargon. They have developed recommendations for health-care organizations to improve communication and supported an educational campaign called Speak Up to encourage patient engagement in their health care (JCAHO, 2007).

- *Uncomfortable side effects:* Patients may not follow instructions because of real or perceived side effects, especially with medications. The patient may be less likely to report them if they are embarrassing, such as impotence or incontinence. In addition, incorrect beliefs such as fear of becoming dependent on medications may cause some patients not to take medications. Noncompliance can become part of a negative cycle because the patient feels embarrassed or guilty for not following through and then begins cancelling appointments to avoid health-care providers.

RELATED CLINICAL CONCERNS

When patients are dealing with an acute crisis, most of their energy will be focused on just coping with the situation at hand. They will not be able to concentrate on learning until the crisis has subsided or they have made adaptations to deal with the situation. During this time, instruction should involve only what is absolutely necessary. You will need to be prepared to repeat much of the information provided as the patient may not remember what he or she was told.

Any physical or mental problem that impairs cognition will also interfere with learning. Depression, hopelessness, social isolation, and cognitive difficulties may contribute to compliance when a serious health problem such as myocardial infarction is diagnosed (Rieckmann et al., 2006).

LIFE SPAN ISSUES

Children

Following a particular treatment plan can be difficult for ill children and their families. Medications may affect behavior, alertness, or school performance.

Incorporating a child's medical care into family life can create many stressors, contributing to noncompliance because the child may not be able to be responsible. It can be time consuming and difficult to administer. Working parents and single-parent families may not have the time to be able to supervise the child or take him or her for follow-up care. Because the child may not be able to communicate his or her needs, medical care can be difficult to monitor.

The presence of attention deficit hyperactivity disorder (ADHD) can contribute to discipline problems that make following recommendations very difficult. DSM-IV-TR (2000) lists a diagnosis of Oppositional Defiant disorder in children and teens. This diagnosis is found in 2% to 16% of children and is characterized by a recurrent pattern of negative, defiant, disobedient behavior that can contribute to noncompliance with health-care instructions.

Parents who refuse to give a child needed medical attention can have legal and ethical ramifications that could be interpreted as negligence or even abuse. Parental autonomy to make decisions for their child may be overridden in the courts if it is determined the child is placed at some risk. In these extreme situations, legal intervention would be required. Further assessment of parental motivation and religious and cultural beliefs that affect the care of the child needs to done before any further actions are taken.

Adolescents

Adolescents are particularly vulnerable to problems with compliance. Their attitude is often related to struggles with maintaining independence and rebelling against adult authority. In addition, any medical regimen that affects body image puts additional demands on the teenager. Also, because the adolescent does not want to appear different from his or her peer group, complying with instructions may be particularly difficult. For example, a diabetic adolescent who is eating lunch with friends may be fearful of exposing his or her dietary restrictions.

Older Adults

Noncompliance is an extremely important issue for elderly people, who experience more chronic illness than the general population. Chronic illnesses often require multiple medications and are often combined with over-the-counter drugs as well as complementary and alternative therapies. Some elderly persons see more than one specialist and have a variety of prescriptions from the physicians they see or may be given contradictory treatment advice. They may become easily confused. Decreased muscle mass and increased fat stores may make individuals more prone to drug side effects. The elderly patient may need more assistance and time to explain instructions. If living alone, the elderly patient may have limited support for encouragement or reminding. Hearing and vision deficits as well as limited manual dexterity caused by arthritis can present other problems. In addition, cognitive impairments including poor short-term memory may inhibit the patient's compliance by causing him or her to forget instructions or how many pills have already been taken.

POSSIBLE NURSES' REACTIONS

- May become angry or frustrated because the time spent with patient seemed fruitless.
- May criticize or judge patient who does not follow instructions.
- May feel that situation is hopeless and makes less effort to communicate with patient.
- May judge self as inadequate or incompetent when patient does not follow instructions.
- May feel responsible for patient's noncompliance. Nurse may have difficulty recognizing that ultimately the responsibility for health care belongs to the patient.

ASSESSMENT

Behavior and Appearance

- Does not follow rules or instructions, demonstrated by:
  - Refusing to take or change medications
  - Continuing unhealthy habits
  - Missing medical appointments
  - Altering medical regimen
  - Challenging the necessity or helpfulness of treatments
  - Leaving facility against medical advice
  - Arguing without constructive resolution
  - Indicating understanding or agreement with treatment plan and then not following through
  - Hiding inability to read or comprehend educational material

Mood and Emotions

- Anger
- Depression
- Resentment
- Irritability
- Anxiety

Thoughts, Beliefs, and Perceptions

- Religious or cultural beliefs in contradiction with compliance actions
- Believes health care should be obtained only when symptoms are blatant or impairing needed activity

- Suspicions concerning motivations of health-care professionals
- Lack of confidence in own abilities
- Denial of health-care needs
- Psychotic thought process or suicidal thoughts
- Belief that one cannot question health-care provider
- Low self-esteem and fear of acknowledging lack of understanding of instructions

Relationships and Interactions

- May avoid sharing information with others about medical regimen
- Tendency to manipulate or control others
- Family not providing needed support
- Inconsistent relationship with health-care team; at times may be very critical of them and other times more positive toward them
- Following instructions from only one particular nurse

Physical Responses

- Deterioration of health because of lack of compliance
- Blood or urine tests showing drug levels inconsistent with reported medication intake; discrepancies in other tests

Pertinent History

- Poor outcomes from previous medical treatment
- Poor relationships with past health-care providers
- Noncompliance in earlier health-care treatments
- Inability to read or write

COLLABORATIVE MANAGEMENT

Pharmacological

Noncompliance for medication regimen is a major health problem. Not following instructions for medications can contribute to safety problems including overdoses. Many side effects of drugs are caused by misunderstandings about how to take medication (Goldberg, 2006). Patients do not take medications for a variety of reasons including fear of side effects, lack of knowledge about the purpose of the drug, denial of the diagnosis, lack of money to pay for medications, and lack of support or reinforcement (Box 12–3).

BOX 12–3
Factors that Influence Medication Compliance

Factors that Increase Compliance:
- Client's perception that illness is severe and medication is needed
- Client's knowledge of illness and treatment
- Moderate level of anxiety (useful worrying)
- Continuity and length of relationship with caregiver
- Return of unpleasant symptoms immediately on stopping medication
- Caregiver optimism regarding use of medication
- Written instructions tailored to patient's reading level provided
- Family support
- Side effect management is addressed
- Patient has easy access to obtaining medications (pharmacy close by)
- Longer acting tablets used where possible to reduce frequency of taking pills
- Client receives positive reinforcement for taking medicaitons
- Self-monitoring tools/diaries are easy to maintain
- Patient obtains health information over the Internet that reinforces need for medication
- Simpler way to take medication provided or fewer number of tablets prescribed

Factors that Decrease Compliance:
- Numerous lifestyle changes required
- Uncomfortable side effects
- Lack of support for compliance
- Fear of independence and recovery
- Lack of immediate return of symptoms if medication is stopped
- Fear of drug dependence
- High-cost drugs or equipment required
- Long period when symptoms are controlled

Source: Adapted from Carpenito-Moyet, L. (2006). *Nursing diagnosis: Application to clinical practice* (11th ed). Philadelphia: Lippincott Williams & Wilkins; Falvo, D. R. (2004). *Effective patient education* (3rd ed.). Sudbury, MA: Jones and Bartlett.

Multidisciplinary Team Communication

To ensure the best chance for patient compliance, a team approach is essential. All health-care providers should be consulted to ensure a cohesive treatment plan and approach that the patient understands. This is a pivotal nursing responsibility because nurses coordinate most of the care provided, both in the hospital and in the home. Discrepancies in instructions from physicians, physical or occupational therapists, pharmacists, or other health-care providers need to be discussed so that the patient is not left to choose whose advice to follow. Understanding factors that may contribute to poor compliance must be communicated to all team members.

NURSING MANAGEMENT

NONCOMPLIANCE evidenced by failure to adhere to medical regimen, failure to keep appointments related to health beliefs, cultural influences, lack of understanding instructions.

Patient Outcomes

- Verbalizes beliefs that influence noncompliance
- Demonstrates adherence to treatment plan
- Expected therapeutic goals realized

Interventions

- Develop a trusting relationship with patient. Communicate interest and openness to patient's needs and beliefs.
- Assess the degree of noncompliance and the underlying reason for it. One common area of noncompliance is in using medications. Many prescriptions are never filled, or they are filled and never used. When seeing a patient in the hospital or in the home, always review the medications the patient has, how they are being taken, and the patient's understanding of why the drug is necessary. Check expiration dates, the name of the physician who ordered the drugs, and the instructions on the labels. Analyze whether the patient is taking more than one drug for the same reason, especially if they were ordered by different physicians. If necessary, encourage patient to bring in pill bottles to doctor appointments so pills can actually be counted.
- Encourage the patient to share beliefs or traditions that affect health care. Demonstrate to patient your interest in learning about these. Do not criticize or belittle these beliefs; rather, communicate your respect for them.
- Ask the patient to share rationale for avoiding the prescribed treatment. Resolve any misunderstanding the patient may have about the treatment, its side effects, or its potential outcome. Avoid insisting that the patient give up his or her beliefs. Never argue with the patient about the value of the beliefs. Instead, explain any negative outcomes that these beliefs may cause with his or her condition.
- In critical situations, the patient may need to be confronted more directly with life-threatening consequences of noncompliance (e.g., taking insulin).

- Enlist assistance of family, friends, caregivers, or, if beliefs are based in a particular culture, others with whom the patient may relate to, to explain the consequences of these actions on the patient's health status.
- Talk with family members about their beliefs about the patient's illness to determine their role in noncompliance.
- Obtain feedback from the patient to ensure that he or she understands the instructions given. Use an interpreter if needed.
- If appropriate, negotiate the best compromise with the patient. Have him or her commit to one or two areas in which he or she will comply rather than expecting the patient to give up all his or her beliefs completely.
- Identify one staff member who has the best relationship with patient to provide information.
- Recognize that it may be impossible to alter the patient's strong cultural or religious beliefs. Understand that in some cases, illness, or even death, may be more acceptable and a higher priority than giving up one's beliefs.
- Encourage patient to share factors that contribute to noncompliance. Ask the patient to explain the rationale for actions taken or not taken.
- Avoid using medical jargon or abbreviations that may confuse or intimidate. Encourage open communication so that the patient will tell you when he or she does not understand something.
- Have patient perform a return demonstration or verbalize his or her routine to determine patient's understanding and determine areas of noncompliance.
- Break down complex regimens into small steps.
- Assess whether other methods of teaching would be more appropriate, such as videos, Web sites, interactive tutorials on the computer, role-playing, pamphlets with more pictures, or pamphlets written at a lower reading level. Minimize any distractions during teaching sessions.
- Incorporate principles of adult learning in educating adult patients. For example, explain rationale, avoid lecturing or belittling the patient, involve patient in discussion, and allow patient to identify ways teaching can be incorporated into his or her lifestyle.

INEFFECTIVE MANAGEMENT OF THERAPEUTIC REGIMEN (INDIVIDUALS) evidenced by acceleration of illness symptoms or verbalized difficulty with regulating or integrating prescribed regimens related to complexity of therapeutic regimen or health care system.

Patient Outcomes

- Identifies factors that contribute to not following medical regimen
- Demonstrates adherence to treatment plan
- Expected therapeutic goals realized

Interventions

- Ensure that the patient is in the best physical and emotional state for learning to occur. Remember to repeat information that was previously given when the patient was dealing with the acute crisis. Avoid teaching if patient is in pain or has other discomforts.
- Take the time to talk with the patient about his or her understanding of the problem, why he or she is receiving this information, and what is expected to be the outcome.
- Demonstrate acceptance of the patient by use of eye contact and touch where appropriate. Take care to avoid critical comments about the patient's situation.
- Set realistic expectation with the patient.
- Assess role of family in patient's health-care regimen. Determine who provides care for patient at home, and determine the caregiver's role in the noncompliance. Observe caregiver's technique if appropriate, and provide information as needed.
- Determine patient's understanding of using the health-care system. Review ways to get appointments, arrange additional care such as home care, and how to contact health-care providers. As needed, check with social service agencies to provide needed transportation, equipment, or other services.
- Help identify ways in which patient can individualize information. For example, if a patient works rotating shifts or travels extensively, you will need to focus your teaching on how to adapt the treatment plan to best fit into his or her lifestyle.
- Identify ways to reinforce patient's self-esteem and sense of competency. Provide positive reinforcement and recognition of patient improvement.
- Incorporate rewards as part of the teaching. For an adult, rewards may include those activities that increase self-esteem and a sense of control.
- Be sensitive to signs that the patient is tired or is losing interest. Reschedule teaching for another time.

INEFFECTIVE COPING evidenced by not doing, partially doing, or revamping treatment plan related to anxiety about illness, inadequate coping mechanisms.

Patient Outcomes

- Verbalizes anxieties and concerns
- Verbalizes acceptance and commitment to the treatment plan
- Demonstrates adherence to health-care regimen
- Expected therapeutic goals realized

Interventions

- Encourage the patient to discuss worries and concerns regarding the illness. Determine patient's understanding of the illness, prognosis, and treatment plan. If patient's understanding is not accurate, review the appropriate information about the condition with him or her.

- Encourage the patient to express feelings verbally rather than act them out through noncompliance.

- Repeat and reinforce teaching. The patient's learning ability may be impaired by anxiety or physical status.

- Give patient some control in treatment regimen. Seek his or her ideas for adaptations that can be made. Identify other areas in patient's life where he or she can exert control. Consider negotiating a contract with the patient to reinforce compliance.

- For the patient who is impatient and perfectionistic, point out the need to develop realistic expectations of behavior changes. For example, he or she may not be able to lose weight and give up smoking at the same time.

- Approach the suspicious patient with the expectation of compliance. Keep directions clear and simple, and always be honest.

- Make an effort to reduce the patient's anxiety before teaching session.

- Reinforce the idea that the patient is ultimately responsible for his or her own health.

- If major life changes must be made, break down expected changes into achievable steps that may be easier to accept and master. Develop a way patient can chart own progress.

- If patient has relapsed, provide encouragement to start again and point out positive steps that were achieved despite the setback.

- Continually assess emotional blocks.

ALTERNATE NURSING DIAGNOSES

Anxiety

Decisional Conflict

Knowledge Deficient

Powerlessness

Self-Care Deficit

Therapeutic Regimen Management, Ineffective: Families

Thought Processes, Disturbed

WHEN TO CALL FOR HELP

- Patient refuses to comply with medical regimen, with life-threatening implications.
- Family or caregiver abuses patient or interferes with patient's compliance.
- Patient uses folk remedies or alternative health practices that complicate current medical condition.
- There is evidence of suicidal or psychotic thinking as reason for noncompliance.
- There is increased staff conflict over dealing with patient's noncompliance.

WHO TO CALL FOR HELP

- Attending physician
- Manager
- Psychiatric Team
- Social Worker
- Educators, Advanced Practice Nurses

PATIENT AND FAMILY EDUCATION

- Determine appropriate materials available to assist in patient education including pamphlets, videos, closed-circuit health education channels in the hospital, or flip charts.
- Determine if appropriate educational materials are available from pharmaceutical and medical equipment companies. Many times, they have excellent materials available at no charge.
- Identify appropriate times to provide education to patient and family. Realize that at times, the patient may not be ready for teaching when the nurse is available. Other alternatives need to be identified.
- Provide information in patient's primary language if possible.
- Before starting an education session, ensure that the patient and family have needed tools to enhance comprehension including glasses, hearing aids, and pain controlled. Patients may be too embarrassed or intimidated to tell you that they need these items.
- Identify other resources, such as diabetes educators, ostomy nurses, pharmacists, or dieticians, to assist in teaching. Be sure to coordinate teaching so that no conflicting information is given.
- Use appropriate adult learning principles for all education (see Box 12–2).

- To promote compliance with prescribed medications educate the patient and family on: potential side effects, what to do if a dose of medication is missed, where to call if concerned about a negative reaction to a drug, keeping of diary of medications taken, and utilization of a pill box.
- If patient and family are using the Internet for health-care information, give information on identifying reputable sites. Encourage patient and family to bring information they are obtaining on the Internet to medical appointments so it can be evaluated. See Box 12–4 for Tips on Teaching Patients About Health Internet Sites. Many sites offer information in several languages as well.

CHARTING TIPS

- Document all identified factors that contribute to noncompliance.
- Use objective, nonjudgmental terms to describe behavior.
- Document the teaching plan and patient goals to ensure that all health-care team members are providing the same information.
- Document all teaching given and patient and family response to the education.
- Document patient's verbalized reason for and effects of noncompliance.

BOX 12–4
Teaching Patients About Health Internet Sites

- Look for sites that are affiliated with a university or professional health-care organization to have more credibility (may include web sites ending in .edu or .org). Many professional and governmental Web sites have specific information written for the layman in easy to understand language, such as healthyminds.org (American Psychiatric Association), National Institutes of Health. Websites ending in .com are generally supported by for profit companies that may influence content.
- Looks for credentials, educational backgrounds, and board certification of those providing the information
- View any site with skepticism where sweeping claims of health or cure are promised
- Check for the date of the posting
- Check for commercial sponsorship of the site–this may influence the information
- Bring copies of website materials to your health-care provider to review and discuss
- Online chat rooms and blogs can provide support but can also expose a person to misinformation

COMMUNITY-BASED CARE

- Refer the patient for home health follow-up to evaluate home situation and its influence on compliance. Inform home health nurses of concerns regarding patient's compliance and any effective or ineffective strategies you have used.
- Identify practical issues that inhibit compliance such as lack of transportation, funds, or insurance. Then seek potential resources for assistance. Involve social worker, case manager, or community resources advisor for assistance.
- Refer to support groups, community education programs, or volunteer support programs, such as Reach for Recovery, or ostomy visitors. These people may provide needed reinforcement or role models for motivation and support. Online chat rooms and blogs can also provide support.
- Ensure that the patient and caregivers have adequate information for follow-up appointments and future treatment and that they have needed phone numbers and resources to call for more assistance.
- Refer patient for follow-up counseling if persistent noncompliance is related to inadequate coping skills or psychiatric disorder.

The Demanding, Dependent Patient

___ Learning Objectives ___

- List the possible causes of underlying anxieties that could escalate a patient's demanding, dependent behavior.
- Select effective interventions for a patient who consistently needs to be the center of attention.
- Identify possible nurses' reactions toward demanding, dependent patients.

Glossary

Dependent personality disorder – *Behavior characterized by a pervasive and excessive need to be taken care of, leading to: submissive and clinging behaviors; fears of separations; a severe lack of self-confidence; difficulty making everyday decisions; difficulty expressing disagreement.*

Entitlement – *An unreasonable expectation that others will provide especially favorable treatment and automatic compliance.*

(Healthy) narcissism – *An adequate amount of self-love, acquired during early childhood, providing a healthy self-esteem without negating the needs of others.*

Hidden dependency – *Dependent behavior that is not obvious. Person may try to coerce others into behaving in ways that meet his or her needs.*

Histrionic personality disorder – *Behavior characterized by pervasive and excessive expression of emotion and attention-seeking behavior.*

Interdependence – *Having the capability for a normal balance between dependent and independent behaviors.*

Narcissistic personality disorder – *Behavior characterized by a pervasive pattern of an inflated sense of self-importance, need for admiration, and lack of empathy for others.*

Regression – *An individual's response to overwhelming anxiety by moving back to a much earlier, more comforting phase of childhood.*

Both demanding and dependent patients can consume an enormous amount of nursing resources. When patients exhibit these behaviors, it is essential to identify the problems early so that efforts are not counterproductive and resources are not drained (Manos & Braun, 2006). Very dependent patients can stir up resentment in caregivers, and that inhibits the setting of limits (Groves, 2004). Setting baseline behavior goals help the patient contain or deal with his or her needs to a tolerable degree for both the staff and the patient and prevent dysfunctional behavior from interfering with the planned healthcare regime. Demonstrating a healthy narcissism is seen when an individual speaks up for him/herself and displays self-care behaviors.

The *demanding* patient consistently wants more than the nurse can or should give and asks for more than is reasonable. A request is usually expressed as an emergency, with absolute insistence that it is a legitimate, rightful claim. The *dependent* patient wants to be taken care of in more ways than is normal for an adult. Unable to function independently or with self-reliance, this individual has a sense of helplessness and powerlessness and either actively or passively expects others to take responsibility to meet his or her needs, make personal decisions, and provide support. Traits of dependency are found in many patients with psychiatric disorders (Sadock & Sadock, 2007).

When a person is hospitalized, a dependent relationship occurs because basic rules of living, such as when to eat, are set by others. An adult with healthy coping mechanisms can usually adjust to this dependency role appropriately. However, the response is not so predictable in individuals who have consistently learned to use maladaptive coping mechanisms throughout their lives or in those whose situational stress have exhausted their normal coping abilities. When the patient deviates too much from commonly expected behaviors, misunderstandings and battles can be generated between the patient and staff. Maladaptive responses can include growing resentment at feeling so helpless, regression to a clinging neediness more characteristic of earlier years in life, fighting and refusing to follow rules, covert expressions of the need to be cared for with an overemphasis on physical symptoms, or relentless demands for affection.

Patients with certain types of personality disorders, particularly dependent, narcissistic, or histrionic types, normally exhibit a relentless demand for attention, and need to be dependent on others. Criteria for each of these personality disorders are listed in DSM-IV-TR (2000). These individuals believe that their views are correct and that others must adapt to them. Because these behaviors are long-standing, they are very resistant to change. Additionally, the stress of illness and hospitalization can cause other individuals who normally function without the need to be demanding and dependent to exhibit these behaviors. This may occur when there is a growing resentment at being helpless or when normal coping mechanisms have been exhausted. This behavior can also be a normal temporary response in an individual faced with adjusting to a chronic condition, such as quadriplegia. An individual may express his or her intolerance for the dependent role by fighting, refusing to follow rules and meet expectations, or by overemphasizing physical symptoms. Patients with dependent personality disorder tend to get others to assume responsibility for major areas of their lives and experience intense anxiety when alone (Sadock & Sadock, 2007).

ETIOLOGY

Psychological theories examine early developmental experiences that inhibit successful independence contributing to demanding or dependent adult behavior and may even result in a personality disorder. For instance, a child may learn that to be heard and acknowledged, he or she must persist in making demands on parental attention. Both inadequately met needs and overindulgence during the first 18 months of life can discourage independence. If the child was not allowed to ask directly for what is needed, he or she may learn to get needs met by having physical symptoms, particularly if extra attention is received only during early bouts of illness, when physical care provided the only expressions of support and nurturing. If the child assumed the caretaker role for an ill parent, he or she may view illness as the main vehicle for obtaining care and assistance.

Patients who feel unloved and worthless or who are afraid to be alone may make frequent requests for the nurse to do things in an attempt to get attention. With attention given, the patient's anxiety decreases, and he or she becomes less demanding.

In hidden dependency, the patient can be very controlling, intimidating, dominating, or possibly even an overly caring caretaker. The patient does not seem obviously dependent but attempts to coerce others to behave in ways designed to meet his or her needs.

Patients with chronic personality disorders have a limited repertoire of coping skills and can respond to anxiety by becoming more dependent and demanding, regardless of whether such behavior is appropriate to the situation. These are also associated with low self-esteem and depression. Contributing factors include demanding, perfectionistic parents and parents living vicariously through their children.

RELATED CLINICAL CONCERNS

Independent decision making and initiative taking can be adversely affected by dementia, depression, hearing and other sensory problems, and limited intellectual abilities. Dependent individuals may use drugs as a method of coping with intolerable feelings of anxiety and helplessness, which can lead to a pattern of substance dependency.

LIFE SPAN ISSUES

Children

Infants are expected to be totally dependent. Younger children are still expected to be dependent in the areas in which they have not yet matured to the point of being able to do things for themselves. As children grow older and physical, psychological, cognitive, and social spheres develop, they are expected to do age-appropriate tasks, make decisions, interact, and exhibit independent behaviors. Children who must be more dependent because of illness or disabilities may have more struggles with these issues.

Adolescents

The struggle with dependence and independence is the hallmark of adolescence. At times teenagers are children and at other times they act like adults. They can have an inflated sense of self and self-importance, with little empathy for others as a natural part of trying to form their own identities; however, this does not mean that they will develop a personality disorder. People in this age group may be influenced more by their peers, who are supports against the pressures of the adult world and its expectations. They often become dependent on peers for recognition and gratification. Parents can become confused by the frequent vacillation between responsible behavior and childlike dependency, especially in earlier adolescent years.

Adults

Dependency can be manifested in fears of leaving the home of origin, difficulties maintaining jobs, and remaining financially dependent on parents. Brief periods of dependency during times of stress can be normal.

Older Adults

As individuals age, they may experience an accompanying increased dependence based on losses in agility, speed, or strength. Some elderly people face illnesses along with the loss of previous support systems. Old friends and relatives may die or become preoccupied with their own growing limitations. Elderly persons who are treated as children incapable of making independent decisions and behavior may eventually respond with dependent and demanding behaviors. However as people age and experience increased frailty, they may need to begin accepting more dependency and assistance from others.

For an older individual with a narcissistic personality disorder, adjusting to physical and occupational limitations can be particularly difficult, often straining family relationships.

POSSIBLE NURSES' REACTIONS

- Nurses have different tolerance levels for demanding, dependent behaviors. Patient may be considered difficult by one nurse but not by another. The extremes of these behaviors are usually considered difficult by all.
- May experience frustration and anger with the constant demands.
- Resentful when patients appear to demonstrate sense of entitlement
- May expect thanks or reward for meeting patient's needs.
- May feel guilty about not meeting all the patient's stated needs and question own competence. May try to avoid the patient.
- May not recognize that giving too much to patients who can do things for themselves is detrimental to the patients' emotional and physical health.
- May confuse appropriate limit setting with being overly harsh and withholding.
- May be punitive or hesitate to be firm with patients because of anger and fear about being punitive. It may also seem easier just to give in to the patient's demands.
- Nurses with strong dependency needs or who are inexperienced may initially overidentify with patients and try to meet all of their demands. May resent giving so much and not being appreciated.

ASSESSMENT

Behavior and Appearance

- Intrudes into personal space and time of others
- Unkempt appearance, either actual inability to provide self-care or an unconscious attempt to get others to provide care
- Demanding assistance although able to do things for self
- Manipulative behavior, such as:
  - Arguing or begging
  - Crying, clinging
  - Calling nurse "mean," "hardhearted," "a bad person," "incompetent"
  - Dwelling on health problems and medical history

- Complaining of feeling used and victimized by others
- Constantly seeking attention, suggestions from others
- Disregard of facility rules
- Regression; wanting to be totally taken care of, fed, repeatedly reassured, or comforted
- Frequent use of call lights
- Repeated visits to nurses' station
- Demands to have physician called several times each day
- Use of family visits to demonstrate helplessness; getting relatives to make demands on staff
- Sense of entitlement

Mood and Emotions

- Frequently angry; may be expressed in passive-aggressive behavior
- Fears being alone or abandoned
- Anxiety

Thoughts, Beliefs, and Perceptions

- Believes that each request is an actual problem requiring instant attention
- Low self-esteem with chronic feeling of helplessness and inadequacy
- Resistant to interpretations that point out reason for behavior (may experience this as an attack)

Relationships and Interactions

- Self-absorbed, with little interest in others' concerns or problems
- Frequently clings to others
- Sometimes nagging
- Fights or reverses roles and becomes a helper to others if unable to tolerate or acknowledge own dependency needs
- Dependent relationships with significant others (SOs), in which other person makes all decisions, answers for patient
- Others dislike caring for or being with patient for long periods

Physical Responses

- Overconcern about health and preoccupied with symptoms
- Frequent requests for and preoccupied with medications, especially for pain or anxiety
- Adverse drug interactions if prescriptions taken from several different doctors who are not aware of each other's involvement

Pertinent History

- Long history of medical problems, some of which linger atypically for an unusually long time or do not quite match patterns of usually diagnosed diseases; does not respond to usual treatments
- Goes from one doctor to another in search for diagnosis and treatment for complaints that show no physical basis
- Multiple hospitalizations
- Unnecessary surgery
- Diagnosed in the past with histrionic, narcissistic or dependent personality disorder

COLLABORATIVE MANAGEMENT

Pharmacological

Multiple medications, perhaps from different prescribers, can generate a host of problematic adverse effects. Psychiatric medicines may also be used. A tendency for dependency may lead to increased risk for dependency on medications. Confusion and lethargy in elderly patients, which can lead to more dependent behavior, can be caused by overmedicating or too many types of medications. A pharmacological review can be helpful in these instances. Antidepressants can be used for depressive symptoms. Anxiolytics for anxiety and panic attacks may be used.

NURSING MANAGEMENT

POWERLESSNESS evidenced by demanding, dependent behaviors related to anxieties generated by illness, disability, and/or hospitalization.

Patient Outcomes

- Displays less demanding, dependent behavior and conveys needs more directly and appropriately
- Provides increased amount of self-care as physical condition permits
- No longer exaggerates physical complaints to gain attention, support, and concern

Interventions

- Assess baseline:
  - Consult with family or significant other to determine if behaviors are normal for the person.
  - Evaluate if the patient is demanding in all situations or only in specific ones and if he or she exhibits this behavior only with certain people.

- Identify the specific behaviors the patient uses to express dependency.
- Determine whether the patient's helplessness is consistent with his or her medical problem or if patient is more independent when not in view of others.

• State limits and rules in advance. Discourage unnecessary or excessive time spent at the nurses' station. Discourage asking for nurses' assistance when the patient is aware that the nurse is on break, at lunch, or leaving at the end of the shift.

• Assess the required amount of assistance the patient needs and provide help when it is needed. Diplomatically point out unreasonable demands: "We're concerned about your overall well-being. In our experience, patients feel more effective and better about themselves when they do as much as they can. Let's discuss what you're realistically able to do right now and what the nurses need to provide."

• Make an extra effort to communicate concern:

- Demonstrate active listening. Sit down rather than stand up during the talk. Repeat statements or reflect feeling being expressed, as necessary.
- Be consistent. If you have told the patient that you will speak with him or her at a specific time and are unable to do so, explain reasons and reschedule.
- Give feedback to demonstrate that you understand what patient is asking for, feels, or needs. Encourage patient to describe his or her fears and anger over the loss of control.

• Explain that identifying each situation as an emergency makes it difficult to determine what is an actual emergency.

• Determine if the patient has had previous bad experiences with health-care providers or institutions. He or she may need reassurance that proper treatment is being given.

• Give support and reassurance to allay fears when first attempting behaviors that will lead to more independence. Assure the patient that you will be available if needed.

• Help patient to distinguish between feeling helpless and being helpless. Provide a progress list of at least one new activity per day, however small, that he or she can do independently.

• Encourage the patient to identify and verbalize real sources of anger. Ask how he or she usually handles anger. Suggest ways to redirect anger into positive activities.

• Encourage patient to make independent choices. Accept different preferences and opinions.

• Do not take an overly directive approach because it can reinforce dependency.

- Identify and point out patient's strengths; provide praise whenever used.
- Determine whether some of the patient's expressed needs are better met by other professionals.

INEFFECTIVE COPING evidenced by demanding, dependent behavior related to continuous and ongoing personality disturbance that hinders ability to do health-care tasks effectively and communicate concerns appropriately.

Patient Outcomes

- Uses less dependent behavior with fewer unnecessary demands for nurses' attention
- Uses appropriate methods to gain attention and support
- Verbalizes appropriate degree of health concerns
- Makes informed choices
- Initiates and carries through tasks

Interventions

- Obtain history from patient and significant others to determine patient's baseline style of interaction before illness or hospitalization. Those who have displayed demanding and dependent behaviors as a lifelong pattern may present more complexities.
- Be aware that patients who have long-standing, ingrained, demanding, dependent patterns will be resistant to change. Be patient and explain limit setting as often as needed.
- Determine realistic expectations for behavioral changes and expect that any changes will occur in small gradual steps.
- If the patient becomes upset because you are not presently able to spend time with him or her, determine a convenient time and provide assurances that patient will have your undivided attention.
- Assess whether the patient is inappropriately using other health-care workers or volunteers or is interacting inappropriately with visitors or other patients.
- Do not personalize remarks made by patients who need to feel superior. If the patient wants to speak only with the charge nurse or doctor, let those individuals explain the limits of their availability.
- Be aware when patients are using seductive behaviors to gain attention, control, or unnecessary assistance. Mild behaviors can be ignored to discourage future use. Persistent behaviors need firm confrontation.
- Assess for the use of manipulative behaviors to gain attention or dependence. Encourage methods to increase self-esteem that can decrease the patient's need for approval from others.

- Analyze behaviors to determine what needs the patient may be expressing when he or she asks the staff to perform tasks that could easily be done independently.
- Point out to the patient ways in which he or she has control of some situations.
- Assess the cause of a problem with independent decision making. If it is caused by a lack of information, provide all the information you can. If the patient always has difficulty making decisions, teach effective problem-solving skills.
- Recognize your own tolerance for demanding, dependent behavior. Ask for assistance or temporary reprieve if necessary. For extremely dependent patients, strive for a balance between rotating staff to help decrease dependency on one nurse and providing consistent nursing care.
- Be especially diplomatic in correcting patient's behavior. Narcissistic patients may react to criticism or defeat with rage, disdain, or counterattack. If this occurs, help the patient regain a perspective on feedback and response.
- Maintain your own perspective when receiving praise from dependent or histrionic patients as well as the devaluing or ignoring of your efforts and contributions by more narcissistic patients, who tend to take all the credit.
- Praise independent and interdependent functioning. Reassure the patient that he or she will not be forgotten nor abandoned by the staff when more independent. Reward less demanding behavior by spending more time with the patient.

ALTERNATE NURSING DIAGNOSES

Anxiety
Decisional Conflict
Self-Care Deficit
Self-Esteem Disturbed
Social Interaction, Impaired

WHEN TO CALL FOR HELP

- When the patient is "burning out" staff with insatiable, unreasonable requests
- When the patient's demands or needs for assistance become so unrealistically prolonged that it impairs staff's ability to adequately care for other patients
- When the patient is not getting good medical care because of staff anger
- If the patient seems resistant to all interventions attempted

WHO TO CALL FOR HELP

- Critical Incident/Employee Assistance
- Psychiatric Team
- Attending Physician
- Manager
- Social Worker

PATIENT AND FAMILY EDUCATION

- Teach decision-making skills, such as problem identification, listing possible solutions, considering possible outcomes of each, and evaluating each outcome. Teach the patient to draw upon past experience and intuition when making decisions. Point out potential stumbling blocks such as choices that lower self-esteem or violate values or goals. Caution the patient that there may not be a perfect solution. Teach the concept of collaborative decision making.
- Teach the patient to recognize personal strengths.
- Explain to the patient that in delegating personal decision making to another, one still must retain personal responsibility for one's own life. He or she will have to live with the consequences of the decision.
- Teach the patient to distinguish situations that require immediate attention from those that do not. Explain that identifying each situation as an emergency makes it difficult to determine what is an actual emergency.
- Teach the patient to identify which problems require assistance. Teach the patient to use frustration as an opportunity for problem solving.
- Teach relaxation techniques.
- Teach the family members to identify when they are promoting dependent behaviors and to examine alternatives. Teach approaches that the staff members have found effective.
- Teach the patient the difference between providing good nursing care and catering to excessive demands.

CHARTING TIPS

- Document specifics of demands and their frequency. Note if they occur at similar times or in relation to similar events.
- Document actual patient responses to specific interventions listed in the treatment plan. Avoid subjective opinions about the behaviors.
- Document frequency of requests for PRN medications.
- Document details of unusual physical complaints.

COMMUNITY-BASED CARE

- Anticipate increased dependency and demanding behavior as discharge from one level of care becomes imminent; reduce anxiety by discussing concerns as early as possible.
- Involve patient in discharge arrangements.
- Anticipate that discharge will probably be a difficult time if the patient will be going to a facility with different caretakers and less staff.
- If patient is going home assess what services patient will need at home and discuss arrangements with patient and family.
- Ensure that patient has specific plans for follow-up appointment with physician.
- Remind patient who is about to be transferred to another level of care to continue to use the methods learned for expressing needs.
- Discuss with the next caregivers the interventions that have been effective.
- If the patient's behavioral patterns continue to significantly impair health care and the patient is distressed about this, discuss the possibility of seeking psychotherapy.
- Communicate patient concerns and behaviors to referring agencies.

13

Problems with Substance Abuse

The Patient Abusing Alcohol

Learning Objectives

- Identify factors that contribute to the etiology of alcoholism.
- Formulate appropriate nursing interventions for patients experiencing problems with alcohol abuse.
- Describe common nurse's reactions to the patient abusing alcohol.
- Describe the characteristics of codependency.

Glossary

Alcohol intoxication – *Excessive alcohol use that leads to maladaptive behavior and at least one of the following: slurred speech, incoordination, unsteady gait, nystagmus, impairment in attention or memory, and stupor.*

Alcoholism – *A complex progressive disease characterized by significant physical, social, or mental impairment directly related to alcohol dependence and addiction.*

Binge drinking – *Pattern of periodic intervals of heavy use of alcohol (usually defined as five or more drinks on one occasion) with intervals of no or little use.*

Blackouts – *Lapses of memory resulting from persistent heavy drinking. During blackouts the person may appear to function normally while drinking but cannot recall events afterward.*

Codependency – *Maladaptive coping behaviors that prevent individuals from taking care of their own needs because they are preoccupied with the thoughts and feelings of another. Also known as "enabling behavior."*

Detoxification – *The process of withdrawal of alcohol from the body through supervised medical interventions to prevent complications.*

Dual diagnosis – *Diagnosis of both a substance dependency and a major psychiatric disorder. May also be called co-occurring or co-existing disorder.*

Korsakoff's syndrome – *Severe memory impairment related to thiamine deficiency from long-term alcohol use. Characterized by confabulation and inappropriate cheerfulness.*

Tolerance – *The need for increasing amounts of a substance to achieve desired effect.*

Alcohol remains the most used and misused drug in America. Alcohol use is socially accepted throughout our culture, is included as part of celebrations, religious rituals, and social occasions, and is often used as a relaxant. Nearly 90% of all American adults have used alcohol at some time in their life (DSM-IV-TR, 2000).

The move from social use of alcohol to alcoholism can occur very quickly in some people and over many years in others. In the past, alcoholism was viewed as a defective character trait, a weakness, or a moral flaw. Since the 1950s, it has been realized that alcoholism is a complex disease that responds to proper treatment. Today, the role of brain dysfunction is viewed as key to etiology.

Studies indicate that about 8% of Americans are dependent on alcohol at any one time and 18% report an alcohol problem at some time in their lives (Kessler, et al, 2005). This includes daily or binge drinking that negatively affects the way one lives. Binge drinking is more common in young adults. Three times as many men as women are reported to have a drinking problem; however, it is suggested that women are more secretive in their drinking behaviors, and therefore, drinking by women may be underreported. Alcohol is often used along with other substances, especially in younger individuals, often to alleviate or enhance the effects of other drugs (e.g., to relax after using a stimulant). Heavy drinkers often have periods of enforced abstinence to try to control the problem.

Alcohol is a central nervous system depressant that produces mind-altering and mood-altering effects. Twenty percent of alcohol consumed is absorbed directly into the bloodstream through the stomach. The remainder moves through the digestive system and is absorbed more slowly. Drinking rapidly on an empty stomach or consuming drinks with higher alcohol content will lead to a more rapid rise in blood alcohol level. One ounce of distilled liquor, 5 ounces of wine, and 12 ounces of beer have equivalent amounts of alcohol. It is known that, given the same amount of alcohol, women have higher blood alcohol concentrations than men, even when size is taken into consideration. This is because of differences in fat and body water content, making women more prone to long-term effects of alcohol. Problem drinking is identified by the National Institute of Alcohol Abuse and Alcoholism (2007) for men as having more than four drinks/day or greater than 14 drinks per week and in women and older men as greater than three drinks per day or more than seven drinks per week.

Alcoholism has a tremendous impact on the individual, the family, and society. Spouses and especially children are particularly vulnerable to become victims of alcohol-related abuse. They may experience violence or emotional and physical neglect, and they may blame themselves for the alcoholic's abusive state. Amazingly, 43% of U.S. adults have been exposed to alcoholism through a spouse or blood relative. Alcoholism is truly a family crisis (National Council on Alcoholism and Drug Dependence, 2002). The impact of alcohol abuse on society includes crime, traffic accidents and fatalities, suicide, industrial accidents, fires, and decreased workplace productivity.

People with major psychiatric disorders may also have an abuse problem if they use alcohol to self-medicate for the psychiatric symptoms. The co-occurrence of a psychiatric diagnosis with alcohol or other substance abuse is very common in the mentally ill population. These patients are referred to as having a dual diagnosis or co-occurring disorder. These patients may use alcohol and other substances to self-medicate the distressing psychiatric symptoms of agitation, anxiety, or hallucinations. Alcohol or abuse of other substances may also trigger a psychotic episode leading to a dual diagnosis. Nearly half of all people with severe mental illness are affected by substance abuse, and 37% of alcoholics have at least one mental illness (NAMI, 2003). Goldsmith and Garlapati (2004) report that 47% of schizophrenics, 56% of bipolar patients, and 27% of patients with major depression have a dual diagnosis. The most common psychiatric diagnoses associated with substance abuse are mood and anxiety disorders, attention deficit disorders, and antisocial personality disorders (Miller & Grady, 2004). Patients with co-occurring disorders tend to have poorer outcomes with treatment of both diagnoses. Acute intoxication or withdrawal from alcohol and/or other substances can complicate accurate diagnosis of a primary psychiatric disorder. These patients require interventions specially geared to this population as they often do not fit in standard substance abuse treatment as Alcoholics Anonymous. Collaboration between the psychiatric treatment team and addiction specialists is essential.

ETIOLOGY

Because alcoholism runs in families, there is current support for the *genetic* and *biological* theories as the cause of alcoholism. Alcoholism runs in families with a four-fold increase in close relatives of the alcoholic (Schuckit, 2006). The risk remains even if the children are not raised in the same home as the alcoholic parent.

The current biological theory for abuse of alcohol and other substances is that intrinsic reward pathways in the brain create a biological basis for craving the substance that induces a sense of well-being. The two main pathways are glutamatergic tracts in the prefrontal cortex and dopaminergic tracts. Each time a drink is taken for persons with altered brain function, an intense state of craving for the substance develops. This theory is the basis for the two pharmacological treatments of alcohol abuse: replacement therapy and neuromodulation. Replacement therapy substitutes the abused chemical with a safer alternative as in detoxification. Neuromodulators interact with the receptor system affected by the substance and eventually decrease the craving (e.g., Naltrexone or Acamprosate for alcohol).

A number of *psychological* factors are recognized as contributing to alcohol abuse. One of the most important looks at the link between depression and alcoholism. Alcoholics may have a higher incidence of depression and low self-esteem. Alcohol becomes a way to relieve those feelings. Each time a drink makes the person feel better, it reinforces this behavior. Difficulty managing anxiety and low self-esteem has led to identification of common coping styles (Table 13–1). Denial is the major defense mechanism used when the person is unable to acknowledge the role that alcohol plays in his or her life.

Alcohol use can severely affect the dynamics of the family relationship. Family members use protective behaviors, sometimes called codependent or enabling behaviors, to control or hide the alcoholic's behavior so that a sense of normalcy can be maintained. Affected family members care for and attempt to control the behavior of the alcoholic at the expense of their own needs. The family does not realize that this type of behavior reinforces the drinking patterns and dysfunctional behavior. Examples of these behaviors include minimizing the drinking, finding excuses for the drinker's alcohol use, attempting to control the drinking by diluting bottles or pouring out liquor, covering up for the drinker's unacceptable behavior, and self-blame for the drinking. Family members and friends of the person abusing alcohol are also at an increased risk of emotional or physical abuse.

Social and cultural factors may also contribute to the development of alcoholism. Certain cultural groups have higher incidences of drinking problems, which may represent genetic factors combined with an increased acceptance of heavy alcohol use. It may be part of socially expected behavior. One's social circle may play a role in how alcohol is used as one observes its use by friends or family to avoid problems, become a risk taker, and so on.

RELATED CLINICAL CONCERNS

Alcohol abuse plays a major role in a variety of health problems including gastritis, liver failure, heart disease, and pancreatitis. Twenty-five percent of admissions to general hospitals are related to an alcohol problem, including being treated for consequences of drinking (National Institute of Alcohol Abuse and Alcoholism, 2001). This statistic supports that need for all healthcare professionals incorporating some form of screening in their assessment. Assessing patients for alcoholism abuse can be helpful to prevent complications from withdrawal post-operatively (Sullivan, Sykora, Schneiderman, Narajo, & Sellers, 1989). Alcoholism is the third leading cause of preventable death in the United States (Kessler et al, 2005).

TABLE 13–1

Common Coping Styles Of Alcoholics

Coping Style	Definition	Behaviors
Denial	Person minimizes or does not acknowledge the problem or the results of the problem even when strong evidence is presented.	<ul><li>"I only have two drinks a day, I could stop any time."</li><li>Refuses to admit drinking problems that are obvious to others.</li><li>Family may participate in denial by covering up the problems created by the drinker.</li></ul>
Projection	Blames others for their drinking and behavior.	<ul><li>Avoids taking responsibility for own unacceptable behavior.</li><li>"My brother is the one with the problem. He drinks more than I do."</li><li>"I'd stop if everyone would leave me alone."</li></ul>
Rationalization	Justifies intolerable behavior by giving plausible excuses.	<ul><li>Excuses reinforce denial.</li><li>"My kids are always in trouble. They make me drink."</li><li>"I only drink beer."</li></ul>
Minimizing	Avoids conflict by reducing the impact of the behavior.	<ul><li>Places less value on the behavior and the impact of the problem.</li><li>"You worry too much."</li><li>"I'm not hurting anyone."</li></ul>
Manipulation	Plays one person against another in order to get one's way or cover up or avoid a problem.	<ul><li>Convinces one or two people that he or she will improve if they will help.</li><li>If he or she fails it is the fault of the helper.</li></ul>
Grandiosity	Maintains a sense of superiority and irresponsibility particularly evident when intoxicated.	<ul><li>Lacks concern for others feelings.</li></ul>

Alcohol is toxic to many major organs, especially the heart and liver. The patient with heart disease who abuses alcohol is at increased risk of complications, including hypertension. Liver metabolism may be compromised, and therefore, drugs metabolized by the liver may need dosage adjustments. Alcohol contributes to complications of diabetes.

Hingson (1993) noted that alcohol is a contributing factor in the following: 50% of trauma fatalities, 40% to 50% of falls, and 30% of motor vehicle accidents. If alcohol problems persist throughout a lifetime, the person will die 15 years earlier on average, with major causes being heart disease, cancer, accidents, and suicide (Rivara, Garrison, Ebel, McCarty, & Christakis 2004; Schuckit, 2006). Suicide assessment needs to be included in depressed patients abusing alcohol. Alcohol abuse also contributes to unwanted pregnancies, workplace accidents, and HIV exposure due to high-risk sexual activity.

LIFE SPAN ISSUES

Neonates

Fetal alcohol syndrome is recognized as being caused by alcohol abuse during pregnancy, when rapidly growing fetal brain cells are exposed to alcohol. The end result can be an infant born with mild to moderate developmental disabilities, hyperactivity, facial malformations, heart defects, and growth deficiencies.

Children and Adolescents

Alcohol use by children and adolescents has shown an alarming increase in recent years. Access to alcohol from the home or from friends can make it readily available. Seventy-seven percent of high school seniors have used alcohol (National Institute of Alcohol Abuse and Alcoholism, 2007). Teens who start drinking at age 15 years are four times more likely to develop alcoholism than those who start at age 21 (National Council of Alcoholism and Drug Dependence, 2001).

When teens are found to be drinking, they need to be evaluated for use of other substances as well as high-risk sexual activity and criminal behaviors (Schuckit & Tapert, 2004).

As with adults, children learn from parents, peers, or television and movie images suggesting that alcohol can be a defense against feelings of depression, low self-esteem, or anxiety. It may also represent an acting out against parental authority or enhance a sense of closeness with peers. Children who grow up in a home where one or both parents have an alcohol abuse problem may have an increased risk of abusing alcohol. However, even those children who intensely dislike their parents' drinking behavior may use alcohol as a coping mechanism because they have not learned more appropriate ones. Children and adolescents who become intoxicated are at increased risk of injury related to motor vehicle and bicycle accidents because they usually do not drink in the home. They are also at increased risk of alterations in growth and development because of nutritional deficiencies and because they often do not learn to deal effectively with normal anxiety and other uncomfortable emotions. Adolescents and young adults are more prone to binge drinking, which has been associated with life threatening effects from alcohol intoxication.

Older Adults

Alcohol abuse is often unrecognized and undertreated in the older-than-65 age group. Our society generally does not view the older population as an at-risk group. Because alcohol abuse is often a life-long pattern, elderly people may continue their earlier struggles with alcohol. Because of changes in metabolism with age, it may take less alcohol to begin to cause intoxication or other problems. Others may start drinking in later life because they face increasing problems, such as isolation, loss of spouse, and changes in health status. Alcohol may produce significant health problems in elderly persons, particularly if they have impaired liver function. Mental changes from alcohol use may be confused with dementia. It is a major factor in falls, burns, and suicide attempts. The brain in older adults is more susceptible to the depressant effect of alcohol, and therefore, depression may mask the signs of alcoholism. Other signs might be unexplained falls, poor nutrition, and self-neglect. Use of multiple medications with alcohol can exacerbate alcohol's effects. Withdrawal programs for this age group may require specialized care because of the increased health risks.

POSSIBLE NURSES' REACTIONS

- May view alcohol abuse as a personality defect or weakness rather than a health problem.
- May avoid, criticize, or reject the patient. This may trigger guilt feelings, and the nurse may try to make up for these feelings by being overly sympathetic.
- May have feelings of disgust for the patient.
- May have unresolved feelings related to a past family or personal history of substance abuse.
- May feel helpless to facilitate change, especially in a patient with a long history of alcohol problems.

ASSESSMENT

Behavior and Appearance

- Signs of intoxication include odor of alcohol, slurred speech, loud talking, loss of inhibition, loss of coordination, and poor judgment
- Sudden onset of signs of withdrawal

- Frequently talks or brags about alcohol use
- Exhibits extremes of behavior from euphoria to irritability
- Justifies drinking or the need to drink
- Refuses to discuss drinking or lies about drinking
- Drinks large quantities of alcohol
- Needs to drink increasingly more to get same effect
- Unable to stop drinking once he or she starts
- Overreacts when questioned about drinking pattern
- Reports drinking a much smaller amount than is accurate
- Suicide attempts
- Two or more affirmative responses to the CAGE questionnaire (Box 13–1) suggests dependence, further assessment required

Mood and Emotions

- Depression
- Remorse after a binge
- Low frustration tolerance
- Anxiety
- Low self-esteem

Thoughts, Beliefs, and Perceptions

- Evidence of defense mechanisms of denial, rationalization, projection, and minimizing
- Thinking about alcohol supply and plans to obtain it
- Blackouts
- Hallucinations

BOX 13–1
Cage Questionnaire

To determine the patient's perception of his or her drinking problem, you may ask the following questions. Two or more affirmative answers strongly suggest dependence on alcohol.

1. Have you ever believed that you should <u>C</u>ut down your drinking?
2. Have people <u>A</u>nnoyed you by criticizing your drinking?
3. Have you ever felt bad or <u>G</u>uilty about your drinking?
4. Have you ever had a drink first thing in the morning to steady your nerves or get rid of a hangover (<u>E</u>ye Opener)?

Source: Mayfield, D., McLeod, G., & Hall, P. (1974). The CAGE Questionnaire: Validation of a new alcoholism screening instrument. *American Journal of Psychiatry, 131,* 1121–1123, with permission.

Relationships and Interactions

- Dependent
- Resentful of authority
- Manipulates others to avoid confrontation, conflict
- Blames others for drinking
- Argues with family about drinking

Physical Responses

- Blood alcohol level (0.08 to 0.10 is legal limit to define intoxication in most states) or positive polydrug panel (may be negative, depending on time since last consumption). Blood level is less useful in elderly people because of altered metabolism. Urine testing can be a less invasive approach.
- Amylase may be elevated if liver damage is present. Blood sugar measurement may indicate hyper- or hypoglycemia. Serum magnesium may be low from alcohol damage to the nervous system. Hemoglobin may be low if bleeding is present
- History of falls, burns, accidents
- May have signs of gastrointestinal bleeding, ascites, or jaundice
- May be underweight and show signs of malnutrition and dehydration
- Korsakoff's syndrome from prolonged thiamine deficiency creates a secondary dementia marked by ataxia, confabulation, and peripheral neuropathy
- Withdrawal symptoms may occur 8 to 24 hours after last alcohol use. Analgesics and recovery from anesthesia can precipitate an acute withdrawal reaction. This emphasizes the importance of quick diagnosis to institute detoxification. Assessment of alcohol use in the hospital can be helpful to reduce risk of complications. See Box 13–2 for Clinical Institute Withdrawal Assessment of Alcohol Scale (CIWA-AR). A score of greater than 15 predicts a severe alcohol withdrawal.
- Withdrawal grand mal seizures can occur in a small group of chronic alcoholics
- Alcoholic hallucinosis when hallucinations develop during the withdrawal period. Most often these are visual hallucinations.
- Alcohol-related delirium (also known as delirium tremens) is a medical emergency with a 20 percent mortality rate if left untreated. Complications include pneumonia, dehydration, electrolyte imbalance, respiratory failure, and status epilepticus (Box 13–3).

Pertinent History

- Previous history of alcohol or polydrug use
- History of heart disease, liver disease, gastrointestinal bleeding or varices
- Psychotic, depressed, or manic behavior

BOX 13–2
Clinical Institute Withdrawal Assessment of Alcohol Scale, Revised (CIWA-Ar)

Patient:_____ Date:_____ Time:_____ (24 hour clock, midnight = 00.00)

Pulse or heart rate, taken for one minute: _____ Blood pressure: _____

NAUSEA AND VOMITING — Ask "Do you feel sick to your stomach? Have you vomited?" Observation.

0. no nausea and no vomiting
1. mild nausea with no vomiting
2.
3.
4. intermittent nausea with dry heaves
5.
6.
7. constant nausea, frequent dry heaves and vomiting

TREMOR — Arms extended and fingers spread apart. Observation.

0. no tremor
1. not visible, but can be felt fingertip to fingertip
2.
3.
4. moderate, with patient's arms extended
5.
6.
7. severe, even with arms not extended

PAROXYSMAL SWEATS — Observation.

0. no sweat visible
1. barely perceptible sweating, palms moist
2.
3.
4. beads of sweat obvious on forehead
5.
6.
7. drenching sweats

ANXIETY — Ask "Do you feel nervous?" Observation.

0. no anxiety, at ease
1. mild anxious
2.
3.
4. moderately anxious, or guarded, so anxiety is inferred
5.
6.
7. equivalent to acute panic states as seen in severe delirium or acute schizophrenic reactions

AGITATION — Observation

0. normal activity
1. somewhat more than normal activity
2.
3.
4. moderately fidgety and restless
5.
6.
7. paces back and forth during most of the interview, or constantly thrashes about

TACTILE DISTURBANCES—Ask "Have you any itching, pins and needles sensations, any burning, any numbness or do you feel bugs crawling on or under your skin?" Observation.

0. none
1. very mild itching, pins and needles, burning or numbness
2. mild itching, pins and needles, burning or numbness
3. moderate itching, pins and needles, burning or numbness
4. moderately severe hallucinations
5. severe hallucinations
6. extremely severe hallucinations
7. continuous hallucinations

AUDITORY DISTURBANCES—Ask "Are you more aware of sounds around you? Are they harsh? Do they frighten you? Are you hearing anything that is disturbing to you? Are you hearing things you know are not there?" Observation.

0. not present
1. very mild harshness or ability to frighten
2. mild harshness or ability to frighten
3. moderate harshness or ability to frighten
4. moderately severe hallucinations
5. severe hallucinations
6. extremely severe hallucinations
7. continuous hallucinations

VISUAL DISTURBANCES—Ask "Does the light appear to be too bright? Is its color different? Does it hurt your eyes? Are you seeing any-thing that is disturbing to you? Are you seeing things you know are not there?" Observation.

0. not present
1. very mild sensitivity
2. mild sensitivity
3. moderate sensitivity
4. moderately severe hallucinations
5. severe hallucinations
6. extremely severe hallucinations
7. continuous hallucinations

HEADACHE, FULLNESS IN HEAD—Ask "Does your head feel different? Does it feel like there is a band around your head?" Do not rate for dizziness or lightheadedness. Otherwise, rate severity.

0. not present
1. very mild
2. mild
3. moderate
4. moderately severe
5. severe
6. very severe
7. extremely severe

ORIENTATION AND CLOUDING OF SENSORIUM—Ask "What day is this? Where are you? Who am I?"

0. oriented and can do serial additions
1. cannot do serial additions or is uncertain about date
2. disoriented for date by no more than 2 calender days
3. disoriented for date by more than 2 calender days
4. disoriented for place/or person

Continued

BOX 13–2
Clinical Institute Withdrawal Assessment
of Alcohol Scale, Revised (CIWA-AR) *(continued)*

The CIWA-Ar is not copyrighted and may be reproduced freely.
Patients scoring less than 10 do not usually need additional medication for withdrawal.

Total CIWA-Ar Score _____

    Rater's Initials _____

Maximum Possible Score 67

Source: Sullivan, J. T., Sykora K., Schneiderman, J., Naranjo, C. A., & Sellers E. M. (1989). Assessment of alcohol withdrawal: the revised Clinical Institute withdrawal assessment for alcohol scale. *British Journal of Addiction, 84,* 1353–1357.

BOX 13–3.
DSM-IV Criteria for Diagnosis of
Alcohol-Related Syndrome

Alcohol abuse—Maladaptive pattern of alcohol use that is manifested by one or more of the following within the same 12 months:

1. Inability to fulfill major role obligations at work, school, and home
2. Recurrent legal or interpersonal problems
3. Reduction or absence of important social, occupational, and recreational activities
4. Participation in physically hazardous situations while impaired, for example, driving a car, exacerbation of a symptom

Alcohol dependence—Maladaptive pattern of alcohol use leading to impairment by three or more of the following occurring at any time during the same 12 months:

1. All criteria for alcohol abuse
2. Presence of tolerance to drug
3. Presence of alcohol withdrawal syndrome
4. Ingestion of alcohol to relieve or prevent withdrawal
5. Taking more alcohol over longer period of time than intended
6. Unsuccessful or persistent desire to cut down or control use
7. Great deal of time spent in getting, taking, and recovering from alcohol

Alcohol withdrawal—Cessation of alcohol use which has been heavy and prolonged and has at least 2 of the following within several hours to a few days:

1. Autonomic hyperactivity (high blood pressure, tachycardia, fever)
2. Hand tremor
3. Insomnia
4. Nausea and/or vomiting
5. Anxiety
6. Transient visual, tactile, or auditory hallucinations or illusions
7. Grand mal seizures

Alcohol-induced delirium—An organic mental disorder with symptoms in excess of the usual withdrawal (formerly called "delirium tremens") or intoxication symptoms that occurs after cessation or reduction of long-term heavy drinking or during intoxication. In someone with a history of substance use, symptoms include

1. Impaired consciousness
2. Changes in cognition including memory, language, disorientation, hallucinations (especially tactile such as feeling bugs crawling on one's body)
3. Develops over short period of time (hours to days) and fluctuates over a day.

Source: American Psychiatric Association (APA). (2000). *Diagnostic and statistical manual of mental disorders—text revision (TR.)* Washington, DC: American Psychiatric Association.

- Suicide attempts
- Blackouts, seizures, or delirium
- Alcohol-related police record, possibly including motor vehicle violations or accidents, physical violence, or child or spouse abuse
- May have history of being abused as a child
- Erratic work record because of alcohol abuse
- One or both parents with history of alcohol problems

COLLABORATIVE MANAGEMENT

Pharmacological

Symptoms from alcohol withdrawal generally start within 4 to 12 hours of cessation of heavy drinking. Symptoms are the most intense on the second day. Protocols for detoxification from alcohol include pharmacologic treatment to prevent or reduce the development of alcohol-related delirium. Sedation with longer-acting central nervous system depressants is substituted for shorter-acting alcohol. Benzodiazepines such as diazepam (Valium) and chlordiazepoxide (Librium) are the drugs of choice because they have anticonvulsant actions and are relatively safe. The drugs are usually administered on a routine basis and then tapered down by 20% to 25% per day until withdrawal is complete—usually about 5 days. Shorter acting tranquilizers such as oxazepam and lorazepam (Ativan) may be used if patient has liver disease. Anticonvulsants may also be needed. Detoxification may be done in an alcohol treatment unit or hospital or at home, if adequate supervision is available. Fluid, vitamins, and electrolyte supplementation is also part of the treatment plan. The inpatient setting needs to be used if the patient is at risk for alcohol related delirium, has multiple comorbidities, or is elderly.

Disulfiram (Antabuse) has been used for chronic alcohol abuse. This drug inhibits impulsive drinking because it produces an extremely uncomfortable physical reaction when alcohol is ingested. The drug is taken daily and stays in the system for 5 days after the last dose. If the patient is exposed to alcohol while the drug remains active, he or she may experience headache, tachycardia, nausea, vomiting, flushing, sweating, and changes in blood pressure, as well as potentially serious reactions including shock and cardiac arrhythmias. Because of the risks involved with using this drug, the patient must have the ability to understand the reaction if alcohol is ingested and give informed consent. The patient must be instructed to avoid inhaling substances that could contain alcohol, such as paint or wood stains, and refrain from using any substances with alcohol, including those with hidden sources such as some mouthwashes, elixirs, skin preparations, or colognes. The drug metronidazole (Flagyl) may cause a disulfiram-like reaction when alcohol is also ingested. Antabuse is best used for the motivated patient who is less subject to impulsive behavior and does not have a psychiatric history.

Acamprosate and naltrexone are also being used to treat alcohol cravings and the physical signs associated with withdrawal. These work as neuromodulators to treat the brain dysfunction causing the addiction. These should be used in conjunction with psychological support. Other commonly used medications include beta blockers, clonidine, and haloperidol (for hallucinations).

Dual-diagnosis patients present a challenge because they usually need to continue to take their psychiatric medications during the detoxification process. These medications need to be closely monitored.

Alternative approaches for withdrawal may include herbs and plants such as chamomile for insomnia, valerian for anxiety (should not be taken with sedatives), and kava kava for anxiety (should not be used with sedatives or alcohol). Multivitamins, thiamine, and magnesium therapy are indicated in chronic alcoholics to prevent neurological complications. Patients must also maintain hydration.

Twelve-Step Program

The Twelve-Step Program of Alcoholics Anonymous (AA) is generally accepted as part of every alcoholic's treatment program. AA's philosophy mandates that the individual become sober and never drink or use mood-altering substances again. The person acknowledges that he or she is powerless over alcohol, is always considered recovering, and is never cured. One drink could cause a downward spiral to heavy drinking. The best outcomes occur when the AA group members are of similar age and cultural background.

AA uses sponsors who have been sober for longer periods to support new members. The alcoholic needs to attend regular, even daily group support meetings and work on the Twelve-Step Program. AA chapters are found in virtually every community in the United States. The only requirement for membership is the desire to stop drinking. AA has been the model for other self-help groups, including Gamblers Anonymous and Cocaine Anonymous. Family members of alcoholics can participate in self-help groups following the same model, including Al-Anon for spouses and friends, Al-a-Teen for adolescents, and Adult Children of Alcoholics (ACoA).

Additional approaches may include behavioral, group, and marital therapies.

NURSING MANAGEMENT

INEFFECTIVE DENIAL evidenced by lack of acknowledgment of alcohol abuse related to impaired ability to accept consequences of own behavior.

Patient Outcomes

- Acknowledges own drinking problem
- Expresses feelings while under nurse's care
- Demonstrates problem-solving skills
- Abstains from alcohol and drug use or significantly reduces intake
- Asks for assistance with drinking problem

Interventions

- Help patient identify disturbing feelings by listening to concerns and helping him or her put labels on possible emotions. Patient may have used alcohol to deny feelings and needs assistance to identify them.
- Foster problem solving. Explore with the patient, the coping mechanisms that are more appropriate than alcohol to deal with the specific causes of stress and anxiety.
- Talk with patient about the normal range of personal emotions.
- Discuss behavioral inconsistencies.
- Maintain a positive attitude. Communicate the idea that patient can overcome his or her problems.
- Work with patient to set realistic small goals for abstaining from alcohol and managing his or her problems. This may require structured planning for how to get through the next day without a drink. Encourage use of readings and meditations.
- Reinforce the Alcoholics Anonymous philosophy of "one day at a time." This means setting a goal of not drinking today rather than thinking about not drinking for the next year.

- Develop a trusting relationship. When the patient feels safe with a staff member, encourage examination of the negative consequences of his or her behavior. Recognize that this relationship could become too threatening to the patient and he or she may try to sabotage it or reject the nurse. This is all part of the struggle to face one's problems.
- If patient states, "I could stop drinking any time," have him or her identify what could be done right now to stop. Look for windows in denial that might indicate the slightest insight and focus.
- Set limits on manipulative behavior. Some patients may have learned to be very charming. The goal of these behaviors is to avoid dealing with the real problems.

RISK FOR INJURY evidenced by disorientation, lack of coordination, or aggressive or disruptive behavior related to acute alcohol intoxication, withdrawal, and/or delirium.

Patient Outcomes

- Remains free from injury while under care of the nurse.
- Sleeps at least 6 hours at night.
- Has reduced incidence of medical complications.
- Exhibits appropriate behavior.

Interventions

- Monitor vital signs, seizures, and changes in mental status closely for 5 days after withdrawal from alcohol.
- Monitor closely for signs of withdrawal and report to physician to begin early treatment. With appropriate management, severe complications can be prevented. Recognize that the patient may be using several drugs, so the signs of alcohol withdrawal may be masked or delayed.
- Follow agency policy or protocol for detoxification for high-risk patients.
- Maintain a quiet, calm environment. Use a soft voice and calm, supportive approach to reassure patient.
- Make sure there is a night light in the room. Institute fall precautions. Encourage staff or family to stay with patient to ensure safety.
- Avoid restraints if at all possible by adequate use of medication.
- If the patient has pain from another medical condition, such as trauma or surgery, be sure to treat the pain. Do not withhold analgesia out of fear that it will reinforce addictive tendencies.
- Institute appropriate precautions if patient at risk for seizures, hallucinations, violent behavior.
- Promote use of relaxation techniques and herbal teas to reduce tension and help with possible insomnia.

- Monitor for complications, including cardiac arrhythmias or diabetes.
- Monitor food intake. Encourage fluids and a high-carbohydrate diet. Discourage use of dehydrating foods and fluids such as coffee, tea, and chocolate. Administer vitamins as ordered.
- Provide emotional support for patient and family.

FAMILY COPING: COMPROMISED evidenced by over-responsible behavior to control the alcoholism related to anxiety in the family system.

Patient Family Outcomes

- Demonstrates assertive response when faced with abusive behavior
- Expresses feelings about the impact of alcohol on the family
- Demonstrates reduced number of behaviors that take responsibility for patient's drinking
- Attends support group meetings

Interventions

- Recognize that alcoholism is a health problem that affects all family members. Monitor response of all family members to patient's behavior.
- Give feedback to individuals about over-responsible behavior. Encourage them to recognize the signs and feelings associated with it. Explain how efforts to contain the patient's drinking merely delay the needed confrontation.
- Assist family members to set limits on the urge to "rescue" the patient. Give suggestions on coping mechanisms to reduce the stress. They need support to accept the idea that they are not responsible for patient's drinking or behavior.
- Educate family members about availability and purpose of group support programs. Talk to them about meeting with a chemical dependency specialist for assistance. Participate in a planned intervention technique under the supervision of the specialist when the patient is confronted by family and friends about his or her drinking problem.
- Give person permission to take care of own needs first.
- Teach the family assertive responses to abuse or criticism from others, especially the patient.
- Encourage them to express emotions, both positive and negative.
- Reinforce the idea that ultimately the individual with the drinking problem is the only one who can control his or her own behavior.
- Recognize the fact that family members may unconsciously sabotage patient's recovery in order to maintain the security of the status quo. Remain as objective as possible and avoid becoming involved in family conflicts.

- Prepare patient for changes in relationships with family and friends that may occur once he or she has stopped drinking. There may be some individuals who no longer like the patient when he or she is sober. Patient needs to reexamine these relationships.

ALTERNATE NURSING DIAGNOSES

Noncompliance
Nutrition, Imbalanced: Less Than Body Requirements
Sleep Pattern, Disturbed
Thought Processes, Disturbed
Violence, Risk for

WHEN TO CALL FOR HELP

- Escalation of aggressive, belligerent behavior to violence
- Need to apply restraints
- Intoxication
- Complications including seizures, cardiac arrhythmias, bleeding, high temperature
- Inadequate staff available to manage behavior
- Presence of increase in psychotic behavior
- Sudden change in mental status

WHO TO CALL FOR HELP

- Addiction specialists
- AA sponsor
- Social Worker
- Security
- Psychiatric Team

PATIENT AND FAMILY EDUCATION

- Reinforce strategies to avoid exposure to alcohol. For example, caution patient to avoid contact with drinking friends. Teach patient to avoid his or her old habits that included drinking, and remove all alcohol from the home. Teach patient and family to read labels of products purchased. Avoid products with alcohol in them such as mouthwashes and cough syrup. Avoid any mood-altering substance that could be used as a substitute for alcohol.

- Provide information about the addictive process and how it affects all aspects of one's life. Review "one-day-at-a-time" philosophy.
- Provide information on any medications being used to treat withdrawal and/or alcoholism.
- Provide information on nutrition and how to address possible vitamin and mineral deficiencies.
- Provide information on side effects of medications used to treat alcoholism
- Provide information to patient and family on managing potential seizures.
- Provide health teaching on the potential of gastrointestinal bleeding and liver disease. Encourage patient to avoid using products containing aspirin.
- Educate patient and family on the hazards of drinking in pregnancy and the effects of alcohol on driving and working.
- Teach strategies to replace alcohol with more healthy activities such as sports, hobbies, and journal keeping.
- Reinforce relaxation measures.
- Prepare patient for need to develop social contacts who do not drink.
- Reinforce education to family on avoiding overresponsible responses.
- Prepare the patient for the fact that intense emotions may be more painful without alcohol. He or she may need extra help at these times.
- Remind patient to tell every physician seen about his or her history to ensure that doctor will prescribe medications appropriately.
- Useful Web sites for patients and families include ncadd.org (National Council on Alcoholism and Drug Dependence) and samhsa.gov (Substance Abuse and Mental Health Services Administration).

CHARTING TIPS

- Document vital signs and any evidence of symptoms of withdrawal and delirium.
- Describe in detail the patient's level of consciousness and mental status.
- Document the patient's response to the medications being used for withdrawal.
- Document the family's response to patient's behavior.
- Document any observations of continued alcohol use.
- Document any actions taken to prevent violent behavior.
- If restraints are necessary, document the type, the time the patient was in restraints, the reason why they were applied, the patient's response to treatment, when limbs were released, and the care given to the patient while in restraints.

COMMUNITY-BASED CARE

- Provide information to patient and family on location and phone numbers for local chapters of AA, Al-Anon, and Al-a-Teen, as needed.
- Encourage the patient and family to begin or continue counseling or provide referral to alcohol counseling programs.
- Communicate information on all medications prescribed for alcohol withdrawal and alcoholism
- Encourage the patient to follow up with medical appointments
- Arrange for follow-up home health visits for patients being discharged from detoxification treatment to home.
- Provide information to referring agencies, such as home health agencies or nursing homes, on patient's drinking patterns and the treatment program.

The Patient Abusing Other Substances

Learning Objectives

- Differentiate between substance abuse and dependence.
- Identify common reactions of the nurse to the substance abuser.
- Describe important nursing considerations of abusing amphetamines, cocaine, hallucinogens, nicotine, opioids, and sedatives.
- Identify nursing diagnoses and interventions in caring for the substance abuser.

Glossary

Binge – *Pattern of periodic intervals of heavy use of substances with intervals of no or little usage.*

Cross-tolerance – *State in which the effect of a substance is reduced because the individual has become tolerant to a similar drug.*

Detoxification – *Process of withdrawal of a drug from the body through supervised medical intervention to prevent complications.*

Drug tolerance – *Need for higher and higher doses to achieve same desired effect.*

Dual diagnosis – *Individual with a mental disorder who is also a substance abuser. The substance is often used to self-medicate to relieve psychiatric symptoms. Also called co-occurring disorder.*

Flashback – *Transient recurrence of a disturbance in perceptions associated with hallucinogens that are reminiscent of those experienced when taking the drug. Sometimes referred to as a "hallucinogen persisting perceptual disorder."*

Polypharmacy – *Taking more than one substance at any given time.*

Substance abuse – *The maladaptive and consistent use of a drug accompanied by recurrent and significant adverse consequences often related to physical hazards, multiple legal problems, and recurrent social and interpersonal problems.*

Substance dependence – *Cluster of cognitive, behavioral, and physiologic symptoms indicating that the individual continues use of the substance despite significant substance-related problems.*

Withdrawal – *Negative physiological and psychological reactions that occur when the drug is reduced or no longer taken.*

Using mind- and mood-altering substances is probably as old as the human race. Today, many people use medications or other substances to relax, sleep, and increase energy. Prescription and over-the-counter psychoactive substances such as caffeine, tobacco, alcohol, pain killers, tranquilizers, and common cold treatments are both socially acceptable and commonly used. It is interesting that we accept these substances to help us feel better but loathe people who are dependent on or abuse drugs. People who eventually become substance abusers also take drugs to feel better, possibly as a way to avoid some problems and stressors. Eventually, though, the need to obtain and use the drug negatively affects all aspects of the person's life, including family, job, friends, and other responsibilities. Many people who use drugs retreat to the company of others who share their lifestyle, beliefs, and drugs. Polydrug use is particularly common, as individuals use one drug to counteract or enhance the effects of the first drug.

There is a significant difference between substance dependence and substance abuse. According to the DSM-IV-TR, *substance dependence* is characterized by a pattern of repeated self-administration of a drug that usually results in tolerance, withdrawal, and compulsive drug-taking behavior. *Substance abuse* is characterized by compulsive use in which the individual continues to use the drug even in the face of problems, including inability to fulfill major role obligations at work, school, or home; recurrent use in situations in which it is physically hazardous; recurrent legal problems related to the substance use; and recurrent social or interpersonal problems related to drug use.

Substance abuse is a major health problem for individuals in all ages and socioeconomic groups; however, abuse rates are highest in the 18- to 20-year-old age group (2004 National Survey on Drug Abuse and Health). At some time in their lifetime, 14.6% of Americans have a substance abuse disorder (Kessler, et al, 2005). The National Survey on Drug Abuse and Health in 2004 found that 9.4% of the population has substance abuse or dependence at any one time, with marijuana being the most frequently used illicit drug. Patterns of use vary in relation to cost and availability. The economic impact of drug abuse is tremendous, including crime, medical costs, accidents, and loss of work days in addition to the resulting family dysfunction.

Methamphetamine (known as crystal meth) has been increasingly abused by young people in recent years. It is more often found in rural and suburban communities. This drug is a long-acting amphetamine that contributes to many antisocial behaviors including violent crime, child abuse, and prostitution. Originally produced in this country in meth laboratories from over-the-counter decongestant pseudoephedrine, it is now smuggled in from other countries.

Anabolic steroids are another relative recent drug of abuse. Used by athletes to increase muscle mass, the pattern of addiction to this substance fits the definition of substance abuse when the individual continues to use the drug despite negative effects.

Substances known as "club drugs" have been popular with young people. These include ecstasy, ketamine, and rohypnal. Rohypnal has been associated with "date rape." When this short-acting benzodiazepine is slipped into an alcoholic drink, the victim becomes incapacitated and unable to resist a sexual assault. Ecstasy (also called MDMA) is a stimulant/hallucinogenic that can destroy neurons in the brain leading to brain damage.

It is estimated that 10% to 15% of nurses suffer from some form of chemical dependency (Raia, 2004). Alcohol is the most widely abused drug followed closely by narcotics. Stressful jobs and a tendency to perfectionism, coupled with a feeling of inadequacy; family history; and knowledge about and access to drugs increase the risk of substance abuse in this population. Because they do not fit the image of an addict, nurses often minimize or deny their problem. Many states have now developed Diversion Programs to provide treatment and rehabilitation confidentially.

ETIOLOGY

The causes of drug abuse are similar to those of alcohol abuse; however, because of the wide range of drugs abused, there are some differences.

Biological theories look at the role of specific brain dysfunction and view addiction as a brain disease. Cravings for drugs are stimulated by two pathways—the glutamatergic tract from the prefrontal cortex and the dopaminergic tract. After using a drug that induces an altered state, brain changes that lead to increased craving for this drug again are created. Cocaine has been studied in more depth than some of the other drugs, and it is believed that there may be a deficiency of dopamine and norepinephrine that creates more of a craving for that drug. With opioids, it is theorized that there may be some abnormality in opioid receptors and endorphins.

Psychological theories view drug dependence as an attempt to adapt to severe emotional distress. Low self-esteem and anxiety become masked under the influence of the drug. Drugs relieve feelings of depression and dependency and may be used to suppress anxiety, particularly after a traumatic event such as rape or violent crime. Individuals with tendencies toward antisocial behavior and difficulties with impulse control and frustration tolerance may use substances as a way to control anxiety that contributes to antisocial behavior. In addition, the role of the family and tendency to codependent relationships (see the preceding subsection on alcoholism for complete discussion) also exist with substance abuse. Drug abusers use many of the same coping mechanisms that alcoholics do, including denial, projection, and manipulation (see Table 13–1). Substance abuse can also be a way to cope with overwhelming traumas such as physical and mental abuse.

Sociocultural views recognize that certain drugs may be more likely to be used, depending on peer group, income, or culture. Acceptable behavior within a group, access to specific drugs, and status related to specific drugs may all be influencing factors. For example, crack cocaine has spread quickly within the low-income groups because of its easy availability and low cost.

As with alcohol, patients with a co-occurring disorder of substance abuse and a psychiatric disorder are very common and tend to complicate treatment for both conditions. See previous section of this chapter on patients who abuse alcohol for more information. The National Alliance for the Mentally Ill (2006) reports that 53% of substance abusers have at least one mental illness.

RELATED CLINICAL CONCERNS

There is no evidence to suggest that an individual will become dependent on drugs by taking analgesics for pain. In fact, McCaffery and Ferrell (1994) report that less than 1% of individuals who take analgesics for a painful condition become addicted to that substance. Individuals who have developed drug tolerance require larger amounts of medications to relieve pain. This should not be confused with addiction.

Individuals with a substance abuse problem may experience withdrawal symptoms when hospital admission prevents them from taking the addictive substance. This is an important consideration when analyzing assessment findings. For instance, when a patient who has been hospitalized and NPO for 2 days experiences headaches and irritability, it may be related to caffeine withdrawal. In certain instances, withdrawal symptoms for more potent substances can increase the risk of complications. For example, the confusion resulting from amphetamine withdrawal may cause a postoperative patient to attempt to get out of bed, tear out tubes and intravenous lines, and possibly fall.

The effects of high-risk behaviors that contribute to HIV, hepatitis, and bacterial endocarditis from infections and shared drug paraphernalia cause additional clinical concerns. Individuals may be more prone to high-risk behavior when under the influence of drugs because inhibitions are suppressed. Intravenous drug use remains a major cause of HIV. Many stimulants and inhalants contribute to cardiac arrhythmias.

Polydrug use combined with alcohol is another common finding in the substance abusing population. For example cocaine users commonly use alcohol to get to sleep or calm down. Complications related to multiple drug use include interactions between drugs and synergistic effect of some drug combinations. Detoxification from multiple drugs requires close monitoring by addiction specialists.

LIFE SPAN ISSUES

Neonates

Cocaine use during pregnancy presents severe problems for the exposed neonate. Cocaine crosses the placenta and can induce premature labor. Complications include lower birth weight, decreased head circumference, preterm delivery, and placental abruption. Long-term problems can include aggressiveness and attention deficit. There is often a lack of prenatal care associated with the pregnancy as well because the mother may be fearful of seeking medical care.

Children and Adolescents

Children and adolescents today are at high risk for exposure to substance use and abuse because of the easy availability of drugs in the schools and community. Peer pressure, experimentation, curiosity, and rebellion, as well as trying to find ways to cope or escape from problems, may be part of the etiology. Alcohol, tobacco, and marijuana are most frequently used. Drug use often begins while experimenting with peers. When the child or teen experiences a sense of well-being and power, drug use continues. He/she may then become drawn into the drug culture and possibly into a gang, which provides a support system for continued use. Children and adolescents are more likely to have abuse problems than dependence disorders. Adolescents who are victims of abuse and gay teens are particularly vulnerable to drugs as a way to cope with painful feelings (Tweed, 1998).

Some of the most common abused substances for children and teens include easy-to-obtain over-the-counter substances like inhalants and cough/cold remedies. Children as young as 7 years have been identified as using inhalants. These are an easily available substance to children and younger teens when household items such as hair spray and aerosol whipped cream can be used. Over-the-counter cold and cough medicine abuse is now rising by 50% per year in teens (Partnership for a Drug-Free America, 2006). Products with dextromethorphan can contribute to hallucinations and out-of-body experiences. Use of anabolic steroids often starts in adolescence when a teen becomes active in school sports and also wants to enhance his appearance.

Signs of substance abuse in this group may be indicated by a change in functioning at school, loss of interest in sports, change in sleep patterns, increased isolation, or change in social network.

Older Adults

Substance use and abuse in elderly people are complicated because they routinely take a greater number of prescribed and over-the-counter drugs and have diminished tolerance to many medications. The individual, family, and health professionals often deny this problem in this age group. This may be because family members and health-care professionals are reluctant to accuse an older person of drug abuse. The signs of abuse may also be masked or mistakenly attributed to the use of another drug the person is taking. The older adult is more likely to abuse prescribed tranquilizers, sedatives (especially benzodiazepines), and some analgesics. Falls, unexplained accidents, increased lethargy, loss of memory and attention span, and unexplained confusion may be signs of a drug abuse problem. Use of illicit drugs is relatively uncommon in elderly people, but it may increase in the future as young and middle-age addicts grow older.

POSSIBLE NURSES' REACTIONS

- May have strong negative feelings, viewing the patient as weak, immoral, or responsible for his or her own problems.
- May fear the patient's manipulative, provocative behavior and potential for criminal or violent behavior.
- May tend to minimize patient's concerns or discomforts because of resentment or fear of being manipulated.
- May distance self from patient because of own discomfort.
- May have a rescue fantasy of being the one to help this patient. The nurse may then become repeatedly disappointed when the patient returns to drug use.
- May view patient's cure as hopeless.
- May allow personal or family experience with substance abuse to influence response to the patient.

ASSESSMENT (See Table 13–2)

Behavior and Appearance

- May talk frequently or brag about using drugs
- May have an in-depth knowledge of drugs and how they work
- Dramatic behavior changes, for instance, may be suddenly euphoric, drowsy, more outgoing
- Wears sunglasses indoors because of photophobia or to hide dilated or pinpoint pupils
- Unpredictable behavior
- Grandiosity, overconfidence

(text continued on page 264)

TABLE 13–2

Comparing Commonly Abused Substances

Drug	Intoxication	Overdose	Withdrawal	Nursing Considerations
Amphetamines, including dexedrine and methamphetamines (crystal meth)	*Signs:* Euphoria, high energy, impaired judgment, anxiety, aggressive behavior, paranoia, panic disorders, insomnia and delusions (often seen with long-term use)	*Signs:* Ataxia, high temperature, seizures, hypertension, arrythmias, respiratory distress, cardiovascular collapse, coma, death	*Signs:* Depression, agitation, insomnia, confusion, vivid dreams followed by extreme lethargy	• Used in weight reduction programs and to treat benzodiazepine abuse. • Tolerance can develop fairly rapidly • User often also using alcohol and other substances to relax • May cause a paradoxical reaction in children
		Treatment: Supportive	*Treatment:* Antidepressants, counseling, suicide precautions	• Remains in urine for up to 3 days.
Cannabis, including marijuana and hashish	*Signs:* Euphoria; intensified perceptions; impaired judgment and motor ability; increased appetite; weight gain, sinusitis, and bronchitis with chronic use; anxiety, paranoia; red conjunctiva	*Signs:* Extreme paranoia, psychosis, delirium	*Signs:* Withdrawal syndrome not recognized in DSM-IV-TR though some report loss of appetite, impaired sleep, restlessness, and irritability	• Most widely used illicit drug. • Impaired judgment may contribute to accidents • Respiratory damage from inhaled substances can occur

Drug	Intoxication	Overdose	Withdrawal	Nursing Considerations
Cannabis		*Treatment:* Antipsychotics		• Remains in urine for up to 7 days. • May exacerbate psychiatric symptoms in mentally ill patients. • May negatively affect fertility. • May therapeutically reduce nausea and vomiting, intraocular pressure, and stimulate appetite.
Cocaine, including crack	*Signs:* Euphoria, grandiosity, sexual excitement, impaired judgment, insomnia, anorexia; nasal perforation associated with inhaled route; psychosis associated with long-term abuse	*Signs:* High temperature, seizures, transient venospasms possibly causing MI or CVA, coma, death	*Signs:* Fatigue, depression, anxiety, suicidal behavior	• Crack is smoked or injected IV; has a rapid onset and high dependency rate • Tolerance develops rapidly • Cocaine is inhaled, snorted or injected IV.

Continued

TABLE 13–2

Comparing Commonly Abused Substances—*cont'd*

Drug	Intoxication	Overdose	Withdrawal	Nursing Considerations
Cocaine		*Treatment:* Supportive	*Treatment:* Support counseling, antidepressants	• High risk of acquiring HIV, hepatitis, bacterial endocarditis, and osteomyelitis from shared IV needles or promiscuous sexual relations. • May be used to control appetite.
Hallucinogens, including LSD, psilocybin, and mescaline	*Signs:* Dilated pupils, diaphoresis, palpitations, tremors, enhanced perceptions of colors, sounds, depersonalization, grandiosity	*Signs:* Panic, psychosis with hallucinations, cerebral tissue damage, seizures, hyperthermia, death *Treatment:* Diazepam or chloral hydrate; quiet environment antipsychotics	*Signs:* None	• Flashbacks can occur for up to 5 years. • Could precipitate a psychiatric disorder in susceptible persons

Drug	Intoxication	Overdose	Withdrawal	Nursing Considerations
Inhalants, including glue, gasoline, cleaning solutions, aerosol propellants like deodorants or hair spray, and paint thinner	*Signs:* Euphoria, impaired judgment, blurred vision, unsteady gait	*Signs:* Psychosis with hallucinations, cardiac arrhythmias, CNS depression, coma, cerebral tissue damage, death *Treatment:* Supportive	*Signs:* None	• Most available substance for younger children. • Intoxication period is brief (15-45 minutes) • Can cause permanent CNS damage • May be difficult to detect specific substance used. • Particularly irritating and/or flammable substances can cause trauma and burns in nose, mouth, and airways.
Nicotine, including cigarettes, chewing tobacco, and nicotine gum or patch	*Signs:* Produces a sense of anxiety reduction, relief from depression, and satisfaction	*Signs:* None	*Signs:* Insomnia, depression, irritability, anxiety, poor concentration, increased appetite	• Because most medical facilities do not allow smoking, inpatients may experience withdrawal symptoms.

Continued

TABLE 13–2

Comparing Commonly Abused Substances—*cont'd*

Drug	Intoxication	Overdose	Withdrawal	Nursing Considerations
Nicotine			*Treatment:* Transdermal nicotine patches in decreasing doses, nicotine gum, nicotine nasal spray, and clonidine for severe anxiety, behavioral modification. Long term smokers may need to remain on nicotine therapy for some time.	• Less than 25% of individuals are successful with first attempt to quit. • Self-help strategies with counselling and nicotine replacement has greatest success. • Monitor for weight gain. • Monitor for hypotension with clonidine.
Opioids, including heroin, morphine, meperidine, Oxycontin, propoxyphene, and codeine	*Signs:* Euphoria, analgesia, drowsiness, impaired judgment, constricted pupils	*Signs:* Dilated pupils, respiratory depression, seizures, cardiopulmonary arrest, coma, death	*Signs:* Yawning, insomnia, anorexia, irritability, rhinorhea, muscle cramps, chills, nausea, vomiting, feelings of doom and panic	• High risk of acquiring HIV, hepatitis, bacterial endocarditis, and osteomyelitis from shared IV needles.

Drug	Intoxication	Overdose	Withdrawal	Nursing Considerations
Opioids		*Treatment:* Naloxone, supportive	*Treatment:* Detoxification, possibly with clonidine for severe anxiety and methadone, naloxone, and/or burenorphine to block euphoria	• May be obtained illegally or through prescription abuse • Monitor for hypotension with clonidine.
Phencyclidine (PCP, angel dust)	*Signs:* Impulsive behavior, impaired judgment, belligerent, assaultive behavior, ataxia, muscle rigidity, nystagmus, hypertension, numbness or diminished response to pain	*Signs:* Hallucinations, psychosis, seizures, respiratory arrest, stroke *Treatment:* Gastric lavage; cranberry juice or ammonium chloride to acidify urine (if awake); quiet environment; haloperidol or diazepam; fluids	*Signs:* None	• Have adequate staff available because behavior is unpredictable and patient may become violent. • May consider using four-point restraints.

Continued

TABLE 13–2

Comparing Commonly Abused Substances—*cont'd*

Drug	Intoxication	Overdose	Withdrawal	Nursing Considerations
Phencyclidine				• Drugs remain in urine for several weeks. • Avoid using phenothiazines because they can potentiate the effects of PCP.
Sedatives, hypnotics, and anxiolytics including barbiturates and benzodiazepines	*Signs:* Slurred speech, labile mood, inappropriate sexual behavior, loss of inhibitions, drowsiness, impaired memory	*Signs:* Hypotension, nystagmus, stupor, cardiorespiratory depression, renal failure, seizures (barbiturates), coma, death *Treatment:* Benzodiazepine antagonist (flumazenil); induce vomiting, if awake; activated charcoal; cardiorespiratory support	*Signs:* Insomnia, hand tremor, agitation, panic disorder, nausea and vomiting, anxiety, tinnitus (with benzodiazepines), seizures, and cardiac arrest *Treatment:* Detoxification using gradually reduced dosages of a similar drug, anticonvulsants, and support and counseling	• Abrupt barbiturate withdrawal can be life-threatening. • Alcohol will potentiate drug effects.

Drug	Intoxication	Overdose	Withdrawal	Nursing Considerations
Sedatives				• Cross-tolerance may develop between alcohol and other CNS depressants. • Detectable in blood and urine. • Shorter-acting benzodiazepines have a greater risk of producing addiction and more severe rebound anxiety than longer-acting ones.
Club Drugs including ecstasy (MDMA), rohypnol, ketamine	*Signs:* Euphoria, muscle relaxation, poor judgment	*Signs:* Confusion, hallucinations, severe anxiety, hypertension, seizures, high temp *Treatment:* Supportive	*Signs:* Not physiologically addictive, but psychologic dependence can cause depression, flashbacks	• Can cause memory loss and brain damage. • Physical response may be exacerbated by dehydration.

Continued

TABLE 13–2

Comparing Commonly Abused Substances—*cont'd*

Drug	Intoxication	Overdose	Withdrawal	Nursing Considerations
Anabolic Steroids including testosterone, stanozolol, oxymetholone	*Signs:* Dramatic increase in muscle mass, irritability, increased blood sugar, acne, edema from fluid retention, unwanted secondary sex characteristics	*Signs:* Liver damage, increased cholesterol, hypertension, paranoia, hostility, hyperactivity, manic symptoms *Treatment:* Supportive	*Signs:* Depression, fatigue, anorexia, decreased libido	• Masculinization of women and feminization of men is common • May be self-injected • Repeated use can produce DSM-IV dependence symptoms

- Disheveled appearance
- In children and adolescents, loss of interest in school, drop in grades

Mood and Emotions

- Mood swings
- Low frustration tolerance, angers easily
- Angry outbursts
- Anxiety, especially associated with discussion of drug use
- Emotional reactions related to change in medication regimen, particularly changes in analgesics
- Depressed; verbalizes self-deprecating thoughts

Thoughts, Beliefs, and Perceptions

- Denies impact of drug use
- Rationalizes that he or she can stop using any time
- Persistent belief that drug is for medical use only
- Obsessive thoughts about drug use and access to drug supply
- Suicidal ideations

Relationships and Interactions

- Change in circle of friends and isolation from family
- Blames others for need to use substances and other problems
- May become more isolated as fears of exposing habit to others increases
- Charming, charismatic, or manipulative with others

Physical Responses

- Needle tracks (raised marks from repeated IV injections) may be seen in antecubital space, wrist, feet, behind knees, or in tattoos.
- Recent injection sites may be red and swollen.
- Abscesses and ulcerations may be present.
- There is evidence of drug(s) in urine testing. Each drug varies as to how long it remains in the body. Check with the laboratory for specifics.
- Pupil response varies from constricted to nonreactive with different drugs.

Pertinent History

- History of withdrawal symptoms, overdosage, complications from past drug use
- Psychiatric disorders
- Family history of drug or alcohol abuse
- Criminal record and other legal problems
- Daily or binge drug abuse or dependence
- History of eating disorders

COLLABORATIVE MANAGEMENT

Treatment for substance abuse frequently requires a multidimensional approach including pharmacological treatment for detoxification, individual and group counseling, Twelve-Step Program, and education. Most treatment can be done on an outpatient basis, except for high-risk detoxification.

Pharmacological

Pharmacology can be used to replace the illicit substance as in Methadone. Pharmacology can also be used to neuromodulate the drug cravings by interacting with the receptor system in the brain affected by the substance. Examples of neuromodulators include buprenorphine and naloxone for opioid addiction. These substances also reduce the physical signs of withdrawal.

Medications are used in detoxification programs for many drugs, including opioids, barbiturates, sedatives, and tranquilizers. They are used to control withdrawal symptoms and discourage continued use of the abused substance. Most are used for only short periods until withdrawal is complete; however, in some cases, they may be used for longer periods to control cravings for the drug. Methadone, a synthetic narcotic that resembles morphine and heroin but does not produce the euphoric effects, is used daily on a long-term basis to treat heroin addiction. Both physical and psychological dependence are maintained on methadone, but the euphoric effects of heroin are blocked. Patients usually make daily trips to a methadone clinic to obtain the drug. Buprenorphine, an opioid with agonist and antagonist action, has been used as an alternative to methadone. Naltrexone also reduces the euphoric sensation from narcotics, and clonidine decreases discomfort during narcotic withdrawal. The newest opioid withdrawal treatment uses Suboxone (buprenorphine and naloxone). Addiction specialists must be certified to prescribe this regimen. Patients on this medication must be monitored closely if they have conditions that require use of analgesics. Administering analgesics could precipitate a withdrawal syndrome. So pharmacology can be used to replace the illicit substance like methadone for heroin addiction.

Benzodiazepines and sedative withdrawal is more risky because of the risk for seizures and delirium. Tapering the dose of the identified or similar drug, along with anticonvulsants and antidepressants, is usually used.

Dual-diagnosis patients may require medications for treatment of their psychiatric diagnosis, but efforts are made to avoid sedatives and tranquilizers. Patients with anxiety or psychotic disorders may be using illicit drugs as a way of controlling hallucinations or anxiety.

Nicotine withdrawal has been successfully treated with nicotine replacement and also the addition of bupripion (Wellbutrin). No effective drugs are currently available for stimulant addiction but research is suggesting modofinil (Provigil) may be helpful.

Complementary approaches to treatment of substance abuse might include acupuncture, biofeedback, and massage. Herb and plant products to treat distressing symptoms may be helpful and include chamomile, valerian, kava kava, and St. John's wort. The last is contraindicated if the patient is taking antidepressants, narcotics, or amphetamines.

Twelve-Step Program

The Twelve-Step Program has been used to treat substance abuse and includes groups such as Narcotics Anonymous, Cocaine Anonymous, and Pills Anonymous. The philosophy mandates that the individual remains free from the substance and acknowledges that he or she is powerless over the chemical. Individuals need to attend group meetings routinely. Sponsors who have been drug free for longer periods provide support for new members. Family members can also participate in self-help groups following the same model.

Counseling

Drug rehabilitation also includes counseling to restore physical and emotional stability, identify the person's usual coping mechanism and work to adopt more effective ones, and develop a sense of self-worth and self-esteem.

NURSING MANAGEMENT

INEFFECTIVE DENIAL evidenced by lack of acknowledgment of substance abuse problem related to impaired ability to accept consequences of own behavior

Patient Outcomes

- Acknowledges substance abuse problem
- Abstains from substance use
- Demonstrates participation in treatment plan

Interventions

- Convey acceptance of patient. Avoid criticizing, preaching to, or attacking the patient to get his or her attention.
- Promote trust by listening to concerns and treating patient as an individual.
- Give patient specific feedback on any behavior that appears drug related. Identify defense mechanisms such as blaming others or rationalizing behavior. Encourage personal responsibility for own behavior.
- Provide information on treatment approaches, such as Cocaine Anonymous (CA) or Narcotics Anonymous (NA).
- Help patient identify and share the possible emotions he or she is feeling.
- Help patient see link between substance use and personal and medical problems. Give the patient the opportunity to identify these, if possible.
- Assist patient to identify ways in which drug use affects daily life. Encourage being specific and honest.
- Set limits on manipulative behavior and realistic consequences for this behavior. Recognize that patient may exhibit charming, charismatic behavior, making limit setting more difficult. Never cover up for the patient or act entertained by drug use.
- Recognize that the drug effects may overwhelm the patient's motivation to stop. However, do not ignore signs of patient intoxication. Become familiar with your institution's policies for suspected drug use such as conducting a room search or confiscating drugs.
- If the patient indicates that he or she wants to participate in a treatment program, immediately contact appropriate resources, such as a social worker, to facilitate admittance to a program.

INEFFECTIVE COPING evidenced by anxiety, withdrawal symptoms, inability to function without drugs in recovery related to inadequate coping skills to manage stressors without drugs

Patient Outcomes

- Demonstrates participation in treatment plan
- Demonstrates alternate coping mechanisms to deal with stress that do not involve drugs
- Verbalizes need to continue in treatment
- Abstains from substance use

Interventions

- Help patient to focus on getting through each day without drugs rather than the overwhelming thought of never using them again.
- Give reinforcement for ability to delay gratification and tolerate frustration. Provide information on possible coping mechanisms to reduce stress and tolerate discomfort. Review alternative ways to cope with anger. Role-play dealing with stressful situations.
- Explain the long-term physical effects of drug use, such as short attention span, that affect daily life.
- Prepare patient for the possibility that family and friends may have difficulty relating to him or her when he or she is not using drugs. For instance, friends may seem to abandon the patient who no longer wants to participate in their drug-related activities. The patient will need to prepare to accept this and work on changing these relationships or developing new ones.
- Help the patient discuss realistic future plans and life changes to make when no longer using drugs. Help to identify steps to achieve these goals.
- Encourage participation in support groups or visits or phone contacts with sponsors.
- Monitor to see if visitors are bringing in drugs.
- Provide information on drug treatment for withdrawal. Emphasize need to remain on medications as prescribed.

RISK FOR INJURY evidenced by disorientation, lack of coordination, or aggressive or disruptive behavior related to substance intoxication, overdose, or withdrawal

Patient Outcomes

- Remains free from injury
- Reduced incidence of medical complications related to substance abuse
- Sleeps at least 6 hours a night

Interventions

- Recognize that many people who abuse drugs can function in society fairly well. Early signs of withdrawal may occur during hospitalization with no access to drug supply. Suspicious symptoms should be assessed carefully so that treatment can be instituted as early as possible.

- Determine which substances the patient has been using. Take a careful history from patient or family and friends (if applicable). Obtain ordered urine and blood for drug screening, and carefully monitor the patient's clinical condition and behavior. Recognize that many patients are using more than one substance, including alcohol.
- Institute fall and seizure precautions, as appropriate.
- Recognize that many substance abusers have poor nutritional habits because of anorexia, emotional changes, or inadequate intake. Monitor food and fluid intake. Encourage adequate fluids and nutrition.
- Administer ordered medications to ease symptoms and monitor for adverse and therapeutic effects. Monitor for signs of aggressive, agitated behavior. Avoid restraints, if at all possible.
- Promote rest and sleep by maintaining a quiet environment and encouraging use of relaxation techniques and herbal teas.
- Patients with painful medical conditions need to have analgesics. The substance-abusing patient may need higher doses of analgesics and benefit from a regular dosing with a long-acting analgesic rather than as-needed administration. This avoids the euphoric effect from the analgesic.

ALTERNATE NURSING DIAGNOSES

Infection, Risk for
Knowledge, Deficient
Self-Care Deficit
Self-Concept, Disturbed
Social Interaction, Impaired
Thought Processes, Disturbed

WHEN TO CALL FOR HELP

- Escalation or onset of aggressive, belligerent behavior or violence
- Change in level of consciousness unrelated to underlying medical condition
- Need to apply restraints
- Inadequate staff available to manage behavior
- Patient demonstrating signs of impairment of substances
- Suspected criminal activity related to drug use, selling drugs

WHO TO CALL FOR HELP

- Addiction Specialist
- Psychiatric Team
- Security
- Social Worker
- Attending Physician
- Sponsor from Twelve Step Program

PATIENT AND FAMILY EDUCATION

- Encourage patient to inform health-care providers about past or present drug use because this information will influence drug and dosage selections for needed medical treatments.
- Use caution when using over-the-counter drugs, diet pills, sedatives, and herbal products.
- Teach family members about need to adjust some aspects of their relationship with patient. Help them to identify possible behaviors that could be reinforcing substance use. Give them specific feedback if you observe any of these behaviors.
- Encourage patient to establish new routines and activities that do not involve drug use. This may include avoiding an old circle of friends and developing hobbies or new interests.
- Provide information on risks of exposure to HIV, hepatitis, and other infections. Encourage patient who is at risk to obtain blood tests to determine exposure, and teach health practices to reduce risk to self and others.
- Help patient recognize potential fears and changes that may occur when he or she changes his or her life to live without drugs.
- Provide information on the health impact of specific substances patient is abusing.
- Provide information on treatment of substance abuse to patient and family.
- Provide information on pharmacological treatment of addiction.
- Educate patient and family on effects of drugs on pregnancy, on the job, or operating mechanical equipment.
- Useful websites for patients and families include drugfree.org (Partnership for a Drugfree America).

CHARTING TIPS

- Document behavior associated with intoxication, overdose, or withdrawal.
- Document any indications of inappropriate drug use.

- Describe patient behavior after visits from family or friends.
- Describe response to treatments.
- Describe pain or anxiety behaviors and need for analgesics or tranquilizers.

COMMUNITY-BASED CARE

- Provide referral information on clinics, hotlines, halfway houses, drug treatment programs, and counseling that assist drug abusers.
- Inform referring agencies of patient's history.
- Arrange for follow-up psychiatric home health visit to reinforce drug treatment program as needed.
- Encourage follow-up medical appointments.

14

Problems with Sexual Dysfunction

The Patient with Sexual Dysfunction

Learning Objectives

- Define sexuality and sexual health for adults.
- Differentiate the major sexual dysfunctions found in men and women.
- Identify therapeutic interventions for common sexual dysfunction
- Describe common nurses' reactions to patients with issues about sexual functioning.

Glossary

Dyspareunia – *Persistent genital pain in either a man or woman before, during, or after sex.*

Female sexual dysfunction – *Includes inhibited desire, orgasmic dysfunction, and vaginismus.*

Gender Identity Disorder – *Strong and persistent cross-gender identification*

Impotence – *Erectile dysfunction or inability to attain or maintain an erection sufficient to complete intercourse.*

Male sexual dysfunction – *Includes inhibited desire, erective incapacity, premature ejaculation, ejaculatory incompetence, and ejaculatory pain.*

Premature ejaculation – *Persistent and recurrent ejaculation with minimal sexual stimulation and before the person wishes it.*

Sexual dysfunction – *A change in sexual health or function that the individual views as unrewarding or inadequate. Sexual dysfunction is usually related to one or more of the following: lack of knowledge or incorrect information; biological or physiological causes, such as diabetes, drug or alco-*

hol use, hormonal disorders; change in or loss of body part; ineffective coping or poor relationships; or organic problems (impotence, premature ejaculation, vaginismus, and orgasmic dysfunction).

Sexual response cycle – *Includes excitement, plateau, orgasm, and resolution. Gender, age, culture, experience, and expectation affect each of these stages.*

Sexually transmitted disease – *Any disease that can be contracted by sexual contact; also called venereal disease. Symptoms range from merely annoying to life threatening.*

Vaginismus – *Involuntary spastic constriction of the lower vaginal muscles.*

Human sexuality is a complex phenomenon encompassing biological, psychological, and sociocultural aspects. Biological aspects include the anatomy and physiology of sexual development and sexual activities; psychological aspects include gender identity, sexual self-concept, and valuing one's self as male or female; and sociocultural aspects include sexual orientation learned from the value systems of family, peers, and community. All of these aspects are interrelated, influencing the individual to experience and value the self as masculine or feminine, seeking and giving affection, and striving to meet basic needs for love and belonging

A sexually healthy person has the following characteristics:

- Behavior agreeing with gender identity (persistent feeling of one's self as male or female)
- Ability to participate in loving and committed relationships
- Physical ability to find erotic stimulation pleasurable
- Ability to make decisions about sexual behavior that are compatible with values and beliefs, cultural norms, and social mores
- Ability to make adjustments in sexual functioning appropriate to limitations and changes resulting from illness, injury, or other events such as unavailability of a partner.

Human sexuality can be healthy, satisfying, and enriching, as defined by the preceding characteristics; or it can be the source of physical and mental distress (LeMone & Jones, 1997; Fergusson, 1999). Sexuality encompasses a person's feelings about himself or herself and how to interact with others. Sexuality and sexual behaviors are influenced by age, knowledge, marital status; resources; values; social, spiritual, and cultural norms; and emotional and physical health (Poorman, 2001).

Society today allows people to experience various types of adult relationships. Once believed to be the legal and moral right only of married people, sexual activity is now considered by many individuals to be acceptable for any consenting adult. More people are involved in relationships that were not considered acceptable just a decade or two ago, such as premarital sex, open marriages, remarried or blended families, unions of never-married adults, single-parent families, and homosexual relationships. Although homosexuality was once considered a mental illness, sexual preferences are now considered a matter of personal choice (King, 1999; Levine, 1999; Torkelson & Dobal, 1999).

All aspects of human sexuality may be affected by acute and, especially, chronic illness. Ill health is one of the greatest detriments to sexual expression, not only because it focuses energies toward recuperation but also because it often lowers an individual's sense of personal worth and attractiveness, and indirectly, sexual desire. The most common dysfunctions in women are arousal and orgasmic dysfunction. Common dysfunctions in men are impotence and premature ejaculation.

A diagnosis of sexual dysfunction is made when an individual identifies a problem with sexuality (not when the caregiver is uncomfortable with the patient's sexual preference) or when antisocial sexual behavior results in harm to others. Individuals have the right to make choices regarding their sexual options and should be offered education about them, such as information on appliances and strengthening exercises for cord-injured patients. However, they do not have the right to inflict discomfort or harm on others (Taylor, 1999). Changing social norms for sexual behavior have recently made deviations from "traditional" sexuality more acceptable. Some individuals who adopt alternative modes of sexuality (e.g., homosexuality) experience little or no conflict internally or externally and thus may not be subject to problems of sexual dysfunction. However, some members of society continue to experience extreme discomfort with less traditional sexual expression (Townsend, 2006).

Gender identity disorders can be manifested by repeated persistent desire to be the opposite sex, cross-dressing, and cross-gender role in play as a child (DSM-IV-TR, 2000). Although rare, this condition requires much sensitivity on the part of health-care providers to accept the person as he or she sees himself or herself. Gender identity disorders may be first observed in childhood as the child maintains persistent interest in being the opposite gender and may eventually lead to surgery in adulthood.

Competence and success in handling problems with sexual dysfunction depend on the nurse's knowledge, experience, and comfort with his or her own sexuality. It can be difficult for some nurses to assess a patient's sexual problems or intervene for inappropriate sexual behavior. It may be useful in these situations to confer with a nurse colleague, especially a nurse specialist or a mental health practitioner with training in sexual counseling (Poorman, 2001). Incorporating a sexual history or assessment can be useful to promote an environment of acceptance for a patient and promote needed education (Smeltzer & Bare, 2004). Nurses are in a key position to help patients cope with sexuality concerns related to serious illness (Wilmoth, 2006).

Nurses should not feel that they need to be sex therapists. They can, however, help resolve some sexual problems created by the patient's illness and the limitations it creates. To be prepared to deal with this aspect of patient care, the nurse should:

- Be knowledgeable about sexuality and sexual norms.
- Use this knowledge to understand others' behavior and reactions to sexuality in health and illness.
- Be aware of differences in cultural and individual attitudes and perspectives regarding sexuality.
- Assist patients' adaptation to an optimal level of health regarding their sexuality.
- Make appropriate referrals for patients with more complex sexual dysfunction.

ETIOLOGY

The human sexual response cycle stages describe the type of responses people have during sexual activity. Sexual dysfunction can occur at any of these stages. There is seldom any single cause of unsatisfying or inadequate sexual experiences.

The National Health and Social Life Survey (2001) has identified that 39% of men and 41% of women have had some type of sexual dysfunction in their lives that has lead to some decrease in well-being. A wide range of common sexual dysfunction including erectile dysfunction and decreased desire can be traced to side effects of medications for common medical and psychiatric illnesses (DSM-IV-TR, 2000). Virtually all antipsychotic and antidepressant medications and a variety of other psychotropic medications can cause disruptions in sexual function. Antihypertensives are also implicated in disorders of sexual desire, arousal, and orgasm (Table 14–1). Illicit drugs and alcohol should not be overlooked in evaluating sexual disorders. Many patients believe that alcohol and other drugs decrease sexual inhibitions, whereas in reality, they decrease sexuality and ability to perform sexually. Major tranquilizers, cocaine, and even tobacco have been implicated in sexual disorders (Finger, Lund, & Slagle, 1997).

Physiological causes of sexual dysfunction include disruption of neural pathways as seen in spinal cord injury or prostate surgery; impaired circulation as seen in diabetes or peripheral vascular disease; and hormonal changes as in testicular or ovarian dysfunction. Physiological factors are likely to be consistent across time and situations, whereas disorders with psychogenic causes are likely to be situation or mood specific. Psychological causes include unresolved internal conflicts, low self-esteem, discordant relationships with current or past partners, feelings of dependency or abandonment, and depression. Sociocultural factors include cultural or religious myths or beliefs that inhibit sexual activity.

TABLE 14–1

Drug Categories that Alter Sexual Behavior

Drug Type	Probable Effects
Antihypertensives	Produce vasodilation and decreased cardiac output, depress CNS; cause impotence in men and decrease vaginal lubrication in women
Antidepressants	Peripheral blockage of nervous innervation of sex glands; may have positive effect because they decrease depression
Antihistamines	Block parasympathetic nervous innervation of sex glands
Antispasmodics/ anticholinergics	Inhibit parasympathetic innervation of sex glands
Sedatives and tranquilizers	Block autonomic innervation of sex glands; may have positive effect as they produce tranquilization and relaxation, may have negative effect influencing libido
Oral contraceptives	Remove fear of pregnancy
Alcohol	In small amounts, may increase libido, in large amounts, impairs neural reflexes involved in erection and ejaculation, chronic use may cause impotence
Opioids	Central sedation causes impotence in chronic users
Cancer chemotherapy agents	May produce temporary sterility or neurotoxicity in men, causing impotence
Estrogen	Suppresses sexual function in men
Diuretics	Chronic use may cause impotence

Source: Adapted from Finger, W. W., Lund, M., & Slagle, M. A. (1997). Medications that may contribute to sexual disorders. *Journal of Family Practice, 44,* 33–34; Carpenito-Moyet, L. J. (2006). *Nursing diagnosis: Application to clinical practice* (11th ed). Philadelphia: Lippincott Williams and Wilkins.

Sexual disorders are categorized by DSM-IV-TR (2000) into six major categories:

1. Sexual desire disorders, including hypoactive sexual desire in men or women, and extreme aversion to genital sexual contact

2. Sexual arousal disorders, including female sexual arousal disorder and male erectile disorder

3. Orgasmic disorders in both men and women, also known as delayed or premature ejaculation in men

4. Sexual pain disorders, including dyspareunia in men or women, vaginismus in women

5. Sexual dysfunction caused by general medical condition and substance-induced sexual dysfunction

6. Paraphilias, which are repetitive sexual fantasies or behaviors involving use of a nonhuman object (fetishism), nonconsenting partners (voyeurism, and exhibitionism), or activity that causes humiliation or harm (masochism, sadism, and pedophilia)

RELATED CLINICAL CONCERNS

In nonpsychiatric settings, most nurses see sexual dysfunction related to medical problems, traumatic injuries, or surgical procedures. Sexual dysfunction may be a temporary concomitant of an illness or treatment, or it may be a permanent consequence of chronic illness or injury. Sexual problems associated with illness or injury can be classified into four groups:

1. Lack of interest in or desire for sexual activity

2. Physical incapacity for or discomfort during sexual activity

3. Fear of precipitating or aggravating a physical illness through sexual activity

4. Use of illness as an excuse to avoid feared or undesired sexual activity

Serious, advanced illness can disrupt sexual functioning due to the presence of fatigue, pain, dyspnea, neuropathies, and impaired range of motion (Lamb, 2006). Surgical procedures resulting in changes in sexual functioning include urologic procedures for prostatic hypertrophy; intestinal surgery for colitis, ileitis, or Crohn's disease; and most other fecal or urinary diversion surgeries for neoplasms. Loss of external or internal body parts or functions; relocation of orifices, such as hysterectomy, mastectomy, colectomy, and cystectomy; and amputations can all lead to changes in both physical and mental components of sexual functioning. How a surgical procedure influences postoperative sexual functioning depends on the:

- Reason for surgery, diagnosis, and prognosis related to sexual functioning
- Significance of loss of childbearing and fertility functions

- Knowledge of anatomy and physiology of sexual structures and functions
- Meaning, assumptions, and values related to sexual identity
- Type and rationale for premorbid sexual activity

The main difference between a health disruption resulting from chronic illness and surgical or accidental trauma is the irreversible effect on nerves, blood vessels, and hormonal supply usually associated with surgery and trauma.

Most of the drugs reported to affect sexual functioning directly (see Table 14–1) act on specific neurotransmitters. There is evidence that the primary neurohormone in mobilizing sexual behavior is dopamine, whereas serotonin is the major inhibitor. Therefore medications that block dopamine receptor sites and drugs that deplete dopamine interfere with central control of sexual function, whereas drugs that depress serotonin concentrations in the brain are expected to stimulate sexual function.

Many sexual responses are mediated through the parasympathetic nervous system; therefore, parasympatholytic or cholinergic blocking drugs may cause impotence in men and problems with vaginal lubrication in women. Orgasm and ejaculation are primarily functions of the sympathetic, adrenergic, and nervous system, and therefore, drugs such as anticholinergics may interfere with potency and orgasm.

Ganglionic blocking drugs, such as antispasmodics, impair both sympathetic and parasympathetic nervous system function. Drugs that stimulate or depress the central nervous system can affect sexuality, particularly antianxiety agents and narcotics and many of the substances used socially such as caffeine, alcohol, cocaine, marijuana, and amphetamines. Many therapeutically useful drugs have some adverse effect on sexual function.

LIFE SPAN ISSUES

Children

Masculinity and femininity are defined culturally. Although chromosomes determine sexual identity before birth and by physical appearance of the genitals at birth, postnatal factors greatly influence the way children perceive themselves and others sexually. Gender identity is usually firmly established by the age of 18 months. In rare cases in which gender was misassigned at birth because of physical abnormality or accidental damage was suffered, it is considered almost impossible to reassign a child to the opposite sex after age 2 years.

Research on infantile sexuality indicates that both male and female infants are capable of sexual arousal and orgasm. By age 3 years, children are very aware of how they are alike or different from their parents. Research supports that early masturbation experiences are seen in 5- to 8-year-old children. By age 10 to 12 years, children are preoccupied with pubertal changes and beginnings of romantic interest in the opposite sex.

Adolescents

American culture has very ambivalent feelings about adolescent sexuality. Although teachers and parents realize the importance of psychosocial development, most want to avoid anything that will encourage teenage sex. Trends in teen sex for the past 2 decades include more teens engaging in premarital intercourse, and the average age of first intercourse is decreasing. Nationally, 16 years is most common age for first sexual experience in boys and 17 years for girls (Sadock, 2005). Recently the previously increasing trend in incidence of teen pregnancy has decreased in most areas of the United States. A major concern at this time is sex education regarding sexually transmitted diseases, birth control, and the development of satisfying, long-term relationships with same-sex and opposite-sex friends.

Adults

During this period of the life cycle, from about age 20 to 65 years, every adult must deal with numerous issues that may lead to temporary or long-term sexual dysfunction. Developing sexual relationships, choosing a marital partner, attitudes about premarital or extramarital sex, infidelity, divorce, remaining single, and raising children are just a few of the issues. After age 45 to 50 years, a decrease in hormonal activity, menopause, and other physical changes in both men and women may decrease biological drives. In general, health-care providers should feel comfortable encouraging both sexes to continue healthy sexual activity during adulthood (Townsend, 2006).

Older Adults

There are many myths and stereotypes about sexuality and older people. The most common barriers to sexual relationship in advancing age is health of the partners and in many cases lack of a partner due to death or illness of a significant other rather than lack of desire (Sadock, 2005). A 2004 study by AARP (2005) found that although the amount of sexual activity generally decreases with age, the amount of sexual interest and ability remains fairly constant. Significant health issues affecting sexuality for older people include fear of heart attack, poststroke dependency, fatigue related to chronic illness, erectile dysfunction related to diabetes and treatment for prostate cancer in men, inadequate lubrication in women, and arthritis causing movement limitations. Surgical procedures that are more common in the elderly persons, such as prostatectomy, mastectomy, hysterectomy, and ostomies, also affect the older adult's sexuality. Institutionalization is a particular problem for elderly people because the staff at such facilities may not understand or be sensitive to the sexual needs of their residents.

POSSIBLE NURSES' REACTIONS

- May be shy or insecure about the sexual aspects of their professional role, even though they are sanctioned to touch others in an intimate and personal manner and to ask personal questions, including questions about sexual matters, related to their patients' health.
- May experience anxiety, even revulsion, when dealing with sexual questions or behaviors while caring for their patients.
- May deny their own or their patients' sexuality by avoiding any verbal or behavioral interaction regarding sexual function, for instance, avoiding subject of sex, responding to sexually oriented questions in a vague manner, or using euphemistic expressions like "private parts" or "down below" when referring to genitalia.
- May use hospital rules to sidestep patients' sexual concerns. For example, may assign male staff members to male patients when sexual behaviors or concerns develop.
- May not recognize or may actually encourage patients' becoming emotionally involved with them.
- May experience pity for patients who are unable to perform some sexual acts after injury such as spinal cord injury. May feel insulted, denigrated, or angered by patient behaviors such as flirting, pinching, and exposing body parts.
- May feel uncomfortable dealing with sexual dysfunction in patients.
- May have a mistaken belief that the seriously ill do not have sexual needs or desires and may show a lack of tolerance and empathy for a patient's sexual concerns during illness.

ASSESSMENT

See Box 14–1 for guidelines for an interview with a patient with a sexual problem.

Behavior and Appearance

- Reluctance to answer questions related to sexual functioning
- Concern over changes in sexual performance, body image
- Withdrawn, isolated, embarrassed
- Inappropriate sexual acting out, such as pinching or teasing the nurse, exposing genitalia, or wearing seductive clothing
- May verbalize changes in functioning caused by illness, injury, or surgery

---

BOX 14–1

Guidelines for an interview with a Patient Having a Sexual Problem

These questions serve as a guideline. Adjustments in the focus and depth of the assessment depend on the nature of the patient's problem and the nurse's level of comfort in discussing sexual concerns.

1. Does patient's current physical condition affect level of sexual function?
2. Does patient have concerns about body image or self-esteem related to illness, injury, or surgery?
3. What does patient know about potential or expected changes in sexual function related to the illness, injury, or surgery?
4. What significance does the physical change or limitations have on the patient's perceptions and understanding of sexual function?
5. What are patient's previous sexual patterns?
6. What does patient's spouse or partner understand and believe about the patient's sexual function and the impact of the illness, injury, or surgery?
7. What is patient's outlook and prognosis regarding sexual function?
8. What is patient's level of comfort and willingness to discuss sexual function with health professional, spouse, others?
9. Would patient and partner benefit from more education, counseling, or therapy?

Mood and Emotions

- Fear about future limitations of sexual performance or attractiveness
- Fear, anxiety, or guilt about sexual abilities or loss of function resulting from illness, injury, or surgery
- Presence of stressors affecting sexual functioning, such as job problems, financial worries, religious conflict, value conflict with family or partner, or separated or divorced partner
- Discomfort over lack of privacy, frequent physical examinations, or invasive procedures
- Depression over lack of sexual satisfaction or loss of relationships

Thoughts, Beliefs, and Perceptions

- Lack of knowledge or incorrect information about sexual functioning
- Change in self-concept or body image caused by illness, injury, or surgery
- Denial or misinterpretation of partner's reactions to sexual functioning
- Denies any concerns about sexual functioning but acts in a sexually inappropriate manner with staff or others

Relationships and Interactions

- Sexual dissatisfaction or decreased sexual desire
- Altered relationship with significant other
- Partner unavailable, unwilling, or abusive
- Poor past sexual relationships, absent or negative sexual teaching

Physical Responses

- Painful intercourse
- Inability to complete intercourse, early ejaculation, impotence in men
- Menopausal changes in women because of age, surgery, or medications (such as chemotherapy) causing vaginal dryness and lack of interest

Pertinent History

- Physical diseases or injuries affecting sexual functioning
- History of depression
- History of sexual abuse or rape
- Alcohol or other substance abuse
- Previous sexual dysfunction, such as impotence, painful intercourse, premature ejaculation, or lack of lubrication in women

COLLABORATIVE MANAGEMENT

Pharmacological

Any patient experiencing sexual dysfunction needs a thorough assessment of all medications being taken. Then alternative drug choices as well as changes in doses and timing can be tried. Hormonal therapy may be appropriate treatment in some cases. For example, postmenopausal women may benefit from estrogen replacement therapy or estrogen creams to reduce discomfort during intercourse. Antidepressants can contribute to sexual dysfunction in some, but in others, they have been known to increase desire and reduce depression. Any medications that would increase patient comfort such as analgesics may also be helpful to reduce pain during sexual contact. Medications to treat erectile dysfunction are now readily available. They include sildenafil (Viagra), tadalafil (Cialis), and vardenafil (Levitra). These medications block the actions of an enzyme that inhibit an erection. These medications do not result in sexual arousal but contribute to an erection in the presence of arousal.

Nonpharmalogical treatments for erectile dysfunction include penile implants. Androgen replacement therapy is now being used to treat reduced sexual desire in women (Cameron & Braunstein, 2004). A variety of herbal products are used by individuals of different cultures to enhance sexual functioning (e.g., ginseng, saw palmetto).

Sex Therapy

A patient may need to seek out individual, couple, or group therapy to treat sexual dysfunction. Many mental health professionals have specific training for sexual dysfunction. In addition, the patient may wish to seek out a professional who has obtained certification as a sex therapist from a national organization.

NURSING MANAGEMENT

SEXUAL DYSFUNCTION evidenced by erectile dysfunction, premature ejaculation, vaginismus, dyspareunia, or other changes in sexual behavior related to illness

Patient Outcomes

- Relates valid, accurate information regarding sexual anatomy and function
- Able to verbalize correct information about previously believed myths and misinformation about sexual matters
- Identifies alternate sexual expressions that are pleasurable
- Discusses sexual functioning using correct information

Patient and Partner Outcomes

- Participate in treatment or practices that mediate problem or facilitate and enhance current sexual functioning

Interventions

- Create an atmosphere of understanding, openness, and acceptance between patient and nurse.
- Eliminate or reduce causes for patient to feel embarrassed while discussing sexual functioning.
- Provide privacy, and be nonjudgmental and supportive.
- Begin with other subjects, such as physical or family questions, then move on to questions on biologic aspects of sexuality, such as age at menarche and onset of sexual development, before discussing sexual behaviors or fears. Focus on general knowledge and expectations before moving on to specific individual concerns.
- Determine patient's knowledge and attitudes about sexuality and sexual function.
- Focus on patient's knowledge of anatomy and functioning of body parts that may be affected by disease, injury, or surgery.
- Pay attention to attitudes and words used by patient.

- Identify any misinformation, myths, or beliefs that may affect patient's adjustment to changes in sexual functioning. Validate correct information and correct erroneous information.
- Accept person's feelings and concerns; explore cultural, social, religious, and parental influences on current beliefs.
- Provide new information appropriate to patient's maturational or educational level; include spouse or partner as appropriate.
- Discuss with patient and partner the various etiologies for specific diagnoses; explain cause of problem, if known; provide information about its treatment and prognosis.
- Explore alternatives such as lubricants, estrogen creams, pharmacological treatment for erectile dysfunction.
- Encourage couple to talk over the effect of dysfunction on their relationship.
- Discuss alternate methods of sexual gratification with patient or partner.
- Refer to a urologist or other specialist for further evaluation regarding surgical procedures for penile implants, or vaginal reconstruction when appropriate.
- Refer for further evaluation, counseling, or therapy, if indicated.

SEXUAL DYSFUNCTION evidenced by impotence, premature ejaculation, lack of sexual desire or arousal or other dissatisfying changes in sexual behavior related to inability to adapt to life stressors, e.g., divorce, death, loss of job, depression.

Patient Outcomes

- Identifies stressors affecting sexual function
- Identifies constructive coping patterns and sexual practices
- Resumes previous sexual activity

Interventions

- Assess for factors causing patient's ineffective coping and their influence on sexual function.
- Help the patient to understand and discuss the relationship between life stressors and poor sexual functioning.
- Help patient to determine which stressors can be changed and which he or she has no control over.
- Discuss the modifications of or changes in ways of dealing with stressors. Assist in problem solving for alternatives.
- Help the patient identify alternative methods to reduce sexual energy when partner is unavailable or unwilling, such as the role of regular phys-

ical exercise, alternative sexual practices (self-stimulation, increased social activities if spouse or partner is absent or deceased). Provide educational materials, as needed.

- Refer patient or partner for further counseling or therapy, as indicated, such as consider referrals to marriage counselor, sex therapist, social services as indicated by patient's specific problems.

INEFFECTIVE SEXUALITY PATTERNS evidenced by actual or anticipated negative changes in sexual activity and/or identity related to changes in or loss of body part or physiologic limitations.

Patient Outcomes

- Shows increased acceptance of change in or loss of body part
- Identifies practices that assist in restoration of sexual function despite change in or loss of body part
- Identifies practices that conserve energy and oxygen requirements for sexual activity
- Discusses change in or loss of body part and its influence on sexual functioning

Patient and Partner Outcomes

- Identifies mutual concerns
- Shows increased acceptance of change or loss
- Identifies and uses practices that assist in satisfying sexual functioning

Interventions

- Determine the level of acceptance or adaptation of the patient or partner to the changed or lost body part or function. Note patient's reactions, such as anger, depression, or denial. Explain normal feelings about loss, grief, and change.
- Convey an attitude of acceptance. Be sensitive to the patient's cues that a concern exists, and encourage any attempts to discuss the problem or fear.
- Respect the patient's need for privacy.
- Facilitate the partner's and family's understanding of patient's condition and concerns.
- Encourage need to share by listening and answering questions.
- Include spouse or partner in counseling and teaching if he or she express readiness. Also include spouse or partner in discussions about fear of future losses, fear of rejection by loved ones, and fear of physically hurting partner.

- Help the patient realize that body changes and losses are acceptable to others by spending time with the patient, appropriate touching, and teaching about care during regular nursing care.

- Ask about strengths of relationship with partner and encourage discussion of alternative sexual activities.

- Do not assume that patient knows about how the illness or injury affects sexuality. Many patients do not ask questions or give any indication at all about their concerns.

- Check to determine whether the patient understands medical terminology by asking for feedback on what he or she comprehends. Use pictures and verbal explanations when providing information or giving instructions.

- Provide information over short, repeated visits so that patient has time to think over what you have discussed and to formulate questions for later clarification.

- Check which medications the patient is taking, and inform the patient about any adverse effects on sexual function.

- Encourage the patient to resume sexual activity as close to previous pattern as physically possible. Teach specific information applicable to individual physical condition:

  - For the patient with an ostomy, provide information on ways to control drainage odor.

  - Refer to enterostomal nurse specialist for assistance with appliances. Refer to other specialists as needed.

  - For the patient with cardiac or respiratory disease, teach techniques for conserving oxygen and reducing cardiac workload.

  - Identify the symptoms that indicate sexual activity should be terminated.

  - Provide information on specific techniques if patient is unable to move legs because of arthritis or spinal cord injury.

  - Teach patient to take pain medication before sexual activity for pain caused by arthritis, cancer, and so on.

- Promote the use of alternative methods of sensory and perceptual stimulation, such as body massage.

- Refer the patient and partner to further educational material, self-help support organizations, and therapy as needed. Many self-help groups offer support related to sexual concerns; these include the United Ostomy Association, Arthritis Foundation, American Cancer Society, organizations for the disabled, and Reach for Recovery.

INEFFECTIVE SEXUAL BEHAVIOR PATTERNS evidenced by inappropriate sexual behavior in the medical setting related to ineffective coping.

Patient Outcomes

- Decreases or eliminates sexual acting-out behavior
- Demonstrates willingness to discuss meaning of behavior and its impact on others
- Demonstrates other behaviors for maintaining sexual identity
- Identifies appropriate ways to meet sexual needs in medical setting

Interventions

- Assess meaning of sexual behavior as release of sexual needs or anxiety, aggression, fear of loss of identity, reaction to change in or loss of body part, or need for closeness.
- When inappropriate behaviors occur, identify what happened before acting out.
- Discuss behaviors with patient, and attempt to understand meaning of behavior to patient.
- Give patient feedback about staff reactions to behaviors. Help patient to understand their impact on other patients and staff. Point out which behaviors are most disturbing.
- Set clear limits with patient about what specific behavior is inappropriate.
- Discuss more appropriate ways for patient to meet sexual needs, such as exercise, reading, or spending private time with partner.
- Ensure that the patient knows that sexual acting out is not needed to maintain nurse's interest or concern as a person.
- Provide time to talk with or give physical care to patient when sexual behaviors are not occurring.
- Provide opportunity for the patient to express feelings about sexual identity and the impact of illness, injury, or surgery on body image and self-concept.
- Discuss and negotiate ways to provide privacy during long-term hospitalization.
- Provide structured activity or active games. If appropriate, ask volunteers to arrange for activities outside the current environment.
- Conduct care plan conference to discuss problem and appropriate interventions. When embarrassed or frustrated by sexually acting-out patient, get backup from other staff members, consultants, or administrator who can assist in setting limits and determining care plan goals.

WHEN TO CALL FOR HELP

- Onset of sexually "acting-out" behaviors inappropriate to medical setting
- Increased staff complaints or conflict over management of patient behavior
- Increased staff anxiety over dealing with sexually inappropriate behavior
- Increased sexually inappropriate behavior in other patients
- Patient's sexual behavior interfering with treatment
- Staff inability to provide needed information or counseling to patient

WHO TO CALL FOR HELP

- Mental health professional
- Social Worker
- Nurse manager or educator
- Psychiatric Team
- Advanced Practice Nurse
- Chaplain
- Attending Physician

ALTERNATE NURSING DIAGNOSES

Coping, Ineffective
Knowledge, Deficient
Self-Concept, Disturbed
Social Interaction, Impaired
Social Isolation

PATIENT AND FAMILY EDUCATION

- Review with the patient and sexual partner, if requested, any effects of medications that may affect sexual function. Reinforce need to report these to physician so that alternatives can be found.
- Teach probable causes and treatment for sexual dysfunction if patient and partner request this information.
- Provide information on birth control and prevention of sexually transmitted diseases, as appropriate.

- Provide information on the impact of surgery, illness, and medication on sexual functioning.
- Ensure patient has needed information about use of special devices and drugs, e.g., penile implants, Viagra.

CHARTING TIPS

- Use objective, nonjudgmental terms to describe the patient's sexual behavior.
- Document the patient's sexual concerns even if you do not feel comfortable providing information or education.
- Document the selected interventions for dealing with inappropriate sexual behavior on the patient care plan for consistency.
- Document the patient's understanding of cause and treatment of sexual dysfunction. Include responses of family members if they are involved in patient education and treatment.

COMMUNITY-BASED CARE

- Consult with physician and inform patient and partner about appropriate resources related to sexual dysfunction.
- Provide referrals to appropriate support groups.
- Inform other health-care professionals of patient's inappropriate sexual behavior if patient is being transferred to another facility.
- Inform patient and partner about expected changes in sexual behavior or dysfunction as disease progresses or patient is rehabilitated.
- Provide referral information for further sexual counseling or therapy if needed.

15

Problems with Pain

The Patient in Pain

Learning Objectives

- Differentiate between acute, recurrent, and chronic nonmalignant and malignant pain.
- Examine the reasons for underassessment and undertreatment of pain.
- Describe important factors to be considered in the assessment of pain.
- Describe the role and routes of opioid and nonopioid analgesics in pain management.
- Discuss the importance of alternative (nonpharmacological) methods of pain relief.

Glossary

Acute pain – *Pain, usually of shorter duration, that acts as a warning and protective mechanism. Usually subsides as healing takes place.*

Addiction – *A psychological process, in contrast to drug tolerance, that involves the repeated use of a drug or drugs for psychological, not medical, reasons. Patients who are psychologically dependent on a drug (addicted) will continue to desire the drug even though the pain is resolved.*

Cancer pain – *Usually placed in a category of its own. Even if it lasts for more than 6 months, it is often treated like acute pain because of its progressive nature. Sometimes referred to as malignant pain.*

Chronic pain – *Pain that lasts beyond the ordinary duration of time that an insult or injury to the body needs to heal. Types of chronic pain include recurrent acute pain with potential for recurrence over a prolonged period, with pain-free intervals between episodes; chronic acute pain, which may* *last months or years, but has a high probability of ending; and chronic, benign (noncancer) pain, which occurs almost daily and has existed for 6 or more months. It is now believed that different mechanisms may be involved in development of chronic pain and it is not just a matter of a longer occurrence of acute pain.*

Drug tolerance – *A physiological response of the body, not under the person's control, in which the drug loses its effectiveness after repeated use. Occurs in almost all patients using opioids longer than 7 to 10 days. Needs to be taken into consideration when determining correct dosage of analgesic because the patient may require increased doses to achieve the same effect.*

Pain – *An unpleasant sensory and emotional experience arising from actual or potential tissue damage caused by a noxious stimulus.*

Pain tolerance – *Duration and intensity of pain that an individual is willing to tolerate at any one time. Pain tolerance changes within an individual from one pain experience to another.*

Placebo – *Any medical or nursing measure that works because of its implicit or explicit therapeutic intent rather than its chemical or physical properties.*

Pseudo-addiction – *Patient behaviors that may mimic drug-seeking behaviors and occur when pain in undertreated.*

Referred pain – *Pain felt at a site other than the injured or diseased organ or body part. The pain of coronary artery insufficiency, for example, is often referred to the left shoulder, arm, or jaw, and pancreatic pain may be referred to the middle back.*

Pain is what the person experiencing it says it is, exists when and where he or she says it does. The patient is the authority about his/her own pain. (McCaffery, 1968)

Pain is a universal experience occurring in all age groups and is the most frequent reason why people seek health care. It is also the most feared symptom (Daudet, 2002). Much progress has been made over the last decade in understanding pain mechanisms and the epidemiology of pain. The subject is important for all clinicians because the frequency and perhaps the severity of pain may increase now that progress in medical science has increased survival through old age and chronic illness, and now affects more people than ever before.

Studies continue to show that pain is underassessed and undertreated by health-care professionals. The American Pain Society (2003) reports that the most common reason for unrelieved pain in the American health-care system is the failure of medical personnel to routinely assess pain and pain relief. The classic study by Marks and Sachar (1973) reported that 73% of hospitalized medical patients experienced moderate to severe pain despite receiving parenteral opioid analgesics. Recent research indicates that nurses and physicians continue to undertreat pain in patients because they do not understand pain management principles, they fear causing the patients' dependence on opioids, and they have poor knowledge of opioids, adjuvant therapies, and the components of pain assessment (McCaffery & Ferrell, 1997). Despite the establishment of federal guidelines on pain management (Agency for Healthcare Policy and Research, 1992, 1994), many patients of all ages still suffer unnecessary pain in all health-care settings and at home (Twycross, 1999; Weiner, Peterson, Ladd, McConnell, & Keefe, 1999; Paice & Fine, 2006). In 2001, the Joint Commission on Accreditation of Healthcare Organizations implemented pain management standards that mandate frequent assessment and appropriate interventions.

Pain is a multidimensional and complex phenomenon, requiring effective assessment and management. Many disciplines are involved in pain management in a variety of clinical settings. Optimal pain management depends on cooperation among the different members of the health-care team throughout the patient's course of treatment (Stratton, 1999).

The nurse usually has the most significant influence on management of the patient's pain because of having the most frequent contact with the patient. Consequently, the nurse is in a unique position to identify the patient who has pain; to appropriately assess the pain and its impact on the patient and family, to initiate action to alleviate pain using available resources, and to evaluate the effectiveness of those actions.

Patients vary greatly in their responses to pain and its interventions, as well as in their personal preferences and expectations regarding pain relief. Therefore rigid prescriptions for the management of pain are inappropriate. An effective pain management program will incorporate the following requirements and principles (McCaffery, 1999; American Pain Society, 2003):

1. Pain intensity and relief must be assessed and reassessed at regular intervals in a consistent manner (Fig. 15–1).

2. Patient preferences must be respected when selecting methods of pain management.

3. Each institution must develop an organized program to evaluate the effectiveness of pain assessment and management.

4. Establishing positive relationships between patients and health-care professionals is an important part of successful pain control. Patients should be informed that information about options to control pain is available and they are welcome to discuss their concerns and preferences with the health-care team.

5. Unrelieved pain has severe negative physical and psychological consequences. Aggressive pain prevention and control can yield both short-term and long-term benefits. Although complete elimination of some pain may not be practical or even desirable, techniques are now available to make pain reduction a realistic goal.

6. Prevention is better than treatment. Pain that is established is more difficult to control. The goal should be reduced pain at all times, with "round-the-clock" medications if needed.

Initial Pain Assessment Tool

Date _____

Patient's Name _____ Age _____ Room _____
Diagnosis _____ Physician _____
                                                          Nurse _____

1. LOCATION: Patient or nurse mark drawing.

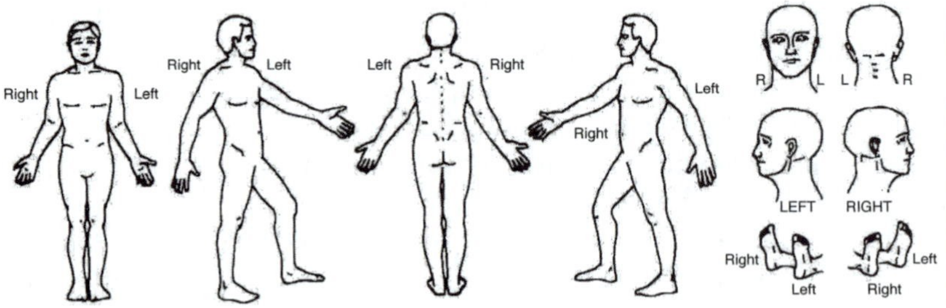

2. INTENSITY: Patient rates the pain. Scale used _____
   Present: _____
   Worst pain gets: _____
   Best pain gets: _____
   Acceptable level of pain: _____
3. QUALITY: (Use patient's own words, e.g., prick, ache, burn, throb, pull, sharp) _____
   _____
4. ONSET, DURATION, VARIATIONS, RHYTHMS: _____
5. MANNER OF EXPRESSING PAIN: _____
   _____
6. WHAT RELIEVES THE PAIN? _____
   _____
   _____
7. WHAT CAUSES OR INCREASES THE PAIN? _____
   _____
   _____
8. EFFECTS OF PAIN: (Note decreased function, decreased quality of life.)
   Accompanying symptoms (e.g., nausea) _____
   Sleep _____
   Appetite _____
   Physical activity _____
   Relationship with others (e.g., irritability) _____
   Emotions (e.g., anger, suicidal, crying) _____
   Concentration _____
   Other _____
9. OTHER COMMENTS: _____
   _____
10. PLAN: _____
   _____
   _____

FIGURE 15–1. Initial Pain Assessment Tool. (*Source:* From McCaffery M., & Pasero C: *Pain: Clinical manual* (2nd ed.) (p. 60). St. Louis: Mosby, with permission.)

ETIOLOGY

The exact mechanism of transmission and perception of pain are not completely understood; however, neurophysiological, psychological, and sociological research has contributed to the formation of pain theories.

The Gate Control theory, originally proposed in 1965 by Melzack and Wall, suggests that pain occurs when smaller diameter type A nerve fibers and very small diameter type C fibers are stimulated. These afferent, or sensory, fibers penetrate the dorsal horn of the spinal cord and end in the substantia gelatinosa. When the sensory stimulation reaches a certain critical point, the "gate" opens and allows nearby transmission cells to project the pain message to the brain. In contrast, the large-diameter type A sensory fibers inhibit pain transmission. When these fibers are stimulated, fast-conducting afferent fibers oppose the smaller fibers' input and activate the substantia gelatinosa "gate" to close, thus blocking nerve transmission.

This theory explains why external methods of pain control work. For example, stimulating the large-diameter type A fibers by massage, applying heat or cold, acupuncture, or transcutaneous electric nerve stimulation (TENS) can override sensory input in the smaller diameter type A fibers and block pain transmission at the gate. Cognitive techniques, such as distraction, biofeedback, relaxation, and guided imagery, operate through the efferent fibers, closing the gate.

In the 1970s, the body's own internally secreted opioid-like substances, called endorphins, were identified. Research found that the brain triggers the release of endorphins, which lock into the narcotic receptors at nerve endings in the brain and spinal cord to block the transmission of pain signals, preventing the impulse from reaching consciousness. This research has helped to explain why pain perception and the need for analgesia can vary greatly from one person to another. Endorphins are depleted with prolonged pain, recurrent stress, and the prolonged use of morphine or alcohol. Endorphin levels are increased during brief pain episodes, brief stress, physical exercise and sexual activity, massive trauma, some types of acupuncture, and some types of TENS, and possibly with placebos. Much of the recent research in this area supports patient-controlled interventions for pain (Ellis, Blouin, & Lockett, 1999).

A number of *neurotransmitters* have been discovered that are found to contribute to the carrying of the pain impulse. These include glutamate and substance P. A number of drugs are being investigated that inhibit binding of excitatory amino acids such as glutamate that normally binds to N-methyl-D-aspartate (NMDA). NMDA antagonists including drugs that contain dextromathorphan and ketamine seem to block the transmission of the pain impulse. This may be one of the mechanisms of actions of methadone.

The multiple opioid receptor theory recognizes that not all opioids work the same way and some cannot be switched back and forth without adverse consequences. There are at least three types of opioid receptor sites in the spinal column. Each type binds somewhat differently with different types of opioids. For example, opioids like butorphanol tartrate (Stadol) or nalbuphine (Nubain) (agonist-antagonist drugs) antagonize the effects of other narcotics like morphine and can contribute to withdrawal rather than pain relief. Knowledge of this theory enhances appropriate selection of analgesics (Ripamonti, Zecca, & Bruera, 1997).

Gender and social and cultural factors also affect the pain response by influencing how the individual interprets pain and how he or she responds emotionally. Through family, social, and cultural values and attitudes, the patient learns which types of pain responses are appropriate within his or her group. Of course, family and social influences change as a child matures. By the time adulthood is reached, the individual may have modified or even rejected many family values or taken on the values of another subgroup. If the patient's values conflict with those of his or her family, additional stress and anxiety may be felt. This may explain why certain patients act differently when family members are present (Fillingim, 2000; Wessman & McDonald, 1999).

Other factors influencing pain behaviors may include the body part involved, the patient's socioeconomic status and religious beliefs, and experience with folk medicine or alternative therapies. A patient's language and vocabulary affect the way in which pain is described. Do not be too quick to assume that you understand what the patient is trying to say, especially if his or her native language and ethnic background are different from yours.

RELATED CLINICAL CONCERNS

Chronic pain is a significant health problem. For example, 10% to 15% of adults in the United States are estimated to have some form of disability from back pain (Borsook, McPeek, & Lebel 1996). One in five Americans suffer from chronic pain (Sternberg, 2005). In addition to disrupting employment, chronic pain can contribute to family problems and social isolation.

Although acute pain is associated with anxiety, chronic pain is more associated with depression. Chronic pain patients are also at higher risk for dependence and abuse of medication because their pain is often not relieved and they begin taking larger doses in hopes of obtaining relief and treating their depression. Health-care professionals may become frustrated and eventually deny the patient the pain medications, making assumptions that the patient is drug-seeking (pseudo-addiction). The chronic pain patient usually requires a multidisciplinary pain team.

The physiological and psychological risks associated with untreated pain are greatest in frail patients with other illnesses, such as heart or lung disease; those undergoing major surgical procedures; and very young or very old patients. Untreated pain can contribute to complications because the patient is unable to cough or deep breathe or get adequate rest or nutrition. Uncontrolled pain in dying patients contributes to the wish to hasten death and is the most frequently stated fear. In patients with psychiatric diagnoses such as depression, schizophrenia, dementia, malingering, and hypochondriasis, pain may be the chief presenting complaint. Treating the underlying psychiatric disorder should lead to reduction in pain. Patients with alcohol or drug withdrawal syndromes need special consideration in their pain management, especially if they also have other medical problems.

Patients with a history of substance abuse are often undertreated for pain leading to increased hospital length of stay, frequent readmissions, and increased outpatient and emergency visits (Kirsh & Passik, 2006; Grant, Cordts, & Doberman,

2007). Long term use of opioids can result in hypersensitivity to pain resulting in further complications. Undertreatment of these patients is often caused by healthcare professionals' misconceptions about addiction.

Each individual experiences and expresses pain in a unique manner, depending on age, gender, culture, and previous pain experience (Box 15–1). All pain is real to the person experiencing it, regardless of its physical or psychological etiology. Each person's ability to tolerate pain is also unique. Depending on the situation, pain tolerance can vary even in the same individual. Anxiety or depression can decrease pain tolerance. Most people with severe or prolonged pain also have emotional changes related to their pain.

About one third of all patients with a diagnosed physical cause for their pain respond to placebos. Nurses should be aware that a positive response, meaning that the patient gets relief after taking the placebo, cannot be used to prove that the pain is psychologically induced. Sometimes just listening to the patient,

---

BOX 15–1
Factors Influencing Pain Tolerance

Factors that may increase or decrease tolerance:

- Past experiences with painful stimuli (e.g., surgery, trauma, illness)
- Knowledge about cause of pain, its treatment, and probable outcome
- Personal meaning of pain (e.g., recurrence of cancer, day off from school or work)
- Knowledge and experience in coping with pain, willingness to try new techniques
- Stress, fatigue, energy levels
- How others treat person when he or she has pain (e.g., secondary gains)
- Available resources (e.g., money for treatment)
- Interactions with healthcare providers (e.g., preventive approach: pain is treated early or patient has to prove that pain is "real" before anything is done to help relieve it)
- Cultural background: some cultures encourage the expression of even mild discomfort, whereas others expect stoic, quiet tolerance of even very severe pain

Factors that usually decrease pain tolerance:

- Disbelief on the part of others
- Lack of knowledge about pain, pain-relief measures
- Fears about addiction, loss of control over pain
- Poor experiences with past pain-relief efforts
- Disability, increasing or long-term
- Fatigue and monotony

acknowledging the pain, and the act of giving a medication can enhance pain relief. Today, it is generally considered unethical for a doctor to prescribe a placebo to treat pain without informing the patient that he/she may be receiving one (Oncology Nursing Society, 1996).

The benefits of adequate and consistent pain management are significant. Benefits include earlier and easier mobilization, shorter hospital stays, increased productive rehabilitation, and earlier return to previous work or lifestyle; or if the patient's condition is terminal, increased comfort and peace of mind. These outcomes should be expected and worked toward with every patient experiencing pain (de Rond, deWit, vanDam, & Miller, 2000; Raines, 2000).

LIFE SPAN ISSUES

Children

As with adults, pain is one of the most feared symptoms in children (Collins & Walker, 2006). Research indicates that younger children, including neonates, may experience some pain more intensely than older children. For children who cannot communicate verbally about their pain, one needs to assess pain by observing physiologic changes, nonverbal behavior, and vocalizations, such as crying or groaning. Consult parents or guardians about how the child expresses pain at home. Knowledge of the child's age, health status and developmental level gives insight into how pain may be expressed (McGrath & Finley, 1999; Twycross, Moriarity, & Betts, 1998; Hunt, 2006).

If painful procedures are needed, be sure they are performed outside the child's room or playroom so that his or her bed, room, and playroom continue to be safe places. If the child is verbal, try to use his or her words for pain when asking about the discomfort. The Wong-Baker Faces Pain Rating Scale is particularly geared to children as well as adults with dementia (Fig. 15–2).

Most dosage recommendations for opioid analgesics in children are not supported by double-blind studies, and underdosing is especially common. Using weight in kilograms to determine doses is useful in many cases when opioids are needed. Initial recommended doses must be viewed as educated guesses and should be adjusted either up or down according to the individual child's response. Toddlers and older children may obtain pain relief from cutaneous stimulation such as massage and TENS and distraction, similar to adults. Adolescents may report more pain than younger children, especially if the pain is chronic.

Older Adults

Pain is not an inevitable part of aging; however, elderly people are at greater risk for many disorders that may result in pain, such as arthritis, cardiovascular disease, osteoporosis, falls, hip fractures, and cancer (Horgas & Elliot, 2004; Barkin, Barkin & Barkin, 2005). Older patients may deny pain more frequently than other age groups because they fear the consequences of admitting pain, such as longer hospitalization or more tests, or they have the mistaken belief that pain

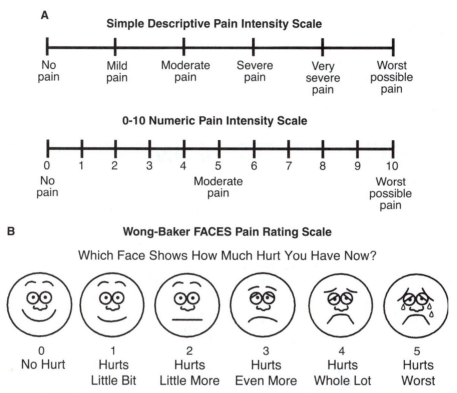

FIGURE 15-2. Pain Rating Scales *(Sources: [A]* Agency for Health Care Policy and Research. (1994). *Management of cancer pain. Clinical practice guideline.* Rockville, MD: Public Health Service, US Department of Health and Human Services (DHHS); *[B]* From Hockenberry, M. J., Wilson, D., & Winkelstein, M. L. (2005). *Wong's essentials of pediatric nursing* [7th ed.] [p. 1259]. St. Louis: Mosby. Used with permission. Copyright, Mosby.)

is normal for their age. Special efforts must be taken to adequately assess pain, especially in confused elderly people. Dementia patients are particularly vulnerable to undertreatment of pain because of their inability to express themselves. Some myths about pain in older adults include that pain is a normal part of aging and opioids cannot be used safely with this population (Curtis, 2006).

Polypharmacy is of special concern in elderly persons. Because of the physiological changes that occur with aging, drug half-life and clearance times are increased. This can lead to increased and unexpected side effects and toxicity, making pain control more difficult in this group. Unrelieved pain may also contribute to confusion and dementia. Adjuvant analgesics must be used with caution in elderly patients because sedation, confusion, and the sedative and anticholinergic effects of many of these drugs can contribute to many other problems. Low starting doses are recommended. Long-acting analgesics may be more likely to cause side effects. A trial of low-dose immediate release analgesics given on a routine basis can be helpful to determine if the dementia patient's behavior is due to pain.

Older adults are more likely to be fearful of using narcotic analgesics owing to long-held beliefs that morphine is associated with death or narcotic use leads to addiction. This can present a significant barrier to effective pain relief. Assess any fears the patient may have regarding taking narcotics. Fear of constipation is also a frequently seen barrier.

POSSIBLE NURSES' REACTIONS

- May rely more on physiological changes or signs such as vital signs, body movement, facial gestures, and other nonverbal behavior than on patients' own verbal reports to assess patient's pain.
- May become insensitive to patient's expressions of pain.
- May have difficulty accurately assessing the patient's pain. Varying opinions among staff members over interpretation of behaviors suggesting pain and selected pain control modalities can lead to very divisive conflicts among staff members.
- May feel extremely frustrated over what can be done to help the patient.
- May fear causing a patient's addiction if the patient requires narcotics for an extended period of time.
- May think that the need for greater pain control is more acceptable for certain types of pain, such as cancer pain.
- May believe that patients will always accurately report pain when they have it.
- May become frustrated over what to do when a patient denies having pain to the physician but continues to request pain medication from nursing staff.
- May feel manipulated by patients who staff members believe are faking pain for the purpose of obtaining more medication.

ASSESSMENT OF ACUTE PAIN

Behavior and Appearance

- Verbalizes pain rating and describes location and character of pain
- Guarded positioning
- Tense or grimacing facial expression
- Rubbing, pulling at, splinting, or protecting painful area
- Fatigued, lethargic
- Crying or moaning
- Restless

Mood and Emotions

- Fearful, anticipating more pain
- Angry, irritable, frustrated
- Depressed, hopeless, withdrawn
- Feeling out of control or helpless about pain if relief is inadequate

Thoughts, Beliefs, and Perceptions

- Wide variations in beliefs about pain, its causes, and methods for relief
- May be confused and unable to concentrate
- Lack of information or misinformation about pain control methods
- Decreased motivation to participate in activities of daily living
- Unwillingness to try alternative pain-relief methods
- Lack of trust in caregivers if pain is not relieved

Relationships and Interactions

- Patient may withdraw socially or have angry outbursts related to pain.
- Secondary gains may influence pain behaviors. For instance, family members may cater to patient's needs more attentively if he or she is in pain.
- Caregivers may avoid the patient because of previous experiences when he or she was in pain, may have feelings of helplessness.

Physical Responses

- Increased blood pressure, pulse, respirations
- Diaphoresis
- Tremors
- Redness and swelling around painful area

Pertinent History

- Previous pain experiences
- Effect of pain on work, sleep, eating, elimination, and sexual patterns
- Previous and current use of narcotics or other analgesics
- Drug or alcohol dependency
- Litigation pending after injury or an accident
- Medical problems, surgical procedures, and injuries

ASSESSMENT OF CHRONIC PAIN

Behavior and Appearance

- Verbalizes pain rating or describes pain
- Presence of pain for longer than expected

- Difficulty maintaining job or other activities
- Frustration, fatigue
- Changes in muscle tone and reflexes

Mood and Emotions

- Depression
- Hopelessness
- Suicidal ideations
- Anger and bitterness
- Preoccupied with pain
- Fear that caregiver will give up on patient and pain problem

Thoughts, Beliefs, and Perceptions

- Fear that pain is intractable and will always affect family, work, social life, finances, and mood
- Perceives others as not believing that he or she is in pain
- Fears losing control over the pain and that the medication will lose effectiveness or be withdrawn before pain resolves
- Has misinformation about effectiveness or alternative pain-relief methods
- Lacks trust in caregivers who do not acknowledge or treat his or her pain

Relationships and Interactions

- Social isolation and withdrawal
- Family or work relationships may have changed since pain became chronic
- Patient's dependency increases with pain
- Patient withdraws from usual activities and friends
- Patient experiences decreased social activities and reduced satisfaction with relationships and diminished sexual interest
- Family experiences fear and frustration about the patient's using pain for secondary gains

Physical Responses

- Anorexia or weight gain
- Impaired mobility
- Insomnia
- Intermittent pain relief with rest; pain recurring with increased stress or certain activities

Pertinent History

- Pain of long duration
- Changes in mood, sleep, appetite, and activity patterns

- Constipation related to prolonged use of narcotics
- Litigation pending after injury
- Prolonged use of medication without effective pain relief
- Physical dependency on pain medications, other drugs, or alcohol since pain became chronic
- Financial problems caused by cost of medical care
- Possible multiple medical complaints, little satisfaction with treatment
- Seeking out numerous doctors for treatment

COLLABORATIVE MANAGEMENT

Pharmacological

Several types of drugs are available to treat pain. Selection is based on the cause of the pain, its intensity and duration, and the patient's response. Mild intermittent pain may be treated with salicylate analgesics, acetaminophen, or nonsteroidal anti-inflammatory agents (NSAIDS). These drugs have specific upper dose limits due to their side effects. More severe, acute pain may need opioid analgesics such as morphine or oxycodone. Determining the most effective medication requires careful assessment of the cause of the patient's pain and his or her perception of the pain and underlying condition. Opioid analgesics generally have no upper dose limits short of side effects.

Factors that influence the effectiveness of medication to relieve pain include:

- Route of administration (Table 15-1)
- Amount and frequency of dosage
- Anticipated onset and duration of action
- Method of drug's action (central versus peripheral)
- Previous experience with medication

The patient experiencing pain needs to be constantly reevaluated to ensure that he or she receives maximal relief with the least potent drug. For instance, a surgical patient may require parenteral opioid analgesics immediately after surgery. As healing occurs, the drug can be titrated to a less invasive method and a lower dose while still maintaining adequate pain control. An equianalgesic list (Table 15–2) gives the dose and route of administration of one drug that produces approximately the same degree of analgesia as the dose and route of administration of another drug. There are many differences among individual patients, so these lists serve only as guidelines to the relative equivalences of various analgesics. Dose and time intervals must be titrated for each patient (Agency for Health Care Policy and Research, 1992, 1994). Patients with chronic pain may need opioids, and the long-acting preparations are particularly useful because they avoid the fluctuating blood levels of analgesics. The World Health Organization Pain Ladder is a useful model to follow for cancer pain (WHO, 2006).

TABLE 15–1

Analgesic Routes of Administration

Oral	Sublingual
• The preferred route • Cost effective • Safe easy administration • Variety of forms (pills, liquid) • Must be able to swallow and absorb	• Easy administration even if patient sedated • Most long-acting products cannot be given this route. • Absorption sometimes erratic
IV Push	**IV Infusion**
• Fast onset for intermittent pain • Short-acting • Less painful than SQ if IV in place • Can be prone to side effects	• Effective for constant pain • Allows for rapid dose titration • Preferred access is central line • Accumulation of drug can contribute to side effects
Patient Control Analgesia	**Subcutaneous**
• Fast onset for intermittent pain • Short-acting • Patient has control • Patient must be awake and able to comprehend instructions	• Faster onset than oral/slower than IV • No IV access needed • May be painful
Subcutanous Infusions	**Rectal**
• Effective alternative to IV drip when no IV access • Only small volume (1-2 cc/hr) can be given.	• Safe alternative to oral • Many oral drugs can be given this route. • Contraindicated in thrombocytopenia, neutropenia
Transdermal	**Epidural**
• Effective for constant pain when stable dose of analgesia needed. • Route of choice if patient unable to swallow, unable to absorb, or is noncompliant. • Can be prone to side effects	• Most effective in intractable pain when traditional routes ineffective • May have less side effects since lower doses used • Requires surgical placement of catheter and more monitoring.

Source: Adapted from Pasero, C., Portenoy R. K., & McCaffery, M. (1999). Opioid analgesics. In M. McCaffery & C. Pasero (Eds.), *Pain: clinical manual* (2nd ed.) (pp. 161-299). St Louis: Mosby.

TABLE 15–2

Opioid Analgesics Commonly Used for Severe Pain

Name	Equianalgesic Dose (mg)		Starting Oral Dose		Comments	Precautions and Contraindications
	Oral	Parenteral	Adults (mg)	Children (mg/kg)		
Morphine-like agonists						
Morphine	30	10	15–30	0.30	Standard of comparison for opioid analgesia. Sustained-release preparation (MS Contin, Oramorph SR) release drug over 8–12 hours.	For all opioids, caution in patients with impaired ventilation, bronchial asthma, increased intracranial pressure, liver failure
Hydromorphone (Dilaudid)	7.5	1.5	4–8	0.06	Slightly shorter duration than morphine	

Continued

TABLE 15–2

Opioid Analgesics Commonly Used for Severe Pain—*cont'd*

Name	Equianalgesic Dose (mg)		Starting Oral Dose		Comments	Precautions and Contraindications
	Oral	Parenteral	Adults (mg)	Children (mg/kg)		
Morphine-like agonists						
Oxycodone	20	–	10–20	0.30		Accumulates with repeated dosing, requiring decreases in dose size and frequency, especially on days 2–5
Methadone (Dolophine)	10	5	5–10	0.20	Good oral potency, long plasma half-life (24–36 hours)	
Levorphanol (Levo-Dromoman)	4 acute 1 chronic	2 acute 1 chronic	2–4	0.04	Long plasma half-life (12–16 hours)	Accumulates on days 2–3
Fentanyl		0.1			Transdermal fentanyl (Duragesic) 25 mcg/hour, roughly equivalent to sustained	Because of skin reservoir of drug, 12-hour delay in onset and offset of transdermal patch; fever increases dose rate.

Name	Equianalgesic Dose (mg)		Starting Oral Dose		Comments	Precautions and Contraindications
Morphine-like agonists	Oral	Parenteral	Adults (mg)	Children (mg/kg)		
					release morphine, 50 mg/day. Oral transmucosal fentanyl citrate available for treatment of breakthrough pain in chronic cancer pain patients already taking around-the-clock opioids. Buccal form of fentanyl (Fentora) now available.	Transdermal patch must be applied to area of body with subcutaneous fat to ensure absorption.
Oxymorphone (Numorphan)	—	1	—	—	5 mg rectal suppository = 5 mg morphine parenteral	Like parenteral morphine

Continued

TABLE 15-2
Opioid Analgesics Commonly Used for Severe Pain—*cont'd*

Name	Equianalgesic Dose (mg)		Starting Oral Dose		Comments	Precautions and Contraindications
	Oral	Parenteral	Adults (mg)	Children (mg/kg)		
Morphine-like agonists						
Meperidine (Demerol)	300	75	Not recommended	Not recommended	Slightly shorter acting than morphine	Normeperidine (toxic metabolite) accumulates with repetitive dosing, causing CNS excitation; avoid in children with impaired renal function or who are receiving monoamine oxidase inhibitors Side effects profile makes this drug unacceptable to use for most pain
Mixed agonist-antagonist Nalbuphine (Nubain)	—	10	—	—	Not available orally, not scheduled under Controlled Substances Act	Incidence of psychotomimetic effects lower than with pentazocine; may precipitate withdrawal in narcotic dependent patients
Butorphanol (Stadol)	—	2	—	—	Like nalbuphine	Like nalbuphine

Source: Adapted from American Pain Society. (2003). *Principles of analgesic use in treatment of acute pain and cancer pain* (5th ed). Skokie, IL: American Pain Society.

Patients on one or more other medications need to be evaluated for possible drug interactions. Drug pharmacokinetics may change because of alterations in cardiac, renal, and liver function; respiratory rate; and gastrointestinal absorption. Fever, sepsis, burns, and shock also affect drug effectiveness. Patients with psychiatric conditions who take antianxiety agents or psychoactive drugs must also be evaluated for possible drug interactions, in particular, the added sedative effects of opioids and many of the psychotropic drugs. Clinicians should be aware that patients in these categories might not respond as expected to pain medication (Borsook, McPeek, & Lebel, 1996).

A factor contributing to undertreatment of pain can be created by the patient who fears taking opioids. Some patient barriers to taking adequate analgesics include fear of side effects (particularly constipation and sedation), and association of opioids with addiction and death.

A variety of herbal products are being used to treat pain, including capsicum ointments, evening primrose for arthritis, and chamomile for migraines. A variety of alternative approaches that may be used include acupuncture, magnet therapy, and biofeedback.

NURSING MANAGEMENT

PAIN, ACUTE evidenced by report of moderate pain, changes in autonomic nervous system (increased heart rate and blood pressure), and reduced ability to perform ADLs related to surgery, injury, or illness

Patient Outcomes

- Reports decreased pain levels
- Identifies previously successful pain-relief techniques to use now to decrease pain
- Identifies and minimizes factors that precipitate or aggravate pain
- Participates in assessment of pain and effectiveness of pain-relief methods
- Demonstrates increased mobility and activity

Interventions

- Perform a thorough pain assessment. Ask patient to rate pain on a consistent scale such as 0 to 10, with 0 being no pain and 10 being the worst possible pain. Determine if the patient can relate more to a visual pain scale (Fig. 15–2). Use the same tool each time you assess that patient's pain. Be sure to determine the patient's perception of his or her pain, previous effective pain methods used, and any misperceptions the patient has about effective pain-relief methods.
- To reduce the patient's anxiety, explain the causes of pain, if known.
- Teach the patient and family about factors that may increase or decrease pain. Try to minimize factors that increase pain perception.

- Teach about any necessary painful procedures before they occur to reduce stress over anticipating the procedure. Patient teaching should include:
  - Basic description of the procedure or test, its purpose, and equipment to be used
  - A description of any sensations likely to be experienced
  - Anticipated duration of procedure and discomfort
  - Measures that can be used to reduce discomfort
- Provide accurate information about analgesics to reduce fear or misconceptions about addiction, tolerance, and physical dependence. Recognize that the patient or family may become anxious when medications are changed. Discuss any changes in medication, dose, or frequency with physician, and plan how to inform the patient about the pain control goals and parameters.
- Provide relief measures at regular intervals rather than on an as-needed basis, even when the pain is still tolerable. Do not expect the patient to wait until pain is unbearable to administer the next dose.
- Use the following approaches when administering analgesics:
  - Determine whether and when to give as-needed medications.
  - Choose the appropriate analgesic when more than one is ordered.
  - Evaluate the effectiveness of administering medications at regular intervals.
  - Monitor responses to administered medications and report promptly any adverse reactions and when they are ineffective.
  - Suggest appropriate changes based on knowledge of the patient and previous response to pain-relief measures.
- Check with patient 30 minutes after administering a pain medication to assess its effectiveness. Include patient in rating level of pain before and after medication or other pain-relief method used. Use the same pain rating scale each time you assess the patient to ensure accurate evaluation.
- Encourage patient's participation in using alternative pain-relief methods such as relaxation exercises or use of heat or cold. Instruct the patient about rigid body position, which can increase pain, and techniques to reduce muscle tension:
  - Select a time when patient is relatively comfortable and able to concentrate so that teaching will be more effective.
  - Use pillows or other supports to splint and support body parts and reduce muscle tension.
- Discuss effects of stress, monotony, fatigue, and distraction on pain perception.
- Provide for privacy for pain expressions if the patient desires.
- Try to limit the number of caregivers interacting with patient and making decisions about pain management.

- Provide opportunities for rest and therapeutic use of distraction, such as visits or watching television, between uncomfortable treatments.
- If patient has a current or past history of drug or alcohol abuse, he or she still needs strong opioids to treat an acute pain problem. Putting this patient on an around-the-clock dosing schedule of analgesics is usually recommended to avoid euphoria. Other suggestions include long-acting analgesics and making a contract with the patient about what medications can be given. Discuss patient's concerns about taking opioids.
- Consult with other staff members or the physician about increased medication at bedtime and before painful procedures to keep pain at tolerable levels throughout the day and to maximize patient's participation in required activities.
- Institute measures to reduce any adverse effects of narcotics. For instance, administer stool softeners and stimulant laxatives (e.g., senna-based products) to combat constipation, antiemetics for nausea, and nonalcohol-based mouthwashes or mouth moisturizers for dry mouth.
- Help the patient to cope with the consequences of pain by encouraging discussion of fears, anger, and frustrations; acknowledge difficulty of situation; and praise and reinforce any efforts to handle pain.
- Consult with pharmacist and physician about alternative opioid and analgesic combinations.
- Consider using aspirin or acetaminophen simultaneously with opioid for maximal effect if appropriate. Also consider use of NSAIDs for peripheral pain.

PAIN, CHRONIC evidenced by ongoing episodes of pain, difficulty performing usual activities, and other effects of chronic pain, such as sleep disturbance or poor nutrition related to effects of illness, surgery, or injury more that lasts beyond the ordinary duration of time that body needs to heal.

Patient Outcomes

- Participates in assessment of pain
- Uses one or more alternative measures to manage pain
- Demonstrates reduced intensity of depression
- Increases participation in activities
- Decreases use of pain behaviors for secondary gain
- Decreases dependence on analgesics when pain controlled

Interventions

- Assess patient's previous and current pain behaviors.
- Encourage the patient to learn and use noninvasive pain-relief methods, such as muscle relaxation, deep breathing, guided imagery, distraction, TENS, and application of heat or cold.

- Incorporate family or caregivers in alternative pain-relief measures.
- Use analgesic medications in conjunction with alternative pain-relief measures to effectively control pain.
- Discuss with physician or pharmacist plan for weaning patient off opioids and onto non-narcotics. Titrate parenteral pain medications and switch to oral doses as soon as possible while ensuring adequate pain control.
- Teach patient and family that oral medication, when prescribed in appropriate dose and frequency, can be as effective as parenteral.
- Administer a loading dose and then maintain a therapeutic drug level of oral medications when first switching to gain the patient's confidence in new treatment.
- Ask patient to participate in evaluation of pain-relief methods by keeping his or her own pain diary.
- Help family or caregiver to recognize and decrease pain behaviors for secondary gain.
- Promote optimal mobility and meaningful activity in patient.
- Assess patient's nutrition and elimination functions related to use of medications and decreased mobility or activity.
- Assess patient's sleep pattern, levels of depression, or other psychological reactions to prolonged pain. Consider use of adjuvant treatments, as indicated.
- Provide the patient and family with the opportunity to discuss fears, anger, and frustration in a private setting. Acknowledge the difficulty of the situation and any of the family's efforts to help the patient cope.
- As indicated, refer the patient for evaluation at a multidisciplinary pain clinic if problems are not improved before discharge.

ALTERNATE NURSING DIAGNOSES

Anxiety
Comfort, Impaired
Coping, Ineffective
Fear
Powerlessness
Self-Concept, Disturbed
Sleep Pattern, Disturbed
Spiritual Distress
Thought Processes, Disturbed

PATIENT AND FAMILY EDUCATION

- Provide information about all pain-relief methods available to the patient. Keep the patient and family informed about changes in treatment plan.
- Teach relaxation techniques (Box 3.2).
- Instruct the patient and family on the use of the pain rating scale.
- Allow the patient to make choices about relief methods used. Involve him or her in assessment of pain; teach how to use pain flow sheet or keep a pain diary, and select appropriate alternative pain-relief measures based on activities and effectiveness of relief methods.
- Initiate teaching with the patient, family, or caregiver related to pain-relief methods to be used after discharge. Review with them the ordered discharge medications, potential adverse effects and how to manage them, what to report to physician, and effective alternative pain-relief measures.
- A useful website for patients and family is www.painfoundation.org/ (American Pain Foundation).

WHEN TO CALL FOR HELP

- Pain-relief measures are ineffective.
- Pain levels increase.
- Patient or family is unwilling to learn about alternative methods of pain relief.
- Psychiatric problems are interfering with patient's use of prescribed pain-relief methods.
- There is increased frustration from dealing with the patient's or family's pain behaviors.
- Analgesics ordered are ineffective and physician refuses to make changes.
- Patient continues or increases use of pain behaviors for secondary gain.
- There are concerns over patient's or family's ability to manage pain after discharge.
- Evidence of abuse of opioids.

WHO TO CALL FOR HELP

- Pain team
- Addiction specialists
- Social Worker
- Palliative Care Team/Hospice
- Attending Physician

CHARTING TIPS

- Include the selected pain rating scale in the assessment and evaluation documentation. Besides the pain rating, document location and description of the pain.
- Use objective, nonjudgmental terms to describe pain behaviors and responses to pain relief measures. When possible, use the patient's own words to describe the pain.
- Document the response to all pain relief measures.
- Document any factors or activities that increase or decrease pain.
- Note all side effects of analgesics.

COMMUNITY-BASED CARE

- Review with the patient, family, or caregiver the patient's progress with pain management since admission.
- If patient is being discharged with prescriptions for opioids, give referrals for local pharmacies that carry these medications.
- Allow sufficient time for the patient to adjust to the change from parenteral to oral administration of pain medications and to practice alternative pain-relief measures before discharge.
- Consult with the physician if patient's pain is not controlled before discharge or if pain is expected to continue for some time thereafter. Obtain a home health referral to assess pain at home and follow up with medication compliance and monitor side effects.
- Instruct the patient, family, or other caregivers on how to use a pain flow sheet or maintain a pain diary at home.
- Suggest that the patient be referred to an appropriate pain treatment center where multidisciplinary treatment is offered.
- Include the selected pain rating scale in all assessment and evaluation documentation.
- Use objective, nonjudgmental terms to describe pain behavior and responses to pain-relief measures. When possible, use the patient's own words when describing the pain.
- Document patient's responses to all pain-relief measures used.
- Document any factors or activities that the patient or family can identify as an increase or decrease in pain tolerance or effectiveness of pain-relief methods.

16

Problems with Nutrition

The Patient with Anorexia Nervosa or Bulimia

Learning Objectives

- Describe the similarities and differences between anorexia nervosa and bulimia.
- Formulate nursing diagnoses and interventions for patients with anorexia nervosa or bulimia.
- Identify common nurses' reactions to the patient with anorexia nervosa or bulimia.
- Describe the complications of anorexia nervosa and bulimia.

Glossary

Anorexia nervosa – *A potentially life-threatening eating disorder characterized by self-starvation in a relentless pursuit of thinness, an intense fear of becoming fat, and delusional disturbance of body image.*

Binge – *Rapid consumption of large amounts of food in a short period of time (usually less than 2 hours).*

Binge eating disorder – *Recurrent episodes of binge eating that lead to feelings of distress. Not associated with purging.*

Bulimia (bulimia nervosa) – *An eating disorder characterized by some of the following: consuming large quantities of food in a short time terminating in abdominal pain, sleep, social interruption, self-induced vomiting, and laxative use.*

Compulsive overeating – *Consuming large volumes of food without purging.*

Eating disorders – *Gross disturbances in the patterns of ingesting food.*
Purge – *Planned or unplanned episode to undo damage of binge, including self-induced vomiting, laxative use, or diuretic use.*

Dieting is a national obsession, especially with women. Numerous fitness clubs are filled with individuals trying to attain the idealized thin, muscular body. Cochrane (1998) reports that more than 50% of American women are on a diet at any one time. Extreme thinness is increasingly common in models and actresses as the idealized image. It seems that it has become accepted behavior to be obsessed with body weight and shape, and to view food as a source of stress. Self-esteem and happiness in young girls are often linked to weight and body shape. Adolescent girls may be rewarded for dieting with either increased social acceptance or praise from parents (White, 2005). When this social influence is combined with certain biological, psychological, and family dynamics influences, it could be the beginning of an eating disorder (Yager & Anderson, 2005). Eating disorders have little to do with simply not eating enough or overeating. Rather, they are psychiatric disorders with substantial emotional and physical consequences.

Anorexia nervosa and bulimia (sometimes called "bulimia nervosa") most commonly occur in young women, and the incidence of these disorders is on the rise. One to five percent of young women suffer from them (Wolfe, 1998). Women and girls are 10 times more likely to suffer from these disorders than men and boys. Male reports of eating disorders may be underreported though (Spader, 2007). Patients with an eating disorder may be treated in psychiatric facilities, but may require admission to an acute-care hospital for treatment of complications or for initial diagnosis to rule out other conditions. There are many similarities between these two eating disorders and long-term anorexics may develop bulimia in later life (Table 16–1).

The term *anorexia* (as in anorexia nervosa) is really a misnomer because this condition has very little to do with appetite. It has more to do with the person's morbid fear of obesity causing obsessive fear of losing control of food intake. In fact, the person is often hungry and views the discomfort of hunger as a reminder of the deprivation he or she needs to inflict on himself or herself. Only in the late stages is appetite actually lost. The distorted body image causes the patient to view himself or herself as fat even though appearing emaciated. No amount of weight loss relieves the anxiety, causing this deadly cycle to continue. Complications can continue for years, even after successful treatment.

The American Psychiatric Association (2000) reports 0.5% to 3.7% of women suffer from anorexia nervosa in their lifetime. Often diagnosed in adolescence, anorexia nervosa is often viewed as representing struggles with autonomy and sexuality. Poorer prognosis is associated with an older age of onset, a lower minimum weight, and vomiting. Purging, which promotes electrolyte imbalance and arrhythmias, is usually combined with compulsive exercise, making a most lethal combination. Successful treatment is measured by weight gain, return of menstruation (usually absent in anorexic women), and reduced number of

TABLE 16–1

Comparing Anorexia Nervosa and Bulimia

	Anorexia Nervosa	Bulimia
Epidemiology	• More than 95% female • Younger adolescent onset • Fairly rare	• 90% female • Young adult onset more likely • 2–3 times more frequent than anorexia
Appearance	• Emaciated • Below normal weight	• Normal or overweight • Weight fluctuations
Family	• Rigid, perfectionistic • Overprotection	• More overt conflict
Behavior	• Introverted • Socially isolated • High achiever • Excessive exercise	• Impulsive • More histrionic, acting out
Signs	• Cachexia • Hair loss • Amenorrhea • Dry skin • Pedal edema	• Dehydration • Chronic hoarseness • Chipmunk facies (parotid gland enlargement)
Prognosis	• 5%–18% mortality rate • Frequent life-long problems with food • Bulimia • Depression	• Death is rarer • Life-long problems with food

compulsive behaviors. Early intervention is associated with improved prognosis. Full recovery of weight, growth and development, menstruation, and normal eating behavior occurs in at least 50% to 70% of treated adolescents (Yager & Anderson, 2005).

Bulimia was officially designated as a psychiatric disorder in 1980 and is harder to diagnose than anorexia. It is more common than anorexia and affects a larger cross-section of the population. Sadock and Sadock (2003) report that the incidence is 1% to 3% of young women. As with anorexia, bulimia is mainly a condition of younger women; however, some studies show that about 10% of bulimics are male (DSM-IV-TR, 2000). Men with bulimia tend to be older at onset. Both men and women often demonstrate difficulties with impulse control, associated with higher incidence of drug abuse and acting-out behavior such as petty crime. The long-term prognosis is unclear because the relapse rate remains high.

Unlike the patient with anorexia, the one with bulimia uses food as a temporary relief of stress, which leads to binge eating. The resulting sense of shame and disgust then causes the patient to purge by induced vomiting or use of laxatives. The cycle of bingeing and purging may begin as a way to lose weight but can become a compulsive behavior.

Bulimia is associated with fewer life-threatening complications than anorexia, but it can lead to chronic conditions including sore throat, dental erosion, and parotid gland enlargement from chronic vomiting. Electrolyte imbalances from chronic use of laxatives, diuretics, enemas, and emetics can occur. A bulimic individual can consume thousands of calories in a short time.

A third eating disorder recently listed in the DSM-IV-TR (2000) is binge eating disorder, which involves eating large quantities without purging. People suffering from this disorder are most often obese or exhibit fluctuations in weight. Weight-loss programs report seeing more clients with this disorder. This disorder is believed to be much more common that anorexia or bulimia.

ETIOLOGY

Individuals with eating disorders report a premorbid history of dieting and attempts to control their weight. What makes this progress to anorexia nervosa or bulimia is unclear, but most likely genetic, biological, psychological, and family factors are all involved. There are many similarities in etiological theories between these two conditions. Both disorders are also significantly associated with depression and family dynamics, in which food plays a large symbolic role.

Anorexia nervosa may have *genetic* influences because there is an increased incidence of its occurrence among daughters and sisters of anorexics. The *biologic* influence may be multifactoral. Research suggests that there is an interrelationship between multiple neurotransmitters, including dopamine that regulates appetite, body size, and fat distribution. Dysfunction of the hypothalamus has also been implicated. Because the symptoms usually begin in adolescence, hormonal changes may be an important contributor.

Psychoanalytic theory suggests that the core of anorexia can be a child's fear of maturing and unconscious avoidance of developmental tasks. By not eating, the person forestalls sexual development and maintains his or her role as child in the family. Other dynamics include perfectionist tendencies developed through demanding, overachieving parents and a profound disturbance in the mother-child relationship. Anorexia gets out of control as the person tries to achieve the perfect image. Many family therapists believe that anorexia symptoms represent a dysfunctional family situation. The patient tries to present a "perfect good girl" image, trying to meet the family's distorted view of perfection. Also, the eating disorder gives the patient a sense of control that counteracts the feelings of loss of control, anxiety, and need to avoid conflict. Some reports indicate that a mother's preoccupation with weight and food can be a source of conflict between mother and child, and the eating disorder becomes a means of control for the child. An overwhelming sense of worthlessness in the child may also be responsible. Comorbid psychiatric disorders include major depression, anxiety disorders, and obsessive-compulsive disorder (Yager & Anderson, 2005).

Specific theories on the cause of bulimia are limited. *Biological* views regard low levels of the neurotransmitters norepinephrine and serotonin as associated with bulimia. Low serotonin is known to increase the need for intake of carbohydrates and is also associated with depression. Bulimia may be related to impaired satiety mechanism.

Family dynamics in bulimia are often characterized by a high degree of conflict, marital discord, and acting out. This may contribute to the patient's developing increased anxiety with intimate relationships and a fear of abandonment and conflict surrounding parental authority. Low self-esteem contributes to feelings of inadequacy and a deep-rooted sense of shame and guilt. Some studies have noted an increased incidence of family members with a history of alcoholism and the possibility of physical or sexual abuse. These individuals are more likely to have comorbid psychiatric disorders, including borderline, panic disorder, and major depression.

RELATED CLINICAL CONCERNS

Anorexic and bulimic patients may have a history of being overweight when young. Anorexics have been noted to weigh more at birth. Bulimics may have a history of anorexia when younger, as well as a tendency for obesity within the family.

Life-threatening complications from anorexia include cardiac arrhythmias, electrolyte imbalance, and cardiomyopathy. Serious bulimia complications can include electrolyte imbalance and erratic blood sugars.

LIFE SPAN ISSUES

Children and Adolescents

Anorexia and bulimia remain a condition generally seen in adolescence and young adulthood. Children as young as 8 years old often admit to preoccupation with diet and atypical eating habits. A sense of self-consciousness and insecurity with one's body is a normal part of growth and development; however, children whose self-esteem becomes more closely tied to satisfaction with their body size tend to become more prone to eating disorders. This is often influenced by the way in which adult caregivers perceive and respond to them. Children who are overweight may experience increased criticism and demands made upon them, leading to low self-esteem. In adolescence, awareness of cultural ideals becomes even stronger. Adolescents may notice that thinner contemporaries have more friends or dates.

POSSIBLE NURSES' REACTIONS

- May feel shocked or disgusted by patient's behavior or appearance.
- May resent the patient because of the belief that the disorder is self-inflicted. This may make it difficult to express empathy, which, in turn, may make the patient feel rejected.
- The nurse may feel helpless to change the patient's behavior, leading to anger, frustration, and criticism.
- The nurse may inadvertently re-create family power struggles with patient by trying to make the patient eat by nagging, cajoling, arguing, or even tricking. This will inhibit a trusting nurse-patient relationship.
- The nurse may feel overwhelmed with the patient's problems, leading to feelings of hopelessness or to the setting of rigid limits to feel more in control of the patient's behavior.
- Many nurses become embroiled in power struggles with these patients, which may trigger angry responses in the nurses.

ASSESSMENT OF ANOREXIA NERVOSA

Behavior and Appearance

- Emaciated
- Tends to cover up body with large clothing in attempt to hide appearance, although some may exhibit thinness with a sense of pride
- Avoids being weighed; may try to manipulate weight by putting weights in pocket
- High achiever in school and work
- Ritualistic behavior surrounding food (such as eating every third bean)
- Spends time with food-oriented activities, such as cooking or shopping for others
- At mealtimes, tries to hide not eating by:
  - Cutting up food to give appearance of less food present
  - Moving food around plate
  - Hiding pieces of food in pockets or under plate

- Exercising obsessively (possibly in secret)
- Using laxatives or foods with a laxative effect excessively
- Not giving a realistic picture of his or her eating patterns

Mood and Emotions

- Has high anxiety associated with mealtimes, weight gain, being weighed, and especially any control issue
- When under stress, may feel need to starve self more
- Experiences feelings of sadness and low self-esteem
- May feel need to punish self for feelings of pleasure
- Denies feelings of sadness or anger and often appears pleasant and compliant

Thoughts, Beliefs, and Perceptions

- Distorted attitude toward appearance, weight, and food that overrides hunger and reason
- Distorted body image: sees self as fat despite others saying that the opposite is true
- Perfectionist, compulsive, rigid
- Seeing self as helpless and dependent; great difficulty making decisions
- Possible mental status changes from malnutrition such as memory lapses, poor attention span, poor judgment, and bizarre behavior
- Denying seriousness of low body weight

Relationships and Interactions

- Introverted; avoids intimacy and sexual activity
- Secretive
- Fears trusting others; needs to be in control

Physical Responses

- Extreme weight loss; weight less than 85% of that expected for age and height
- Cachexia
- Fatigue
- Amenorrhea
- Hair loss; presence of lanugo (fine body hair covering)
- Low pulse rate, low blood pressure, low body temperature
- Chronic constipation
- Dry skin
- Altered laboratory values including low hemoglobin and hematocrit (or high if dehydrated), hypokalemic (especially if using laxatives or diuretics), high blood urea nitrogen (BUN), and serum creatinine
- Insomnia

- Consuming large volumes of fluid to distend stomach, which may lead to hyponatremia
- Pedal edema related to malnutrition
- In late stages, may exhibit arrhythmias and congestive heart failure
- Pathological fractures caused by bone loss from estrogen deficiency and ovarian dysfunction

Pertinent History

- Involved in activities in which small size is important, such as ballet or gymnastics
- Uses food-oriented coping mechanisms, such as stopping eating or excessive eating, to deal with stress
- Family history of depression, eating disorders

ASSESSMENT OF BULIMIA

Behavior and Appearance

- Weight is normal, slightly overweight, and fluctuating.
- Routinely goes into the bathroom shortly after meals.
- Eats normally or sparingly when with others, and binges in private. Purging behaviors may follow, including self-induced vomiting, laxative or diuretic misuse, fasting, or excessive exercise.
- May appear normal without obvious problems.
- Functions normally.
- Behavior is sometimes histrionic or impulsive.
- Tends to act out.

Mood and Emotions

- Binge triggered by some emotional stress; initially some relief of anxiety during the binge but tension slowly increases as feelings of remorse and guilt build
- Purge in response to feelings of remorse and guilt
- Anxiety over appearance and weight
- Anxiety around mealtimes as patient fears loss of control
- Feelings of anxiety, depression, self-disgust

Thoughts, Beliefs, and Perceptions

- Perfectionist
- Preoccupied with appearance, weight
- Self-critical

- Very aware that own behavior is abnormal
- Feels powerless over binge-purge cycle
- Believes he or she is unable to change
- Suicidal thoughts

Relationships and Interactions

- Overt conflict within family
- Goes to great lengths to keep binge-purge behavior a secret from others
- Generally social and gregarious, with a strong need to be accepted by others
- Sexually active

Physical Responses

- If bingeing: abdominal pain, malaise, fluctuating blood sugars.
- If vomiting, chronic hoarseness, parotid gland enlargement causing chipmunk facies, dental caries, loss of enamel on teeth, skin changes over dome of the hand (if use finger down throat to induce vomiting). Use of ipecac to induce vomiting can induce cardiac symptoms including palpitations, chest pain.
- If abusing laxatives, abdominal pain and diarrhea.
- Other symptoms may include dehydration, hypokalemia, and cardiac arrhythmias.

Pertinent History

- Anorexia nervosa as a teenager
- Drug or alcohol abuse (especially cocaine as a way to control appetite)
- Involvement in activities in which weight must be kept down such as modeling, ballet, athletics

COLLABORATIVE MANAGEMENT

Pharmacological

The Agency for Healthcare Research and Quality (2006) found that medications were of limited value in treatment of anorexia. Antidepressants, particularly fluoxetine (Prozac), and other selective serotonin reuptake inhibitors (SSRIs) have been used in patients with clinical depression, anxiety, and obsessive-compulsive symptoms for both anorexia and bulimia (Yager et al, 2006). Fluoxetine in higher doses has been helpful in bulimia. Some antidepressants and atypical antipsychotic drugs also cause weight gain as a side effect. Antipsychotic medications may be used in patients who are extremely obsessive compulsive. Tricyclic antidepressants and monoamine oxidase inhibitors are generally not used in anorexia because of increased side effect profile in malnourished individuals.

Antianxiety medications have also been useful. Bulimics have also been treated with lithium and phenytoin (Dilantin). Anorexics may resist taking medication just as they do food, and it becomes another part of the power struggle to get the patient to comply.

Over-the-counter diet aids and herbal products may be used in the hopes of promoting weight loss.

Dietary

The dietary regimen for the anorexic patient generally involves a slow, steady weight gain of no more than 3 pounds per week (Yager & Anderson, 2005). Too-rapid weight gain can put undue stress on the heart and precipitate complications. Management by a clinical dietitian or nutrition support team is essential. These patients need careful assessment of their nutritional needs. In severely ill patients, malnutrition must be treated before any improvement from psychotherapy can be expected. For life-threatening situations, aggressive nutritional interventions are required. This may include enteral feedings with nasogastric or gastrostomy tubes or total parenteral nutrition. Some patients do well with these aggressive measures because they are relieved that they do not need to make decisions about food. Others may react with resentment and feel an increased loss of control, causing the patient to take more drastic control measures such as increasing exercise, using laxatives, or changing the drip rate or solution being infused. Bulimic patients need dietary education and supervision to control weight. Patients who have bariatric surgery need close nutritional monitoring and special attention to vitamin and mineral intake.

Psychiatric

Individual and group psychotherapy is essential in treating patients with bulimia and anorexia nervosa. Because patients with both conditions also commonly exhibit troubled family relationships, family therapy is also needed. The treatment plan for anorexia nervosa may include a behavior modification and cognitive therapy program. Patients are given rewards for any weight gains and increased restrictions for any weight loss or self-destructive behaviors. To increase the chance of success, patients should participate in developing the treatment plan. Written contracts that clearly explain the patient's behavioral expectations have been effective.

Bulimics may also benefit from keeping a diary of their food intake, feelings, and binge-purge behaviors. Patients who are hospitalized in the acute setting may benefit from evaluation by a psychiatrist.

NURSING INTERVENTIONS

NUTRITION IMBALANCED: LESS THAN BODY REQUIREMENTS evidenced by weight loss, avoidance of food, excessive exercise, hiding food, self-induced vomiting related to self-starvation, binge-purge cycle.

Patient Outcomes

- Increased oral intake (anorexia nervosa)
- Weight gain at rate of no more than 2 pounds per week or per prescribed treatment plan (anorexia nervosa)
- Reduced incidence of strenuous exercise (anorexia nervosa) and/or purging (bulimia)

Interventions

- Recognize that patient may be very defensive about eating behavior and attempts to keep it secret. Mealtimes may be very stressful. Create environment of acceptance to encourage a trusting nurse-patient relationship.
- If personnel are available, stay with patient during meals to be sure food is actually eaten. Create a social atmosphere rather than a supervisory one.
- Give patient as much control as possible around eating behavior. Encourage him or her to select some foods. Set limits, however, on length of mealtimes. Lengthy mealtimes tend to increase anxiety and acting-out behaviors.
- Monitor food and fluid intake. Measure urinary and fecal output. Assess skin turgor. Do this in a matter-of-fact manner. Avoid power struggles or criticism. For example, note what patient has eaten without scowling or making demands. Recognize that telling a patient, "You have to eat more" will create tremendous anxiety and probably lead to defiance. For the patient at home, recognize that monitoring food intake and controlling bingeing may be more difficult and require a commitment from family members.
- Weigh patient regularly, using same scale. Treatment plan may include setting a minimal safe weight range that must be maintained. This can remove the power struggle from mealtimes because patient knows what is expected.
- Set limits on dysfunctional behaviors such as strenuous exercise and use of bathroom after eating.
- Set limits on time spent alone in the bathroom after meals. Also insist that patient wait at least 30 minutes after eating before using bathroom.
- Present meals without threat, coercion, or criticism. Recognize that arguing about food will only increase the problem. In addition, avoid cajoling or tricking patient into taking more calories.
- If you suspect that patient is trying to sabotage the treatment plan, talk openly with patient about your concerns. Be aware that patient may have a need to hide food to give impression that he or she is eating.
- Reinforce the idea that patient can avoid more aggressive interventions, such as tube feedings, by meeting acceptable minimal weight standards,

per treatment plan. For example, patient may need to gain 2 pounds a week. This can be a way for patient to maintain control because he or she can decide how to accomplish it.

- For the patient who binges and/or purges, assess specifically what the patient does including method of self-induced vomiting, laxative, or diuretic use.

DISTURBED BODY IMAGE evidenced by inaccurate perception of appearance and morbid fear of obesity related to distorted thoughts and inability to perceive body size and physical needs realistically.

Patient Outcomes

- Verbalizes more realistic perception of his or her body
- Refers to body in a more positive way

Interventions

- Encourage patient to express feelings, especially about the way he or she thinks about or views himself or herself.
- Avoid overreacting to self-deprecating comments patient may make about his or her body. Recognize that these feelings and images are very real to the patient. For example, the patient may dwell on having "fat" legs even though they may be very normal or even emaciated looking. Listen to patient, and explore how the fear of fat creates distress. For example, "I understand you see yourself as fat; however, I do not see you the same way." Avoid responding to patient's self-deprecating remarks by minimizing the patient's statements.
- Encourage discussion of positive personal traits, especially regarding patient's body image.
- Encourage patient to dress attractively and to use makeup and jewelry, as appropriate.
- Avoid insincere compliments about patient's appearance.

INEFFECTIVE COPING evidenced by bingeing-purging behavior, obsessive behavior around food related to disturbance in impulse control.

Patient Outcomes

- Verbalizes feelings to others while in care of the nurse
- Demonstrates reduced number of behaviors that would sabotage treatment plan
- Demonstrates more adaptive coping mechanisms while in care of the nurse
- Participates in decision making

Interventions

- If patient is panicked over personal feelings or behavior, remain calm and help patient focus on ability to remain in control. For example, patient may feel panicked over a weight gain and want to exercise or purge. Help patient focus on short-term goals that he or she can achieve. Identify one area over which the patient has some control. Reinforce coping abilities.

- Communicate support and empathy to patient. Be nonjudgmental to encourage sharing of feelings and coping mechanisms. Demonstrate acceptance by use of support and concern to help the patient feel lovable and accepted.

- Recognize the importance of developing a trusting relationship with patient. One or two staff members who attempt to develop a therapeutic alliance with patient can be particularly helpful. Recognize that patient may be very angry about entering treatment program. Developing a trusting relationship will take time. Show acceptance by use of touch, and if appropriate, talking about interests. Avoid just focusing on food.

- Be consistent in treatment plan. All staff members need to be aware of how to handle sabotaging of plan, such as hoarding food or self-induced vomiting.

- Listen for signs of perfectionist thinking and explore ways to challenge unrealistic expectations. Recognize that patient may have very rigid, fixed beliefs.

- Encourage patient to make small decisions. This tends to empower the patient and assists in imparting a sense of control and accomplishment.

- Assess patient for depression, suicidal risk, and substance abuse, and intervene as appropriate.

- Be aware of the family's role in patient's behavioral responses. Patient may need help in seeing himself or herself as a capable person outside the family unit.

POWERLESSNESS evidenced by feeling out of control in presence of food related to inability to control bingeing and vomiting cycles.

Patient Outcomes

- Reduce incidence of bingeing and purging
- Able to describe triggers for bingeing and purging

Interventions

- Educate about the binge and purge cycle and how it perpetuates itself.
- Explore with patient the triggers that bring on desire to eat excessively. Once triggers are known, explore alternative ways to address them as in call a friend, write in diary, exercise.

- Explore the signals the patient feels that lead to purging. Encourage him/her to write down feelings at that time.
- Encourage keeping a calendar of tracking symptoms and feelings.
- Challenge irrational thoughts that may take over when tension is building toward binging.

ALTERNATE NURSING DIAGNOSES

Anxiety
Denial, Ineffective
Family Coping: Compromised
Fluid Volume Deficit
Knowledge, Deficient
Self-Mutilation, Risk for
Sexual Dysfunction
Thought Processes, Disturbed

WHEN TO CALL FOR HELP

- Patient expresses suicide thoughts or makes a suicide attempt.
- There is evidence of psychotic thinking, hallucinations, or severe obsessive-compulsive behavior including repetitive obsessive thinking.
- There are signs and symptoms of severe malnutrition or serious complications including cardiac symptoms, hypokalermia, or renal impairment.
- Patient demonstrates signs of substance abuse.
- Staff is in conflict over treatment plan.

WHO TO CALL FOR HELP

- Psychiatric Team
- Dietitian
- Internist
- Social Worker
- Attending Physician

PATIENT AND FAMILY EDUCATION

- Provide information on the long-term effects on the body of anorexia nervosa and bulimia.
- Involve family in what symptoms to identify and report. Review with them how to deal with self-destructive behaviors so as not to reinforce them.
- Provide information on the Twelve-Step Program as in Overeaters Anonymous for dealing with addictions if appropriate. This is helpful for some people with eating disorders.
- Review nutritional information and recommended dietary program.
- Teach stress management and relaxation techniques to reduce anxiety, especially at mealtimes or when feeling need to binge-purge.
- Educate patient and family on the need to continue long-term treatment.
- For patients who use self-induced vomiting, encourage adequate dental care.
- Reinforce need for close medical supervision.
- Teach central line care and tube feeding administration, as appropriate.
- Provide education on health effects of laxative and diuretic abuse.

CHARTING TIPS

- Document intake and output.
- Document description of behavior at mealtimes, purging behaviors.
- Document description of interactions with family.
- Document patient's verbalization about his or her body image.
- Document all self-destructive behavior.
- Review assessment of potential complications, for example, cardiac status.

COMMUNITY-BASED CARE

- Psychiatric follow-up is essential, including family therapy. Referrals need to be made for appropriate treatment.
- Refer for adequate nutritional support follow-up if appropriate, including management of enteral feedings and central line care. If patient is being followed by a home health agency, encourage referral to dietitian. Home health agency social work and psychiatric home health referral may also be helpful to encourage compliance with psychiatric care, for family support, and for behavioral management.
- Refer patient and family to support groups, if available.
- Refer patient to dental care follow-up if patient is vomiting.
- Refer patient to Overeaters Anonymous, if appropriate.

The Morbidly Obese Patient

Learning Objectives

- Differentiate obesity from morbid obesity.
- Identify potential lifestyle restrictions and prejudices faced by morbidly obese persons.
- Describe effective interventions to enhance self-esteem for these patients.
- Identify common emotional reactions of nurses to the morbidly obese patient.

Glossary

Bariatric surgery – *Surgery performed on morbidly obese to achieve restriction in food intake.*

Body mass index (BMI) – *Describes body weight relative to body fat. It is calculated by dividing weight in pounds by height in inches squared, then multiplying by 704.5.*

Chronic obesity – *Life-long overweight condition with few fluctuations.*

Developmental obesity – *Obesity that began in childhood or adolescence and is often associated with problems of self-concept.*

Ideal body weight – *Standards based on actuarial tables of height and weight.*

Morbid obesity – *A condition in which an individual is 100 pounds or 100% over his or her ideal body weight or body mass index of greater than 40.*

Obesity – *Having an excess of adipose tissue and being at least 15% over ideal body weight or body mass index of greater than 30.*

Pickwickian syndrome – *Extreme obesity in which demands of body size on a small chest wall lead to cardiovascular and respiratory changes, including hypoxemia, cyanosis, reduced vital capacity, and pulmonary edema.*

Reactive obesity – *Obesity that starts later in life and is the result of maladaptive coping styles at times of stress such as death of a loved one or leaving home.*

The cultural ideal of the thin body has no greater dichotomy than the image of those with extreme obesity, also known as morbid obesity. Although aesthetic preferences for body size and shape vary from culture to culture, today the thin, fit body is idealized for both women and men in America. Prejudice against the obese has a significant impact on anyone with a serious weight problem, but morbidly obese people often face outright discrimination.

The American population has been steadily gaining weight over the last 30 years. Currently two-thirds of Americans are classified as overweight and 30% as obese (National Health and Nutrition Examination Survey, 2000). Extreme or morbid obesity is seen in only a small percentage of the population, but its impact on health care is great because of the multiple medical complications caused by this condition. BMI is now the standard used to determine obesity because it is more reflective of body fat percentages than the older ideal body weight tables.

Morbid obesity affects all ages and races, although it is much more common in lower socioeconomic groups. Obesity is equally distributed between men and women. Potential health problems include a wide range of chronic conditions, including hypertension, cardiac problems, diabetes, respiratory insufficiency, and joint and back disorders. Risk of death increases with a BMI greater than 30. Nutritional deficiencies are also extremely common because the obese person may lack a well-balanced diet or experience protein deficiencies related to crash dieting. Obesity is not classified as a psychiatric disorder in DSM-IV-TR, but because of the emotional factors associated with it, it may be considered under the psychiatric diagnosis Psychiatric Factors Affecting Medical Conditions (Townsend, 2006).

Society often views these individuals as undesirable. They may be abused by strangers and treated with contempt by family members. Even health-care professionals may view them as emotionally disturbed, even though there is no increased incidence of psychopathology in morbidly obese people. Others may view these individuals as lazy, unkempt, and lacking in self-control. Many experts promote viewing these individuals as having a chronic illness rather than a cosmetic problem.

Morbidly obese people face discrimination particularly in the workplace because they are viewed as less healthy, less diligent, and less intelligent than their thinner peers. Certainly, with this kind of reaction, it is no wonder that these people often experience poor self-esteem, feelings of isolation and helplessness, and loss of control.

Morbidly obese individuals often have subjected themselves to many weight-loss strategies, only to regain the weight, which increases the stress on the body. Some studies suggest that individuals whose obesity has persisted for more than 5 years have very limited success with treatment.

Obesity is a complex issue, and any weight-loss program needs to include a multidisciplinary approach. Successful weight-loss programs need to include medically supervised diet and exercise programs, and emotional and social support. When these measures have been unsuccessful, some people pursue surgical interventions, called bariatric surgery. Although many types of surgery for obesity have been tried, the most successful today is the vertical band gastroplasty, in which a smaller stomach pouch is created through gastric stapling (Weber & Clavien, 2006). Another procedure is the lap band adjustable gastric banding system which is done laparoscopically. An access port is created to adjust the band to restrict or increase food intake. These procedures are generally considered only for people with a BMI greater than 40 or those with BMI over 35 with serious medical complications related to weight.

Some educators have noted that fewer than 50% of health-care professionals advise obese patients to lose weight (Goldsmith, 2000). Some reasons for this low percentage include discomfort about addressing the subject, lack of time to talk with the client, and a belief that this recommendation will not make any difference. Yet a client is three times more likely to try to lose weight if he or she is advised to by a health-care professional. However, extremely obese people may avoid regular medical care because of shame about their weight.

ETIOLOGY

Extreme obesity is a complex problem, and its etiology is probably multifactoral. Most often it begins early in life.

The *biological* view considers that early onset is related to childhood development of large-size adipose or fat cells. The cellular hypertrophy results from increased food intake and decreased energy expenditure. Other factors may include impaired hunger-satiety mechanism in the hypothalamus and endocrine disorders, leading to slower metabolism or changes in insulin or cortisol production. The set point theory focuses on the body as being programmed to maintain a certain level of fat stores. This could explain why some people gain weight so easily. *Genetic* studies have found that 60% of obese subjects have at least one or both obese parents (Galzis & Kempe, 1989). A protein called leptin has been identified to contribute to delayed satiety in some people.

Psychoanalytical theory views obesity as an expression of an intrapsychic conflict that occurred during the oral stage of psychosexual development. Unmet needs and stress in an infant can lead to overeating to decrease anxiety, express hostility, and compensate for lack of love. Unmet oral needs may contribute to behaviors such as being demanding and impatient. Weight can provide a shield against intimacy. This can explain why individuals who lose large amounts of weight without adequate psychological support may experience intense anxiety and feelings of vulnerability.

Learning theory looks at how overeating occurs in response to tension, stress, or boredom. This can be a learned behavior from childhood, when parents used food as a source of reward and attention. Increased obesity has also been found in people with a history of sexual trauma. Large size can be an unconscious mechanism for defense against an abuser. Binge-eating disorders may also be present. These individuals may use food as escape from stress and depression. Problems with bingeing are the most common reason for seeking counseling associated with being overweight.

Sociocultural factors must be included because food and eating are such important parts of our society. Social customs are often centered on food. Mealtimes may be an important part of family life and family traditions.

RELATED CLINICAL CONCERNS

Sedentary lifestyle, possibly related to a medical condition that limits mobility, is a significant factor in developing morbid obesity. In addition, treatment regimens for some conditions may increase the risk of severe obesity. Steroids can quickly contribute to increased adipose tissue development, and some antidepressants, antipsychotics, and estrogens can cause weight gain.

Obesity is particularly associated with heart disease, hypertension, and increased total cholesterol.

LIFE SPAN ISSUES

Children and Adolescents

The rate of childhood obesity has dramatically increased in the past 30 years. At least 15% of American children and adolescents are obese (National Health and Nutrition Examination Survey, 2000). Obesity in childhood is linked to obesity in adulthood (developmental obesity). In addition, obesity in adults in the child's life contributes to childhood obesity. The child may learn to use food for comfort, solace, reward, and love. Some other contributing factors include more sedentary lifestyles with emphasis on television and computers, fast foods high in calories and fat, and reduction in sports programs in schools. Obese children are often seen by others as sloppy, less intelligent, lazy, and less likeable. Obese children are often victims of teasing and social isolation, adding to poor self-image and causing these children to retreat to food as a coping mechanism. Poor self-image often remains throughout life regardless of the person's educational or vocational success. Childhood growth spurts may resolve some overweight tendencies, but other children go on to be morbidly obese. Weight loss in children must be approached cautiously to prevent nutritional imbalances.

Older Adults

A past history of obesity is the major contributor to obesity in elderly people. An increased sedentary lifestyle as a result of failing health or medications, or poor nutrition because of low income, low energy, or depression also contribute.

POSSIBLE NURSES' REACTIONS

- May view patient as sloppy, lazy, weak, lacking impulse control, mentally ill
- May feel overwhelmed and hopeless with patient's problems
- May resent the demands placed on the staff with the increased workload created by patient's size and need for special equipment
- May tend to focus on patient's size rather than view him or her as an individual with unique feelings
- May feel guilty for these negative feelings

ASSESSMENT

Behavior and Appearance

- Binge eating, secretive night eating, hoarding food
- Repeated dieting
- Dressing in large, oversized clothing
- Sedentary lifestyle, may avoid chance to exercise
- May exhibit night eating syndrome with cycle of insomnia, increased hunger, eating large amounts, morning anorexia

Mood and Emotions

- Depression
- Difficulty being assertive
- Guilt, shame associated with overeating
- Strong emotions that trigger need to eat
- May feel hopeless, overwhelmed, out of control
- Unrealistic expectations, leading to disappointment

Thoughts, Beliefs, and Perceptions

- Finds many powerful meanings in food, such as comfort, love, and security
- Distorted body image
- May see self as thinner, possibly indicating denial, or larger than true self
- May respond to external cues and thoughts rather than hunger in deciding what and when to eat
- If weight is lost, possible fears of success or intimacy on an unconscious level when patient can no longer hide behind the weight

Relationships and Interactions

- May lack social skills
- May avoid social situations for fear of rejection
- May cover feelings of rejection by joking

Physical Responses

- Hypertension
- Diabetes
- Arthritis, trauma to joints and back
- High serum cholesterol

- Cardiac disease
- Malnutrition
- Fatigue
- Dyspnea on exertion
- Pickwickian syndrome includes sleep apnea, daytime somnolence related to carbon dioxide retention, and symptoms of congestive heart failure

Pertinent History

- Multiple attempts at weight loss
- Childhood obesity
- Chronic illness
- History of obesity and sedentary lifestyle

COLLABORATIVE INTERVENTIONS

Pharmacological

The drug traditionally used in weight-loss programs is amphetamine. It is included in many over-the-counter "diet pills" even though they have been of limited benefit in suppressing appetite. In addition, they frequently have adverse side effects, including hypertension, stroke, and renal failure. Antidepressants such as sertraline (Zoloft) and fluoxetine (Prozac) have a side effect of anorexia and have been used with success in long-term weight-loss programs. They also reduce irritability associated with depression.

Searching for weight-loss drugs is the focus of much research. New weight loss drugs include sibutramine (Meridia), which suppresses appetite by blocking serotonin and norepinephrine; and orlistat (Xenical), which reduces absorption of 33% of dietary fat. In 2007, orlistat was released as an over-the-counter version called Alli. Both drugs have significant side effects that limit their use including depression and anxiety. Phentermine, an appetite suppressant, has been available for many years and is used in many over-the-counter weight-loss products.

Administering any medications to morbidly obese people requires extra caution because some may require dose adjustments. Some medications may need to be given in higher doses because of the increased body weight, whereas other drugs, such as theophyllines, may need to be administered in lower doses because the metabolism of the drug is affected by the patient's lower protein or higher fat stores. Check with the pharmacist for specific information on the chosen drug. The route of administration can also affect absorption and distribution of the drug. Drugs administered intramuscularly may not be absorbed if the needle does not reach the muscle. If the medication is deposited in fat tissue, its absorption is slowed and onset of action may be delayed. Intravenous administration may be the most effective route. Because IV access is often difficult, central line insertion may be the most efficient.

Dietary

Beginning and maintaining a weight-loss program in morbidly obese people requires close medical and dietary supervision. It must be remembered that even large persons can still be malnourished, and proper balance in the diet must be addressed. A complete nutritional assessment needs to be done. Patients with medical problems require very close supervision to maximize outcomes.

NURSING MANAGEMENT

SELF-ESTEEM, DISTURBED evidenced by negative self-image, feelings of powerlessness related to feelings of self-degradation and response of others to the obesity.

Patient Outcomes

- Verbalizes positive traits about self
- Verbalizes concerns to nurse
- Demonstrates fewer self-critical remarks
- Participates in self-care

Interventions

- Avoid preaching or criticizing about need for weight loss; these approaches will only increase patient's negative feelings and sense of hopelessness and powerlessness.
- Provide privacy and treat patient with modesty. Be aware that patient may be extremely sensitive to having body parts exposed.
- Have extra help available before turning or ambulating a patient to prevent falling and help patient feel more secure.
- Have adequate-sized and reinforced equipment such as wheelchairs and beds to avoid embarrassment of squeezing patient in to accommodate your equipment. Check to see if patient has own custom wheelchair. Have family bring clothing from home if hospital gowns are inadequate.
- Recognize that patient may feel very anxious about being stared at by strangers, particularly in a hospital situation. Prepare other departments for patient's appearance and needs.
- Listen for cues as to how patient views self and appearance. If patient makes self-deprecating remarks, explore these feelings. Focus on positive traits other than body size. Patient does not need to be reminded of his or her large size.
- Give patient the opportunity to share feelings. He or she needs to be viewed as an individual and encouraged to identify feelings.
- Explore use of makeup, hairstyle, and dress, as appropriate, to increase feelings of self-esteem.

- Encourage the patient's participation in treatment plan to avoid passivity. Provide encouragement to make decisions about all aspects of care. Work with patient to problem-solve ways to maintain participation.
- Assess patient's support system and encourage his or her involvement.

NUTRITION, IMBALANCED: MORE THAN BODY REQUIREMENTS evidenced by morbid obesity related to excessive intake, emotional factors, or altered health maintenance.

Patient Outcomes

- Begins to identify feelings or thoughts that contribute to overeating
- Demonstrates changes in eating patterns
- Identifies one short-term goal to attain
- Demonstrates nonfood-related coping mechanisms

Interventions

- Assess patient's condition and priorities of care before assuming that treatment plan should include weight loss. Patient must be involved in deciding if weight loss is a realistic objective at this time. Patient motivation is essential to the success of a weight-loss program.
- Obtain baseline weight. Identify scales adequate to handle patient's weight beforehand. Also, consider using two scales or, in the hospital setting, use a bed with adequate built-in scales.
- Assess the patient's eating patterns and typical daily intake. Provide a supportive environment so that patient can feel secure to be honest. Recognize that patient may feel need to minimize his or her intake.
- Assess patient's knowledge level about eating patterns. Be alert to beliefs held about weight and weight loss by patient and family. For instance, patient may say that the entire family is "fat" or "it's genetic."
- Assess skin and mobility. Patient may be prone to skin breakdown and complications related to poor mobility or hygiene.
- Identify coping mechanisms to deal with stress and anger that do not involve food, such as taking a walk, deep breathing, or talking to a friend. Give patient feedback on alternative coping mechanisms and identify the link between stress and desire to eat.
- Focus on short-term goals to identify successes in weight loss or improved mobility. Help the patient identify nonfood rewards when goals are met.
- For the patient at home, explain that removing easily accessible high-fat and high-calorie foods from the house will lessen temptation.
- Assess family involvement. Recognize that family can consciously or unconsciously sabotage weight-loss plans by exposing patient to old eating habits. Encourage the family to eat foods similar to those eaten by the patient for shared meals.

ALTERNATE NURSING DIAGNOSES

Activity Intolerance
Body Image, Disturbed
Coping, Ineffective
Gas Exchange, Impaired
Health Maintenance, Ineffective
Noncompliance

WHEN TO CALL FOR HELP

- Patient experiences serious complications from diabetes, hypertension, or heart disease.
- Patient expresses desire to start a potentially dangerous quick weight loss program.
- Patient exhibits signs of severe depression or self-destructive behaviors.
- Patient demonstrates signs of substance abuse.

WHO TO CALL FOR HELP

- Weight loss specialists
- Internist
- Psychiatric Team
- Social Worker

PATIENT AND FAMILY EDUCATION

- Provide information on starting an exercise and weight-loss program.
- Strongly encourage patient to maintain medical supervision for any weight-loss or exercise program.
- Provide information on behavior techniques for weight loss, such as eating slowly and serving smaller portions.
- Teach patient to become more aware of body signals of hunger and satiety.
- Teach appropriate exercises within patient's ability. Explain that even minimal exercise, such as short walks several times a day, can help reduce weight and promote health.
- Teach patient how to monitor for possible complications such as diabetes and cardiac problems.
- Give family information on weight loss, nutrition, and ways to support patient's health.

- Consider focusing education on reducing medical complications and increasing activity rather than just weight loss.
- Teach coping mechanisms to reduce anxiety that do not involve food.
- Encourage patient to continue in psychosocial support program after weight loss is achieved to learn skills to deal with new image.

CHARTING TIPS

- Document baseline weight, mobility, and skin condition.
- Document response to activity.
- Document eating patterns.
- Note coping mechanisms in response to stress.
- Note indications of motivation regarding treatment.

COMMUNITY-BASED CARE

- Provide referral information to support groups such as Weight Watchers or Overeaters Anonymous as appropriate.
- Encourage nutritional and medical follow-up.
- Assess whether patient needs assistance with transportation to medical care.
- Provide information to home health agency or other health-care providers on patient's special equipment needs and other concerns.

17

Problems Within the Family

Family Dysfunction

Learning Objectives

- Differentiate between traits of functional and dysfunctional families.
- Discuss the role of systems theory related to the family.
- Describe the signs of caregiver role strain.
- Identify effective nursing interventions to help the family cope with the illness of one of its members.

Glossary

Extended family – *Family network beyond family of origin, including step-parents, grandparents, aunts and uncles, and others.*

Family – *Two or more individuals who depend on one another for emotional, physical, and economic support*

Family dysfunction – *A family that develops ways of interacting with one another that leads to impaired functioning, both among the members and outside the family boundaries.*

Family of origin – *Family into which one is born or adopted.*

As the basic unit of society, the family is the most important influence on shaping who we become. The traditional nuclear family, with two parents and child or children, has undergone tremendous changes in the last few decades, and some of these changes will affect generations to come. Changes from 20 years ago include increased likelihood to be smaller, presence of multiple wage earners, required child care assistance, and the presence of stepchildren. According to the most recent U.S. census data available, less than 25% of all U.S. families fit the description of a traditional nuclear family. This is down from 44% in 1960. The 2000 U.S. census showed a 25% increase in female single-parent households and a 62% increase in male single-parent households since the 1990 census. Single-parent households represent the single biggest change in U.S. family life. Changing economic needs, changes in women's and men's roles, and a decreased tendency to accept unsatisfactory relationships have contributed to a high divorce rate and significant changes in family structures. Economic changes in the United States have been a major contributor to the changing American family. This is seen in more women working, the need for childcare, young adults still living with their parents, and senior adults moving in together or with other family members (Casper & Haaga, 2005).

Another new trend is the great increase of never married mothers (Casper & Haaga, 2005). Single-parent households, stepfamilies, childless couples, and a variety of combinations of cohabiting individuals are increasing. These new family constellations are increasingly accepted in our society (Friedman, 1998; Thornton & Young-DeMarcko, 2001; Harmon Hanson, 2005). The increasing presence of immigrants from a variety of countries also influences families with linguistic diversity and cultural conflicts between generations.

Stresses caused by relationship adjustments can influence one's health status. Also, a change in the health of any member of the family can create family disorganization or even a crisis when roles, patterns, or routines must be restructured. Anger, guilt, and denial may all occur as the members try to adapt.

Even in families that function satisfactorily, an illness may cause a tremendous crisis as the family shifts life patterns to meet the demands created by the illness. A family member may need to take on the added demands of being a caregiver to an ill person at the same time as he or she is handling other major family responsibilities. Even the healthiest functioning family may enter a crisis period in response to a devastating illness or death. Relatives may need to move in, which changes the social structure of the family, or the family may need to outlay large amounts of money to provide extended care, affecting the family's future goals. Changes in health of parents and siblings from one's family of origin and extended family may require helping with caregiving.

Because of the impact illness has on the family and the family members have on the patient's recovery, members need to be involved in the patient's treatment plan. Family response can represent a major source of stress to the nurse as family conflicts and dynamics are acted out. Family members' own fears, lack of sleep, conflicts with each other, and loss of emotional support can all contribute to their sense of isolation and possible mistrust of healthcare professionals.

ETIOLOGY

Bowen's *family system theory*, developed in the 1950s, views the family as a homeostatic system of relationships. This theory remains generally accepted. A change in functioning of one member results in compensatory changes in the other members in an attempt to maintain equilibrium. For example, when a family member becomes ill, other members will adapt to fill the roles of the ill member while he or she is sick. The family system is always changing as it adapts to internal and external stimuli in its attempt to remain stable.

All families have unwritten, covertly expressed rules, such as "conflict is wrong," and roles, such as "Dad makes the final decision." These covert roles are often more obvious when the family copes with stress and often requires an enormous amount of adjustment when roles must be reversed. For example, if the father, who makes all the decisions, becomes ill, a normally dependent member may accept more of the decision-making responsibilities, reversing the established roles. If past relationship problems do not support the changes, family members may exhibit unhealthy behaviors such as anger (possibly directed at the hospital staff) and guilt. The illness can also exacerbate any relationship problems among other family members.

In stressful situations, family members may exhibit behaviors that seem to temporarily help the relationship while they focus on the current crisis, reducing the anxiety and intensity of existing relationship problems. Some of these attempts at solutions can create more stress for a family member. At times, one member is identified as the "problem" and the rest of the family focus attention on that member and his or her problem. This is called scapegoating and allows the family to avoid confronting the real conflicts within the family. For example, parents with marital relationship problems may focus their attention on their child's behavior problems rather than their own.

Breakdown in family function occurs when dysfunctional communication is predominant and rules of communication are ambiguous (Goldenberg & Goldenberg, 2004).

RELATED CLINICAL CONCERNS

The family can play a key role in how a person responds to illness. Support and love from family may encourage a patient to concentrate on healing and strengthen his or her will to survive. In some families, however, the sick individual may be viewed as dependent and unacceptable, reducing his or her will to survive and remain a burden to the family.

LIFE SPAN ISSUES

Children

The family represents the young child's whole world. The family ideally gives the child a supportive environment in which a sense of trust and seeing one's self as a separate, competent person is developed. As the child grows, the world expands outside of the family, exposing him or her to new ideas, conflicts, and inconsistencies. Separation from this comfort can create an enormous amount of stress for both child and family.

Other outside factors may influence this separation anxiety. Because more and more children are being cared for by babysitters or in day care, adjustment to an environment outside the home may be less stressful. However, if the child has experienced a loss of a loved one, such as through death or divorce, separation may be even more stressful.

The great increase in the number of stepfamilies has created new, compli_ cated relationships. Children must adapt to new family members, yet maintain relationships with parents, siblings, and others. The last few decades have also seen an increase in the number of single fathers and men involved in child rearing.

Middle Age

Sandwiched between caregiving for younger family members and older family members can create added burdens at a time of life when the individual had hoped to be free of extra responsibility. Bringing in parents or other older relatives into the home can create more burden, especially if they have health concerns. However, these older adults can also contribute to the family for emotional and possible financial support (Casper & Haaga, 2005).

Older Adults

With today's longer life expectancies, older people are more likely to become incorporated into new families as they remarry, cohabitate, or maintain some type of group living situation. Adjusting to a new spouse's family at an advanced age can be a challenge because adult children may be ambivalent, or even resentful, about their parent's new relationship. These new relationships can create some major relationship problems within the families and may result in very difficult situations when the parent becomes ill.

The need to care for sick elderly relatives is also a source of family relationship problems. Today, because many families do not have one member who stays at home and has the ability to care for an ill parent, caregiving can become a tremendous burden, both physically and financially. The caregiver may be faced with overwhelming guilt and, possibly, anger. An ill parent may be viewed as an intrusion into a family already overwhelmed with caring for the children with both parents working. If an elderly person with a chronic illness is admitted to the hospital, it is essential to assess how well the family is coping with the situation and how well they are able to care for the elderly person. In the home, be aware of what family members are trying to verbalize. Sometimes they would like more assistance but hesitate to ask for it because they are too afraid or feel guilty.

POSSIBLE NURSES' REACTIONS

- May anticipate problems with all families because such problems are so common
- May resent the disruption in routine that may result when family members want to be involved in patient care
- May feel uncomfortable in the presence of family members acting out their conflicts
- May resent the family's criticisms, which may be their attempt at maintaining control of the situation
- May relate patient's situation to personal family conflicts, possibly causing uncomfortable feelings
- May become overinvolved with a patient's family and experience the emotional highs and lows related to patient's progress and family response
- May incorrectly view a family as dysfunctional if their relationship styles differ from the nurse's past experience in a family
- May feel overwhelmed with dysfunctional family's problems

ASSESSMENT

Each family exhibits unique behaviors related to the normal roles established within the family. Some of the common problem behaviors are listed in the following section.

Behavior and Appearance

- May exhibit behaviors that isolate others from family interactions.
- Change in behavior patterns when in the presence of various family members.
- May exhibit a defensive response to staff members.
- May consistently place blame on others.
- May exhibit a lack of empathy toward the ill family member.
- May exhibit a lack of congruence between verbal and nonverbal communication.
- Some family members may be open and realistic about diagnosis, treatment, and prognosis, and others may deny any problem, blame the staff members for the problem, or avoid the patient altogether.

Mood and Emotions

- May exhibit contradictory, confusing, or inappropriate reaction to the situation

- May be unable to express or display feelings
- May avoid emotional situations

Thoughts, Beliefs, and Perceptions

- Family may indicate inaccurate or unrealistic beliefs about the patient's condition or prognosis or one's ability to provide adequate care.
- Family may be operating on the basis of myths or inaccurate beliefs that impede care.
- Family may think it is wrong to share concerns with others.
- Family may focus on personal reactions to the patient rather than objectively viewing the patient's needs.

Relationships and Interactions

- Roles among family members may be rigid.
- Individual family members may do anything to placate others to prevent an angry response or rejection.
- Family may have difficulty managing conflict.
- Family may be in a state of constant conflict.
- Family may pay undue attention to the ill family member.
- Family may appear to get along well when the history suggests that relationship problems have existed in the past.
- Family members may evade opportunities for communication.
- Family may avoid visiting or having contact with the patient.
- There may be inappropriate or miscommunication among family members. Communication may be unclear, nonspecific, or indirect.
- One family member may take the lead in defining the needs of the patient and family, or several members may jockey to assume the lead role.

Pertinent History

- History of child abuse, domestic violence, elder abuse, or family conflict
- History of psychiatric illness or substance abuse
- Recent losses or deaths in the family and past significant losses or trauma

COLLABORATIVE MANAGEMENT

Family Therapy

Family therapy can be an important treatment to assist the family under stress. When problems such as a psychiatric disorder, abuse, marital conflict, and substance abuse are present, a therapist can assist the family in dealing with the current stressor and finding more long-term solutions to their relationship or adjustment problems. Therapists may meet with all the family members or limit meetings to a few key members. Young children can also be included.

Social Services

Social service agencies can investigate needed support services for families in distress on either a long- or short-term basis. They can direct the families to agencies that may provide additional finances or extra help, such as Meals on Wheels.

NURSING MANAGEMENT

INTERRUPTED FAMILY PROCESSES evidenced by inability to meet demands of its members, avoidance of making decisions, inappropriate communication between members related to impact of ill member on family system, dysfunctional family processes.

Patient and Family Outcomes

- Participates in treatment planning and care of ill family member
- Identifies resources available to assist family in coping
- Acknowledges diagnosis and prognosis of ill family member

Interventions

- Identify the family constellation, patterns of family interactions, and family leaders. Assess the ways in which the family members interact with each other and the patient's response to family involvement. Determine from the patient whom he or she considers closest family and recognize that this could be close friends rather than relatives. Avoid making assumptions about whom the patient wants involved.
- With a large family, consider asking them to identify one member who will get the information on the patient's condition and take the responsibility to share it with the rest of the family. This avoids the need for multiple calls for information.
- As appropriate, ask the patient whom he or she wants to be involved.
- Involve these family members in treatment plan. Inform them of what is happening according to patient wishes. Take the time to orient family to agency routines and visiting hours.
- Identify family support systems within the family.
- If family members exhibit disruptive behaviors, evaluate the underlying reasons. Talk with patient and family to determine the cause.
- Analyze the family's ability to care for the patient and what they need to know when caring for the patient at home. Encourage family involvement in basic care needs if acceptable to patient. Involving the family in the care can help the patient accept his or her condition. For example, having the spouse care for a condition such as a colostomy can give the patient a sense that he or she is not disgusted by patient's body.
- If patient does not want family informed of his or her condition, talk with patient to identify reasons and fears. Not including the family may

be a way of maintaining denial. Respect the patient's wishes, but continue to talk regarding the risk of social isolation. If patient is seriously ill, one person will need to be identified who knows his or her wishes.

- If family wants information withheld from the patient, discuss their fears. Point out that hiding the truth is not helpful to the patient. Dishonesty inhibits future trust and communication. Help family acknowledge their fears. However, recognize that certain cultures have strict rules concerning sharing bad news with loved ones, especially a parent. Avoid becoming angry at this situation and alienating the family. The family could distrust the healthcare team and block communication channels.

- Regularly assess the family's awareness of patient's condition and expectations for recovery and future treatment. Avoid use of medical jargon.

- If the family seems to avoid involvement in the patient's care or treatment plan, determine the reason. Consider giving them one task to do at a time to encourage their involvement without being overwhelmed.

- Encourage the family to verbalize their feelings about the illness. Respect their need for privacy to express emotions. Encourage family to leave patient's room to discuss areas of conflict. Use open-ended questions to promote sharing of feelings and concerns about problems with family interactions.

- Allow flexibility in visiting, if possible. Recognize the need for family members to spend the night and for young children to be allowed to visit. As needed, set clear limits on disruptive behavior, and limit the number of visitors to reduce stress and fatigue on the patient. Encourage visitors to coordinate who will visit on certain days and times.

- As needed, organize a care conference with family members to discuss patient's care needs and any conflicts the family and staff may be having. Avoid having too many staff members in attendance because this could intimidate family. Focus on reassuring the family of the care and concern of the staff for the patient. Consider involving physician, social worker, or clinical nurse specialist to help intervene if conflicts continue.

- Acknowledge and facilitate family strengths. Promote self-esteem of individual family members by acknowledging their skills and influence on patient ("Your spouse really perks up when you visit").

CAREGIVER ROLE STRAIN evidenced by difficulty performing caregiving activities, inability to meet other family responsibilities, depression, and anger related to multiple losses and burdens associated with caregiving responsibilities.

Patient and Family Outcomes

- Expresses frustrations assertively
- Provides safe care to patient
- Maintains personal needs along with caregiver needs
- Identifies resources available for assistance

Interventions

- Assess caregiver's ability to meet the demands of the patient's care. Identify coping mechanisms and support systems available.
- Allow caregiver the opportunity to share feelings and concerns away from the patient. Reinforce the need to express concerns and emotions. Give caregiver permission to express negative feelings, such as anger and resentment. Provide supportive, safe setting to do this. Reinforce the idea that negative emotions are normal to reduce feelings of guilt.
- Encourage caregiver to be assertive in asking for assistance. Reinforce that others may not know what caregiver's needs are. This is especially important if the caregiver tends to demonstrate martyr behavior.
- Be aware of outside stressors on family members influencing their reactions. Fatigue and working long hours with an ill family member can contribute to ineffective coping mechanisms. Talk with them about possible resources to reduce stress, including enlisting other family members to help, reducing expectations, and hiring outside help.
- Assess caregiver's expectations. Encourage caregiver to have realistic expectations of what he or she can do.
- Remind the family that past conflicts do not disappear even when someone is ill. When family members must spend long hours providing care, resentments can increase. Encourage the family to concentrate on dealing with the immediate stressor while taking steps to work on unresolved conflicts once the situation has resolved sufficiently.
- Encourage the caregiver to develop a routine to care for his or her own needs of sleep, eating, and socializing to effectively care for the patient. Enlisting other family members or hiring outside help can provide the needed break. If the caregiver is unable to get out, help him or her identify ways of maintaining contact with friends by regular phone calls, letter writing, and e-mail.
- At times families "promise" a loved one they will never put him or her in a nursing home. Talk openly about how these promises are sometimes made without realizing the full scope of the situation.
- Give caregivers recognition for the good job they are doing.
- Be alert to caregivers' signs of increasing distress including depression, suicidal risk, hopelessness, and signs of potential physical and emotional abuse of the patient.

ALTERNATE NURSING DIAGNOSES

Anticipatory Grieving
Ineffective Family Coping: Compromised
Knowledge, Deficient
Noncompliance

Sexual Dysfunction
Sleep Pattern, Disturbed

WHEN TO CALL FOR HELP

- Indication of family not acting in the best interests of the patient, such as taking patient out of hospital against medical advice or pushing inappropriate treatments.
- Any indication of abuse within the family must be reported per agency policy and state law.
- Indications that patient is not being cared for adequately include poor hygiene, pressure ulcers, poor nutrition, and dehydration.
- Be alert for destructive behavior within the family, such as substance abuse, attacking each other, or demoralizing patient.

WHO TO CALL FOR HELP

- Social Worker
- Local Family services agencies
- Child or Adult Protective services agencies

PATIENT AND FAMILY EDUCATION

- Provide specific information about patient's illness and care needs, such as pamphlets, videos, and other patient education materials. Make sure these materials match family members' reading level and language.
- Review with family members what to expect from patient's illness and how it may affect communication and coping within the family. Let them know that family problems can get either worse or better during this time of stress.
- Reinforce the need for family members to maintain own self-care routines and to be aware of signs of stress that may lead to them being sick.
- Provide information on support groups and group education programs as well as appropriate Web sites.
- Work with caregivers to develop routines that will make the care as easy as possible. For example, setting up the patient's room at home on the first floor of a two-story house will reduce the caregiver's need to go up and down stairs all day.
- Prepare family for possible course of the illness and anticipated changes in care.
- If the family is planning to hire help, provide suggestions on identifying and managing possible problems, such as the attendant not showing up for work on time or not caring for patient appropriately.

CHARTING TIPS

- Describe which family members visit the patient and the interactions that occur.
- Document information on family structure, which family members patient lives with, and care resources available.
- Document teaching given to family and include their response to any education given.
- Describe caregiver's ability to provide patient care.
- Document family awareness of the patient's condition and diagnosis.

COMMUNITY-BASED CARE

- Involve family in the discharge plan early in the treatment.
- Consider a home health referral after the patient is discharged from the hospital to assess caregiver's ability to provide care.
- Provide specific referrals for additional help in the home or alternate care options.
- Provide specific information on appropriate support groups, such as for family members of people with Alzheimer's disease, stroke, or drug abuse. Also give information on hotlines or other agencies that may be useful.
- Make sure social worker is involved; consider social work evaluation in the home as well.
- Refer family to a family therapist, if appropriate.
- Identify appropriate equipment that will be needed in the home to provide care (for example, oxygen, hospital bed, and wheelchair). Assist in making arrangements for delivery or refer to social service.
- Communicate with home health agency regarding family communication problems and conflicts that may affect care.

Family Violence

Learning Objectives

- Identify suspicious signs of child abuse, domestic violence, and elder abuse.
- Discuss common traits of victims of any type of abuse.
- Discuss common traits of abusers.
- Identify common nurses' reactions to abuse.

Glossary

Abuse – *Willful infliction of physical injury or mental anguish or the deprivation by the caregiver of essential services.*

Domestic (intimate partner, spouse abuse) violence – *Intentionally inflicting or threatening physical injury or cruelty to one's partner.*

Economic abuse (fiduciary) – *Using another's resources for one's own personal gain without permission or making the victim financially dependent on the abuser.*

Family violence – *At least one family member is using physical or sexual force against another that leads to physical or emotional injury.*

Incest – *Any type of exploitive sexual experience between relatives or surrogate relatives before a victim reaches 18 years of age.*

Neglect – *Deliberate deprivation of necessary and available resources, such as medical or dental care.*

Physical abuse – *Deliberate violent actions that inflict pain or nonaccidental injury.*

Psychological (emotional) abuse – *Deliberate and willful destruction or significant impairment of a person's sense of competence by battering the victim's self-esteem and inhibiting normal psychosocial development.*

Sexual abuse – *Using the victim for sexual gratification when the victim is unable to resist or consent. This includes rape and developmentally inappropriate sexual contact, incest, and using a child for prostitution or pornography.*

Shaken-baby syndrome – *When an infant is violently shaken by the extremities or shoulders, usually out of frustration and rage over the child's incessant crying.*

Family violence may be America's number one public health issue, yet many nurses caring for victims of this type of violence are often unaware that it is occurring within the families of their patients. Child abuse, domestic violence (also called intimate partner abuse), and elder abuse can lead to life-long emotional and physical problems for the victims and tears away at the very fabric of society as a whole. Carson & Smith-DiJulio (2006) note that 50% of all Americans have experienced violence in their family. It occurs in all segments of society. Family violence is often part of the history of violent criminals and runaways.

Victims are often too fearful or ashamed to report abuse, become adept at hiding the signs, or use massive denial to convince themselves that the abuse is not that bad, so that a violent family situation often goes unnoticed by outsiders. Health-care professionals must be vigilant to recognize the overt and covert signs of abuse. Every state mandates that suspected child abuse be reported, and some states are enacting similar laws for domestic violence and elder abuse. The Joint Commission on Accreditation of Healthcare Organizations (JCAHO) now also requires that standards for identifying and providing services to victims of child abuse, domestic violence, and elder abuse be in place (2001). Nurses in all settings must be alert to signs of abuse. Home health nurses in particular are in a key role to identify abuse within a patient's family.

Child abuse includes physical and emotional abuse, neglect, and sexual abuse, and occurs at all socioeconomic levels. Although statistics are difficult to attain, it is estimated that at least 1 million American children are victims of abuse and neglect each year (2006 Center for Disease Control and Prevention). The youngest children (less than 4 years of age) are the most vulnerable and the most likely to die from abuse or neglect. Reported cases of child abuse have steadily increased over the last few years, but many cases are not reported. Children are a most vulnerable segment of the population because they depend on others for all their needs. Parents are the most common abusers. Shaken baby syndrome is a form of child abuse that contributes to infant deaths each year (Center for Disease Control and Prevention, 2006).

Many states have passed laws for safe surrender sites of newborns if a mother is unable to keep her child. Rather than abandoning an infant, mothers can leave the infant at community locations that often include hospitals and fire stations. Many at-risk teenagers who might be pregnant are often not aware of this law, so community education that reaches teens in their communities must be provided to prevent abandonment and often death of these infants.

Victims of child abuse are at an increased risk of becoming abusers as adults. Even though the child may hate the abusive situation, he or she never gets an opportunity to observe healthy parenting or to learn adaptive coping mechanisms to deal with frustration without violence. Other long-term effects include low self-esteem, high risk for substance abuse, tendency toward depression, difficulty trusting in close relationships, and violent lifestyle including crime. An early sign of child abuse in the victim can be abuse of family pets by the child. Children may try to deal with the situation by controlling another being or seeking an outlet for their anger through a more vulnerable victim. Incarcerated youths are frequently victims of child abuse and neglect (National Council on Child Abuse and Family Violence, 2004).

Girls are the most frequent victims of sexual abuse. Eighty percent of sexually abused children know their abuser, and about 50% of cases involve a parent or caregiver (Mulryan, Cathers, & Fagin, 2000). Long-term effects of sexual abuse include fear of intimacy, sexual problems, eating disorders, and an overwhelming sense of powerlessness. Victims may block out the memory of these incidents until later in life, when a major event or trauma triggers memory recall. Exploiting children in pornography has been increasing with access to the Internet.

Domestic violence most often refers to men abusing their female partners. However, women abusing their male partners or abuse within homosexual couples does occur. This is an enormous societal problem. Like child abuse, domestic violence is found at all socioeconomic levels. It accounts for 22% to 35% of emergency department visits for women (Shea, Mahoney, & Lacey, 1997). Victims of abuse may endure physical, emotional, and sexual abuse. The abuse may increase when the woman becomes pregnant if the abuser perceives competition from the baby. The battered woman syndrome refers to the common personality characteristics of these victims. These women are often economically dependent on their spouse or partner, exhibit very low self-esteem, and believe that they somehow deserve the abuse. Pediatricians may be the first to identify this victim because the woman often will not seek medical attention for herself but will seek it for her children. In addition, many times when there is domestic violence in the home, the children are victims of abuse or neglect. The National Council on Child Abuse and Family Violence in 2006 reports that women are more likely than men to be killed by someone they know and one third of female homicide victims are killed by their intimate partner (as compared with only 4% of men). The victim of the abuse may also be the killer in retaliation for past abuse.

One of the most frequently misunderstood factors in domestic violence is why these women remain with the abusers. It is important to understand that they often feel trapped and have little money, resources, or support, and fear being killed or losing custody of or potential injury to their children. Permeating all these factors is the overwhelming sense of powerlessness.

Elder abuse includes neglect as well as physical, sexual, and emotional abuse. Exploitation of the person's financial reserves by family, hired help, or strangers is also considered abuse. This can occur in the home or in residential facilities. Gray-Vickrey (2000) notes that elder abuse affects 10% of the geriatric population. This problem is greatly underreported and will continue to increase as the population grows older. One problem in reporting it is the inconsistency of laws defining elder abuse. Some states do not include neglect or psychological abuse in their definition, so it is essential to be aware of how elder abuse is defined in the state where you are working or reside. Because the abuser is often the victim's caregiver, even including the elderly spouse, victims rarely report the abuse. They fear reprisals or abandonment because they are dependent on the caregiver. Society's lack of interest in elderly people may add to the underreporting. Caring for a loved one with a cognitive impairment increases a caregiver's risk for engaging in abusive behaviors (VandeWeerd, Paveza, & Fulmer, 2005). Elder abuse can also be difficult to detect by professionals because common signs such as bruising and skin tears may be common in older populations. The patient with dementia is particularly vulnerable because he or she is unable to speak up or will not be believed because of his or her intermittent confusion.

ETIOLOGY

There are similarities in all types of family violence (Table 17–1). A family history of abuse remains a common thread, particularly in child abuse and domestic violence. Childhood exposure to abuse increases a general sense of low self-esteem and reduced ability to deal with frustration, as well as lack of role models to learn to interact in a healthy relationship. Another similarity is the presence of a vulnerable victim.

TABLE 17–1
Characteristics of Victims

Type of Victim	Characteristics
Child	• Incest generally begins after 9 years of age • Self-blame for family conflict • Low self-esteem • Fear of parent or caretaker • Cheating, lying, low achievement in school • Signs of depression, helplessness • One child sometimes singled out in family due to being labeled as "difficult," product of unwanted pregnancy, reminds the parents of someone they dislike or even themselves, prematurity (inhibited parent-child bonding)
Spouse/Domestic partner	• Low self-esteem • Self-blame for batterer's actions • Sense of helplessness to escape abuse • Isolation from family and friends • Views self as subservient to partner • Economic dependence on abuser
Elder	• Older than 75 years of age • Mentally or physically impaired • Isolated from others • Female

Various theories examine what causes a person to abuse another.

Psychological theory suggests that abuse provides the abuser with a sense of power and prestige that boosts his or her self-image. The abuser hates the vulnerable powerless feelings within himself or herself and is able to block them out by creating (transferring) these denigrated feelings in others.

Sociocultural views examine the role of violence in our society. With easy access to weapons and the frequent exposure to violence from the media, potential abusers can identify violence as a socially acceptable coping mechanism. Another contributing factor is that abusers are often isolated with limited resources for assistance. Alcohol and substance abuse by the abuser also contributes by lowering impulses and inhibitions and reducing sensitivity to the impact of their behavior.

Additional traits that contribute to child abuse include a parent who sees himself or herself in the child, the child not meeting parent's expectations, and the parent's viewing the child as being there to satisfy the parent's needs. At times, a parent has no tolerance for normal child behaviors, such as crying, because of the past experience of being unable to express these needs in childhood. So the child's normal behavior reminds the parent of his or her own unmet childhood needs and unresolved anger toward his or her own parents. There is also a very high correlation with drug and alcohol abuse in this parent. The other parent is usually aware of the abuse but remains unable or unwilling to intervene. That parent may unconsciously deny the existence of abuse and is often a victim of spousal abuse. Stepparents may also be abusers as hostility toward the new mate or previous spouse is projected on the child. Incest in the family may be related to sexual problems between husband and wife. Long-term effects for child abuse victims include low self-esteem, difficulty trusting others, anxiety, anger, phobias, depression, and eating disorders.

Domestic violence tends to escalate when the abuser is intoxicated. He or she often displays tremendous jealousy and fears losing the partner. At the same time, the abuser may blame the partner for his or her own problems. Inflicting injury on the woman gives the male abuser a temporary sense of power and esteem. Other factors contributing to domestic violence include the victim's lack of financial support, belief that the children need both parents, and lack of a social support system.

As noted earlier, elder abusers are often caregivers. These abusers often have limited coping mechanisms and limited support, and are emotionally and financially dependent on the elderly person. Most often, they live with the elderly victim. At times, family members can become abusers as resentment toward the elder's dependency increases, or as retribution for the elder's perceived earlier failures as a parent.

Walker (1979) identified the cycle theory of family violence. This theory includes the following stages:

1. *Tension building stage:* Minor incidents of pushing, shoving, and verbal abuse occur.
2. *Acute battering stage:* Built-up tension is released by the abuser on the victim, leading to more brutal and uncontrollable abuse. Afterward, the abuser often does not remember the intensity of the incident. The victim is often able to remember the incident in detail without the emotion.
3. *Honeymoon stage:* The abuser has a sense of remorse that leads to a period of apology, and attempts to make up for the abuse by presents, special treats, and affection. The victim is finally receiving the love and attention she or he so wants and desperately desires to believe there will be no further abuse. This may allow the victim to forgive the abuser and even drop legal proceedings or plans to report the abuse. Unfortunately, this stage is usually short lived and, without intervention, becomes even briefer over time. The intensity and frequency of the cycle and severity of injuries tend to increase over time.

RELATED CLINICAL CONCERNS

Neurological impairment and substance abuse can trigger the abuse cycle by disinhibiting impulse control in the abuser. Illness may be a risk factor to becoming a victim. Resentments may build from caregiving responsibilities when the potential victim is dependent on the potential abuser. In addition, more violence may be inflicted on the developmentally challenged child.

Early dementia may go undiagnosed by the primary care provider unless adequate screening is done, along with communication from family who may be seeing the early signs (Cotter, 2005).

POSSIBLE NURSES' REACTIONS

- The most common reaction is anger and disgust directed at the abuser. These strong negative feelings can cloud the nurse's assessment and judgment, and interfere with selecting appropriate interventions for the abuser.
- The nurse may feel great sympathy for the victim.
- The nurse may also feel anger toward the battered woman who displays powerlessness. May blame her for staying with the abuser or being helpless and become angry if she does not take advice offered.
- The nurse may feel overwhelmed with the family's problems and helpless to change them, especially if the possible victim denies abuse.
- The nurse may feel intense sadness and distress, which could lead to the wish to save or "rescue" the victim. The nurse may act out these feelings by making promises to the victim that in reality cannot be met or could create an unsafe situation for both of them. This could isolate the victim even more.
- Because abuse may be so upsetting, the nurse may deny evidence or refuse to believe it, especially sexual abuse.
- The nurse may fear reporting abuse because of fear of getting involved, possible legal implications, or reprisals from abusers. The nurse may not want to be responsible for displacing the victim from the family. (Note: most states have Good Samaritan clauses in abuse laws that protect healthcare professionals from liability in reporting.)
- Abuser may intimidate the nurse.
- The nurse may identify with the victim or abuser if he or she has had personal experience with abuse.
- May participate in a conspiracy of silence with others to avoid addressing potential problems.

ASSESSMENT OF CHILD ABUSE (See Box 17-1 for General Warning Signs of Abuse)

Child Behaviors and Symptoms

- History of injury inconsistent with child's developmental level (for example, baby turning on hot water)
- Failure to thrive; dull or inactive demeanor
- Signs of malnutrition, poor hygiene, or lack of health care
- Fears discussing how injuries occurred
- Lack of reaction to frightening events (for example, being given an injection) as child has learned to hide fear
- Unusual injuries such as cigarette burns, rope burns, spiral fractures from twisting injury, bite marks
- Unexplained retinal hemorrhage, subdural hematoma—can be a sign of "shaken baby syndrome"
- May demonstrate magical thinking that doctor or nurse will know family secret
- Fear of returning home
- Apprehension when hearing a child cry because he or she thinks another child is being hurt
- Antisocial behavior, such as lying and stealing
- Wearing inappropriate clothing that covers bruises
- Bruises or bleeding in external genitalia
- Torn, bloody underclothing
- Pain on urination or frequent urinary tract infections
- Abnormal discharge or odor in genital area, indications of sexually transmitted diseases
- Pregnancy in adolescent
- Sudden onset of sexually related behavior, such as excessive masturbation, age-inappropriate sex play, or overseductive behavior
- Child being given a variety of gifts or privileges
- Change in behavior including depression, anxiety, regression, running away from home, substance abuse, decline in school performance, inflicting abuse on family pets or other animals

Parental/Abuser Behaviors

- Exaggerated or absent reaction to child's injury
- Failure to show empathy for child
- Inconsistent explanations of injuries
- Care sought for child's minor complaints but not for more obvious illness

- Demands to take child home if pressured for answers or refuses hospitalization
- Explanations not matching injuries; attempts to blame the child
- Nonabusing parent refusing to acknowledge even obvious abuse

ASSESSMENT OF DOMESTIC VIOLENCE

Victim

- Injuries to head, abdomen, breasts, genitalia
- Injuries while pregnant
- Patterns left by item used to cause injury such as rope or teeth
- Frequent urinary tract infections
- Mother of abused child
- History of rape
- Lack of care for own chronic illness
- Demonstrates guilt for seeking treatment
- Use of alcohol or tranquilizers to cover hurt
- Indicates acceptance of violence as a way to maintain family
- Socially isolated with limited financial resources and family support
- Implies a sense of deserving abuse
- Stress-related complaints of headaches, insomnia, nervousness
- Wearing clothes and makeup to cover bruises
- Denies abuse or gives explanations that do not match injury

---

BOX 17–1
General Warning Signs of Abuse

- Delay in seeking treatment for injuries, minimizing injuries
- History of being accident prone
- Pattern of injuries not accidental looking, for example, identical burns on bottom of feet, identical injuries on both sides of head
- Multiple injuries in varying stages of healing
- Conflicting stories from victim and abuser about cause of injury
- Inconsistency between history and injury
- Unusual, even bizarre explanation for injuries
- Repeated visits to emergency rooms or clinics
- Previous report of abuse
- Patient reporting abuse
- Patient fearful of caregiver or partner
- Visits variety of doctors, emergency rooms for treatment

Abuser

- Minimizes injuries even when they become life-threatening
- Speaks for victim or does not let him or her speak
- Controlling, angry
- Does not want victim to be alone with healthcare providers
- Tends to isolate victim by eliminating his or her social support system
- Insists on taking patient back home even if inappropriate
- Criticizes or humiliates victim in front of others
- Access to guns, other weapons
- Abuses family pets
- Rationalizes actions ("she deserved it")

ASSESSMENT OF ELDER ABUSE

Victim

- Evidence of malnutrition, dehydration, poor hygiene, pressure ulcers, not receiving needed medical care
- Unusual injuries such as twisting fractures, cigarette burns on face or back, perforated eardrums from being slapped
- Evidence of sexually transmitted diseases, unusual genital injuries
- Deterioration in mental status including confusion and depression
- Sudden lack of funds in person who previously had resources
- Frail, dependent, possible mental impairment requiring care from family member or hired help
- Extreme dependency, attachment to new caregiver
- Evidence of inappropriate use of restraints

Abuser

- Often lives with victim, lacks resources to live elsewhere
- Refusal to allow diagnostic tests, hospitalization
- Much younger than patient
- Cashes victim's social security or pension checks
- Sudden, intense involvement with patient with little input from other family members
- Evidence of drug or alcohol abuse or mental illness
- Expects dependent elder to meet his or her needs
- Caregiver overwhelmed with patient's care needs, demonstrates frustration and resentment, isolated with limited assistance
- Elderly spouse with dementia
- Coerces senior to change will to his or her benefit
- Shows no guilt or rationalizes actions

COLLABORATIVE MANAGEMENT

Psychotherapy

Individual and group psychotherapy are often used to treat both victims and abusers. For the victim, individual therapy may focus on the damage done to self-esteem and facing and resolving intense emotions toward the abuser, as well as toward others who may have tolerated the abuse (often the other parent in child abuse). The victim should be removed from living with the abuser before entering treatment to reduce the fear of retaliation. In domestic violence, therapists often recommend that the couple separate for a period of time before starting treatment.

Children who are suspected victims of sexual abuse need to be evaluated by therapy professionals in this specialty. Repressed, traumatic events of the past, such as childhood sexual abuse, may also be uncovered during therapy as an adult. This repressed abuse could be influencing the patient's current life without his or her knowledge. However, this is very controversial because repressed memories have been found to be inaccurate. Group therapy may also allow the victim to learn from other victims and develop assertive skills.

More intensive psychotherapy or psychiatric treatment may be required for the abuser if psychopathology is suspected.

Because family violence is a symptom of family dysfunction, family therapy is often part of the overall treatment plan. When children are in the home where abuse has occurred, they must be part of the healing process. In addition, support group programs are available for both victims and abusers.

NURSING MANAGEMENT

FAMILY COPING: DISABLING evidenced by child abuse related to history of abuse in the family, lack of resources, isolation.

Child Outcomes

- Remains free from injury or neglect
- Seeks comfort and assistance from nurse

Parent Outcomes

- Seeks assistance for abusive behavior
- Demonstrates nurturing behavior toward child
- Refrains from abusive behavior

Interventions

- Establish a trusting relationship with child and parents. Avoid threatening behavior or criticizing parents in front of child. See Table 17–2, Interviewing an Abuser or Abuse Victim.

TABLE 17–2
Interviewing an Abuser or Abuse Victim

Do	Don't
Conduct the interview in private.	Conduct the interview with a group of interviewers.
Be direct, honest, and professional.	Try to prove abuse by accusations and demands.
Be understanding.	Display horror, anger, shock, or disapproval of the abuser or the situation.
Be attentive.	Place blame or make judgments about the abuser or the victim.
Inform the patient before making the referral to child or adult protective services and explain the process.	Allow the victim to feel "at fault" or "in trouble."
Assess for risk of danger and help reduce that risk before discharge.	Probe or press for answers the victim is not willing to give.
For Children	
Tell the child that the interview is confidential. Use age-specific language. Ask the child to clarify his or her meaning or words you do not understand. Tell the child whether any future action will be required.	Force the child to remove clothing.

Source: Reproduced with permission: Smith-Dijulio, K., & Holzapfel, S. K. (1994). Families in crisis: Family violence. In E. M. Varcarolis (Ed.), *Foundations of psychiatric mental health nursing*. Philadelphia: WB Saunders.

- Observe parent-child interaction closely, especially when both are under stress. Observe caring and feeding behavior. In the home, observe sleeping arrangements and environmental conditions.
- Recognize that the child very often will not betray his or her parents. Even in the worst situations, the child may fear losing the only security he or she knows and consequently, will deny any problems.

- Involve the child in treatment plan to increase his or her sense of control.
- Demonstrate support, acceptance, and affection of the child. Reinforce child's self-esteem by positive feedback and recognition.
- If child needs discipline, discuss punishment, and clarify that no physical abuse will be used. Consider referral for psychiatric or play therapy evaluation to better understand what is being expressed.
- Encourage play. Be aware that child may be better able to express feelings through play.
- Reinforce parent's strengths, and acknowledge importance of continuing medical care for the child.
- Reinforce positive parenting behavior. Role-model caregiving behaviors for them.
- Avoid hostility toward the parents. At the same time, maintain the child's safety. If child is at risk for being taken inappropriately by parents, have staff remain in attendance with security nearby and inform the parents of your reasons for doing so.
- If sexual abuse is suspected, child needs to be evaluated by appropriate professionals, including psychologist, pediatrician, gynecologist.
- Be aware of agency policy and state laws on reporting suspected child abuse. Contact supervisor and/or social worker to implement appropriate reporting. Participate in collecting evidence, as indicated, and ensure that proper procedures are followed.
- Be sure that supervisors, physicians, and social services are informed when a suspected abuse is reported.

FAMILY COPING: DISABLING evidenced by domestic violence related to vulnerable victim, abuser with family history of abuse, isolated, limited resources, and/or intense jealousy.

Victim Outcomes

- Acknowledges the abuse
- Identifies options to escape abuser
- Remains in treatment even if pressured to not obtain care

Abuser Outcomes

- Seeks assistance for abusive behavior
- Refrains from harming others

Interventions

- Establish a trusting relationship with the victim. Avoid displaying shock or disgust at the story. Encourage victim to share fears and concerns. Ask specific questions to avoid a vague response.

- Assess the victim's safety. If there is a risk, implement agency security policies, as appropriate. If victim is in the hospital, restrict phone calls and visitors. Consider a pseudonym for the patient's name. For patients at home, determine need to involve the police and information on legal restraining orders. If there are children in the home, determine their risk of injury. Be aware of state and agency policies for reporting domestic violence.
- Reinforce victim's self-esteem. Identify positive traits and coping mechanisms. Encourage victim to talk about accomplishments and goals.
- Encourage victim's participation in treatment plan including follow-up with medical appointments. Help victim take control of some areas of his or her life and make some decisions.
- If possible, identify available support systems and determine their awareness of family's problems. Encourage patient to involve some people who can help. Support maintaining regular social contacts.
- Encourage realistic evaluation situation. Do not reinforce denial or avoidance.
- Be aware that during the "honeymoon stage" the victim may not be willing to discuss abuse. Describe the cycle of abuse to the victim. Give the victim written information on resources to use at another time.
- Encourage problem solving. Challenge him or her to identify realistic options, and reinforce all efforts to be assertive.
- Encourage talking about events that led up to the abusive event. Dispel any myths of guilt or responsibility for causing or deserving the abuse.
- Be sure that supervisors, physicians, and social services are informed when a suspected abuse is reported.

FAMILY COPING: DISABLING evidenced by elder abuse related to multiple stressors associated with elder care.

Elder Outcomes

- Identifies resources available for assistance
- Remains safe and without injury
- Continues to receive adequate health care

Caregiver Outcomes

- Identifies resources available for assistance in patient care
- Demonstrates more effective coping mechanisms
- Provides safe care to the elderly patient

Interventions

- Assess the elderly patient's condition and determine the role of caregiver in providing adequate care. Patients with pressure ulcers, dehydration, lacerations, and bruises need to be evaluated; however, be aware that these may occur unrelated to abuse or neglect.

- If abuse is suspected, talk with patient and caregiver separately. With the patient, listen to his or her description of the caregiver and any complaints he or she may have. Then verify the information, if possible, with the caregiver, other family members, or health-care providers. Establish a trusting relationship with the caregiver by acknowledging positive accomplishments, as well as the stress of caregiving.

- If signs of abuse occur in a long-term care facility, observe patient care routines and the care of other patients. Note the use of restraints and the quality of hygiene provided. In the home, if patient is being left alone while restrained, action must be taken immediately to stop this unsafe practice.

- Provide education to staff in long-term care on identifying and preventing abuse or neglect.

- Recognize that patients with altered mental status may falsely accuse caregivers of abuse. However, every accusation must be evaluated.

- Encourage the patient to be as independent as possible by remaining involved with family and friends, having his or her own telephone, and having neighbors check his or her status regularly. Appropriate independence will also promote self-esteem and self-reliance. Even in the highly dependent patient, it is important to maintain the individual's sense of control.

- Encourage problem-solving skills in patient and caregiver. Promote their abilities to find alternate solutions under stress.

- If patient is in an unsafe environment, implement agency policies and state laws as appropriate to determine reporting mechanism and action. If patient refuses to leave environment, determine patient's ability to make decisions. Involve physician and/or social worker as needed. Consider psychiatric evaluation. Involve family and friends if needed to encourage patient action.

- Determine caregiver's stress level and determine if additional resources are available and would defuse the situation.

- Be sure that supervisors, physicians, and social services are informed when a suspected abuse is reported.

ALTERNATE NURSING DIAGNOSES

Caregiver Role Strain
Family Processes, Interrupted
Knowledge, Deficient
Noncompliance

Parenting, Impaired
Post-Trauma Response
Powerlessness
Rape-Trauma Syndrome
Violence, Risk for

PATIENT AND FAMILY EDUCATION

- Teach effective parenting skills, including appropriate discipline. Abusive parents need skills in disciplining children without violence and often need to learn acceptable outlets for their frustration.
- Incorporate assertive skills to teach potential victims, including young children, to speak up when rights are violated and learn to say no.
- Teach family members the signs of abuse and how to report it.
- Family members need guidelines for hiring caregivers and selecting assisted living situation.
- Teach older adults how to avoid abusive situations by maintaining active social network, and to seek legal advice before allowing anyone to take their possessions or manage their finances. The American Association of Retired Persons has written guidelines to avoid elder abuse. These can be accessed through the Web site www.aarp.org.
- Teach a victim of domestic violence to identify a plan in advance to leave home when needed. This plan should include having a place to go, setting aside money, and implementing security measures for victim and children.
- When children must be removed from their home, prepare them for the emotional grief response that may occur when they are separated from their parents. No matter how bad the home was, children will still grieve. Be sure they understand that they are not being punished.
- Suspected abusers need information on alternative ways to resolve conflicts. If appropriate, refer them to counselors who specialize in abuse and can educate them on the role of substance abuse and violence.
- Review with victims and abusers the need to involve family and friends for assistance.
- Ensure pregnant and at-risk teens know about safe surrender sites in the community where newborns could be safely dropped off if decision made not to keep the infant. (National Crime Prevention Council website can give more information at ncpc.org.)

CHARTING TIPS

- If abuse is suspected, carefully document, possibly with photos, any evidence of wounds, injuries, or poor hygiene. Follow institutional protocols carefully if called upon to participate in evidence collection.

- Document the nature of interactions between victim and abuser.
- Note victim's reaction to the abuser, especially when discharging patient.
- Document victim's report of abuse.
- Document interventions made, including reporting abuse and maintaining patient safety.
- Document any discrepancies between the victim and potential abuser's explanation of injuries.

WHEN TO CALL FOR HELP

- Aggressive, belligerent behavior escalates to violence.
- Presence of abuser leads patient to fear of violence or of being kidnapped.
- Abuser is intoxicated.
- Abuser intimidates patient or staff.
- Victim leaves healthcare agency to return to unsafe environment

WHO TO CALL FOR HELP

- Social Worker
- Protective Service agencies
- Security/law enforcement

COMMUNITY-BASED CARE

- Provide written information on appropriate resources, including parenting support groups such as Parents Anonymous; parenting education programs; shelters; safe houses; 24-hour local crisis hot lines for abuse or National Child Abuse Hotline (1-800-4ACHILD); and National Organization for Victim Assistance (800-TRY-NOVA). If abuse is suspected and patient denies it, provide the information, and encourage patient to keep it in a safe place. For elder abuse, contact the local Adult Protective Services. Many Web sites are available for assistance including National Clearinghouse on Child Abuse and Neglect (www.ncadv.org), National Council on Child Abuse and Family Violence (www.nccafv.org).
- Additional Web sites include www.preventchildabuse.org and www.acf. dhhs.gov/programs/cb/
- Provide information on legal referrals and security measures. If police are involved, reinforce information they give to patient.

- If victim is staying in abusive situation because of fear of leaving family pet, give information on local humane societies that can help with animal care if the victim leaves the home. Veternarians may become aware of abuse when a family pet is injured.
- As appropriate, refer patient for counseling or family therapy.
- Refer for home health follow-up to assess home environment. Inform all referring agencies of concerns about abuse.
- Vocational counseling information may be helpful to the domestic violence victim.
- Anticipate caregiver needs in the home and provide adequate support and equipment.
- Discuss day-care options for children or elderly people.

18

Problems with Spiritual Distress

The Patient with Spiritual Distress

Margaret L. Mitchell, RN, MN, MDIV, MA, CNS

Learning Objectives

- Define spiritual distress.
- Identify some life events and physical changes that may precipitate spiritual distress.
- Differentiate between religion and spirituality.
- Identify effective interventions for dealing with an individual experiencing spiritual distress.
- Describe common nurses' reactions to patients' spiritual distress.

Glossary

Chaplain – *Clergyperson who has a formal relationship with a particular healthcare organization.*

Religion – *A system of beliefs, worship, or conduct. Generally refers to formal, institutionalized practices.*

Spiritual distress – *A disturbance in the belief or value system that is a personal source of strength and hope; may be accompanied by an inability to carry out religious practices, possibly creating even more stress because the individual cannot use spirituality to cope with stress.*

Spiritual leaders – *Officers and persons who provide spiritual support, including chaplains, priests, ministers, rabbis, monks, pastors, elders, deacons, mullahs, or hajjis. There is a wide and diverse range of spiritual practitioners with a number of different titles.*

Spirituality or worldview – *Beliefs of individuals permeate all areas of their life and influence attitudes, beliefs, values, and health.*

All people have a spiritual dimension, regardless of whether or not they participate in formal religious practices. Spirituality allows us to transcend the self and connect with people, our surroundings, and powers outside of ourselves. Spirituality can give meaning to life and impact the ability to trust, love, and forgive. People need to find meaning beyond their current suffering. This allows them to make sense of that situation (Kellehear, 2000). Spirituality is uniquely human; it is universal and innate (Taylor, 2006). One of the difficulties with the Western view of spirituality is that a separation is made between the "spiritual" and "physical" realms. Other cultures, as well as alternative medicine are less inclined to have such a rigid delineation between these areas. Religion is different from spirituality, although it is complementary. Religion gives us tradition, ritual, and a specific doctrine. Spiritual distress is an existential crisis in which the beliefs or values around which the person has organized his or her life are threatened. Various events along the health-illness spectrum as well as outside crises could result in an episode of spiritual distress. The events of September 11, 2001, for many, resulted in spiritual distress, because life as it had been known could no longer be counted on to be predictable. This also can be experienced on an individual or family basis as the result of illness or major change in health. Parents' belief system may be shaken when they learn that their child has an incurable illness or will not recover from an accident. For individuals, it can be learning of a life-threatening illness. When people are faced with these situations, you may hear them say, "Life will never be the same" or "How can I go on living?" The very foundation of their life as they know it is threatened. They may no longer feel safe and able to go about their everyday activities. Some may question their belief in God or other higher power.

Spiritual distress may manifest itself in many different ways. Individuals are a complex combination of biological, psychological, sociocultural, and spiritual parts, all interacting and affecting all other aspects of the individual's life. An insult to one's spiritual dimension can affect every other dimension of the individual and influence the patient's experience of illness.

Spiritual distress occurs when a person believes that life no longer has meaning or purpose, or experiences a sense of hopelessness. Like many other entities that can be viewed on a continuum, spiritual distress may be a temporary, transient phenomenon in a response to a specific stressor or it may be a longer reaching event prompting the individual to question or reexamine assumptions and priorities. In a few rare instances, extreme spiritual distress may indicate psychopathology. One aspect of spiritual distress is what Mary Elizabeth O'Brien (2003) terms as spiritual pain. This includes a perception of loss or separation from God; the experience of evil or disillusionment; a sense of failing God–the recognition of one's own sinfulness or shortcomings and failings; a perception of a lack of reconciliation with God; and a sense of loneliness of spirit. An example of this is a woman, early in the AIDS epidemic, who following childbirth was given a transfusion of HIV-infected blood. The mother developed AIDS. Her religious community was quite conservative and taught that HIV was God's punishment for those who disobeyed God. This patient and her family experienced not only spiritual pain from a sense of separation and judgment from God but also ostracism from her religious community.

In many ways, spiritual distress can follow a similar pattern to the grief response. Grief over small losses may be short-term, and with proper support, recovery will be rapid. Great losses affect the individual more profoundly and can be seen in changes in the person's mood, affect, energy level, interest in life, and somatic condition. In the most extreme pathological grief, in which individuals are not recovering, their ability to carry out activities of daily living is greatly reduced and may sometimes require psychiatric hospitalization. Individuals experiencing similar events such as death of a close family member may respond in a myriad of ways.

Both grief and spiritual distress deal with loss. The major difference is that spiritual distress disrupts the meaning that governs a person's life. There may be a perceived or real deterioration or collapse in his or her relationship with a divine Supreme Being, or with persons who represent the Supreme Being. According to O'Brien, there can be a deep sense of hurt stemming from feelings of loss or separation from God, a sense of personal inadequacy or failure before God and profound loneliness of spirit (2003).

The presence of stressors does not necessarily predict or cause spiritual distress. The Chinese character for crisis, which is a combination of the symbols for danger and opportunity, helps one to understand this. For some individuals, a stressor or crisis, such as a life-threatening illness or tragedy, can ultimately become the source of a tremendously positive experience. Although they readily acknowledge that they would have never chosen such events, they ultimately view them not as traumatic events but as opportunities for growth. In some ways, it parallels a wilderness experience. The arduous physical demands allow an individual to transcend his or her immediate surroundings and experience a sense of empowerment that results in the person being better equipped to handle the challenges of life.

Nurses may feel uncomfortable or experience conflict when providing spiritual support if the patient is religious and the nurse is not or if the patient's expression of spirituality differs from that of the nurse. In addition, nurses may experience conflict with a patient's belief system, as with a Jehovah's Witness patient who refuses a life-saving blood transfusion. These are normal responses to the unknown. How one responds to a patient's spiritual needs depends both on one's education and background. It is important, however, not to evaluate the patient's value system by personal standards. According to Stephenson, Drauker, and Martsolf (2003), some individuals find it easier to describe their spiritual life in terms of relationships and connections and disconnections. Relationships, which were used to describe life stories of persons in hospice, applied equally to others as well as God.

The increased cultural and religious diversity of our society has led to much more diversity of religions in our health-care institutions. Nurses must be open and more sensitive to religious customs that may be foreign to them. Being present for Hindu prayers, respecting the practices of an Islamic patient, and observing death rituals for an Orthodox Jewish patient are all examples of this. Nurses may need to seek out information on appropriate behaviors for religious groups that are foreign to the nurse.

Patients' responses to illness have been found to influence nurses' own spiritual beliefs. In a 1994 study by Taylor, Amenta, and Highfield, oncology nurses ranked their patients as a major source of spiritual nurturing. Nurses, however, may have difficulty providing spiritual care because of lack of skill, time constraints, or fear of being criticized by coworkers. For nurses uncomfortable with religious language and concepts, it may be helpful to approach spiritual distress from a cultural framework. In 1999, the Joint Commission for Accreditation of Healthcare Organizations (JCAHO) added a standard on determining spiritual support services for patients on their admission to healthcare institutions. JCAHO current standards (2007) continue to emphasize spiritual care with particular emphasis on spiritual care for dying patients. Hospice care requires incorporation of a spiritual assessment and offering of chaplaincy services as part of the Medicare Hospice Benefit. Nurses who work or have worked in this type of setting have more exposure to working closely with chaplaincy and may be more comfortable with addressing spiritual distress. There are many ways that nurses can assist in spiritual caregiving as part of routine nursing care (Box 18–1).

BOX 18–1
Nursing Activities to Promote Spiritual Caregiving

- Promote spiritual readings
- Advocate for finding a spiritual leader of patient's faith
- Active listening
- Instilling hope
- Clarifying values
- Touch
- Encouraging meditation and prayer
- Supporting religious rituals
- Promoting being with nature
- Advocate for institution to provide spiritual reading material, religious objects (prayer books, Sabbath candles, incense).

Source: Based on information from Taylor, E. J. (2006). Spirituality and spiritual nurture in cancer care. In R. M. Carroll-Johnson, L. M. Gorman, & N. J. Bush (Eds.), *Psychosocial nursing care along the cancer continuum* (2nd ed.) (pp. 117–131). Pittsburgh, PA: Oncology Nursing Press.

ETIOLOGY

Spiritual distress occurs when particular stressors or life events threaten the individual's belief system and affect biological, psychological, sociocultural, and spiritual aspects of life. These stressors may be unique to the individual, or they may be similar to reactions experienced by others after certain shared events such as September 11, 2001. The crisis may have a variety of causes, including loss of a significant person, employment, position, or status; financial reversal; major illness or loss of a body part, or a change in self-image. In some cultures, it may also result from shame. However, what is lost is not as important as the value that the individual ascribes to it.

Cognitive theory looks at the effect of beliefs on feelings, and psychodynamic theory helps one understand the underlying process of spiritual distress. For instance, a great deal of spiritual distress can be experienced, even to the point of affecting physical health, when a person believes that he or she can never be forgiven. A person's belief in the ability to be forgiven may be associated with his or her perception of how others show approval. The individual may accept forgiveness from God or a higher power in the same manner as forgiveness was accepted from parents because the relationship with God or a higher power is often similar to the relationship with one's parents.

Psychological theories look at the various dynamics that can result in spiritual distress. A person with a high degree of inner strength, or ego functioning, may experience less spiritual distress in response to a loss than one who has a lower level of ego functioning. The way in which one normally adapts to crises and changes will also influence the risk of spiritual distress. Persons who are inflexible may have more difficulty accepting major changes. Similarly, individuals who are prone to anxiety may feel overwhelmed in the face of major change and have difficulty dealing with it.

Crisis theory considers not only the normal changes in life and life event stressors but also looks at the impact of disaster or massive crisis on the individual. Faith or a belief system may help a person to cope with a crisis, but if the crisis is of a high magnitude, the person may feel that his or her belief system is challenged or inadequate and may be of little help.

One of the hallmarks of a disaster or massive crisis, such as a devastating hurricane, earthquake, or crash of an airplane, is the enormous sense of an individual's loss of control and extreme feelings of vulnerability. There may be a sense of betrayal, and the events may be expressed as not being "right." The individual may reveal a sense of how things "should" be, his or her expectation of the world. The sense of betrayal and anger may be expressed in spiritual terms such as "How could God let this happen?"

A sense of mastery over one's environment, highly prized in American culture, is threatened when a major crisis occurs. When an individual no longer feels safe in usual activities, a feeling of unease can spread to other areas of life.

RELATED CLINICAL CONCERNS

Although identifiable traumatic events may precipitate spiritual distress, it is important to be aware of physiological conditions that may exacerbate the situation. Illnesses associated with increased sense of vulnerability and the possibility of death (particularly cancer) may lead to heightened spiritual awareness. Similarly, a patient's moving from aggressive treatment to hospice care may be accompanied with a number of spiritual issues as one's mortality can no longer be denied. Pain, suffering, and severe side effects may affect spiritual life. Patients may also have a reduction in the energy they need for their usual means of spiritual coping, such as praying and attending religious services. Advanced, serious illness may stimulate a patient's wish to repair past relationships and seek forgiveness for past wrongdoings. Spiritual beliefs may support or promote these actions.

Although there is no clear relationship between specific disease entities and spiritual distress, a spiritual state can be influenced by biological changes, such as changes in neurotransmitters, endocrine levels, or blood chemistry. Just as there are differences in coping mechanisms, there are differences in the way in which the individual as an organism responds to illness. Even when an event appears to be a precipitant for spiritual distress, biological factors could also be at work. A complete physical assessment and supporting tests can help determine these biologic factors. Also there is interplay between the physical disorder and mental well-being. An individual who has not had mental illness or spiritual distress in the past, may be affected by both physiological changes that impact things such as moods and a general sense of well-being, as well as the emotional impact of dealing with change and loss.

Spirituality and cancer has probably been studied the most. A diagnosis of cancer can contribute to spiritual distress because the person questions the presence of a higher power, seeing the disease as a punishment for past wrongdoings. It can also strengthen faith, provide motivation for increased use of prayer and self-exploration (Taylor, 2006).

LIFE SPAN ISSUES

Children

Because the belief systems of young children are not as developed as those of adults, children may not be able to adequately verbalize their sense of spiritual distress. Instead, they may present with such physical symptoms as weight loss, failure to thrive, and reversal of developmental milestones. Most frequently their stress is in response to loss of a parent or caretaker or a major change affecting a parent or caretaker. The child can sense the distress of the parent. For example, a young child may not fully understand the impact of death, but he or she can sense, and be negatively affected by, the tremendous distress the loss of a child or spouse can cause his or her caretaker. The child often responds by being more clinging or dependent at times of crisis.

Signs of distress in older children may be subtle. Some children experiencing depression may act out in different ways. Behavioral problems may be exacerbated. It is important to pay attention to subtle changes in a child, such as a lack of interest in usual pursuits, withdrawal or isolation, or a decrease in school performance. One of the most traumatic events for children is loss of parents or siblings by death or divorce. Children may mistakenly believe that they personally caused the loss of the parent and may not comprehend other dynamics at work. Children's spiritual or religious beliefs are strongly influenced by those of their parents. More questioning of parental values tends to occur when the child becomes an adolescent.

Adolescents

Adolescents are generally more able to articulate distress, but they may be hesitant to confide in an adult. More aware of the complexities of life and often having a strong personal moral code, they may be traumatized by the failings of an idealized parent. Loss of parents, siblings, classmates, or acquaintances by death, divorce, or relocation can be tremendously stressful events for the adolescent. Youths whose sexual orientation differs from parental or societal expectation may either act out or experience their crisis in secret. Another traumatic event includes sexual exploitation by peers or adults. Even though sexual activity during teen years is rising, it may be exceedingly traumatic for the individual. Teens, especially girls, must deal with the dilemma of pregnancy and the changes it will make in their lives and those of their parents. Teens are also vulnerable to life's tragedies such as the death of a parent, or loss of a peer due to accident or suicide, which can lead to questioning of spiritual beliefs and loss of hope.

Because adolescents are so impressionable and idealistic, they are very vulnerable to the influence of cults and religious conversions. The beginning recognition that life is not as ideal and perfect as they once believed may cause individuals to lose hope and question their former spiritual beliefs. And if they unite with a particular belief system, because of their developmental stage, it would be anticipated that they may see things in absolute terms as "all or nothing" or "black and white". They may be as receptive to ideas that there may be a mixture of good and bad, or positive and negative attributes.

Middle Age

Promoting spirituality in the family and active participation in religious community with possible leadership roles may be important in this stage of life. Multiple responsibilities may affect a person's time and energy to achieve and meet all the expectations.

Older Adults

Later life is a period characterized by extremes. There is tremendous variety in functioning. For some, a significant change in physical or sensory functioning may affect their view of self and their spiritual beliefs. Many individuals experience the death of a spouse and friends and changes in residence. Some may depend more on their spiritual life as their acquaintances diminish and limitations grow. Spiritual distress in older people often includes questions regarding the afterlife, values, and reflections on the satisfaction and accomplishments of their lives. Forgiveness related to past wrongdoings by themselves or others may become more important.

Religious teachings from childhood may become more important for some in later years as people face changes and losses. However, sometimes attending worship services and participating in religious practices may be more difficult to accomplish because of illness and fatigue or because of changes in mobility or logistics of transportation. It may be that with age they do not have the same level of independence and autonomy that they had during their younger years. The later years can be difficult for those who have not had any particular religious beliefs and have not been affiliated with any religious body.

POSSIBLE NURSES' REACTIONS

- May not feel comfortable or adequately prepared to help patients with spiritual concerns.
- May be influenced by their own background, beliefs, values, and experiences, which may differ from those of the patient.
- May react negatively or judgmentally, or distance themselves from patients whose beliefs, practices, lifestyles, or cultures differ from their own.
- May focus attention on religious content rather than assessing other issues that may be the cause of anxiety.
- May attempt to change or argue with religious content of patient's beliefs.
- May confuse religious with spiritual beliefs.
- May feel powerless when unable to help patients with spiritual concerns. Nurses may distance themselves from patients to cope with their own feelings of inadequacy.
- May not understand the meaning of the loss from the patient's spiritual perspective and may try to reassure the patient in ways that are not effective or meaningful.
- May resent clergy because of their closeness and ability to meet some patients' needs.
- Conversely, out of feelings of fear and inadequacy, may refer patients to the chaplain too quickly rather than attempt to deal with the concerns.
- May reassure patients based on their own knowledge of illnesses and fail to hear the patients' concerns.
- May feel judgmental about individuals expressing spiritual concerns or practices, especially if those concerns are unfamiliar to the nurse.
- May feel anxious when encountering unfamiliar practices.

- May feel so stressed, overworked, or overwhelmed by the physical needs of the patient or their own workload that they do not consider the spiritual dimension.
- May have trouble setting personal limits on the role of the nurse and spiritual beliefs.

ASSESSMENT

Spiritual assessment is required as part of the overall patient assessment by JCAHO. There are a number of models. One model for spiritual assessment is called the HOPE Assessment as discussed in Chapter 3. Spiritual assessment provides the basis for the spiritual plan of care and for communication about the care provided. The purpose of the assessment is to find out how a person finds meaning and purpose in life and identify the concomitant behaviors, emotions, relationships and practices. Fitchett (2002) points out that spiritual assessment is an ongoing process. As the nurse becomes better acquainted with the patient, there is the opportunity to develop a more comprehensive assessment and possibly revise a previous assessment. See Box 18–2 for suggestions on questions to ask in a spiritual assessment.

Behavior and Appearance

- Often has religious items or literature at bedside
- Frequently quotes from the Bible or other spiritual literature
- May display exaggerated religious rituals or behavior such as reading the Bible excessively rather than talking
- May appear withdrawn and preoccupied with own beliefs, unable to focus on conversations and events in immediate environment
- Makes constant reference to religious themes in conversation
- Asks frequent questions such as "Is this God's will?" or "Why is God letting me suffer?"
- Lethargic; may exhibit a lack of interest in surroundings
- May be overtly or passively suicidal
- Frequently questions others about their spiritual beliefs
- States that spiritual beliefs are no longer comforting
- Behavior changes, such as increased alcohol use or acting out

Mood and Emotions

- Highly anxious
- Denies emotions or concerns

BOX 18–2
Assessing for Spiritual Beliefs

Initial Assessment

1. What is your source of strength and hope and meaning?
2. What is your religious affiliation, and how important is this in your life? Any recent changes?
3. Is there a clergy person available to you while in the hospital?
4. Are there any religious or spiritual practices that are important to you while in the hospital?
5. Are there any religious or spiritual articles that are important to you while in the hospital?
6. Is there any spiritual literature that is important to you while in the hospital? Is there any religious music which is particularly significant to you?

Advanced Assessment

1. Has being sick or in the hospital made any difference in your feelings toward God or in your beliefs?
2. What has bothered you the most about being sick or in the hospital?
3. What helps you the most when you are afraid or in need of special help?
4. What religious or spiritual idea or concept is most important to you?
5. What did your family believe? What was meaningful and important to them?
6. What exposure, if any, did you have to religious or spiritual beliefs as a child? Has that changed? How?
7. Have your religious interests arisen gradually or out of a crisis?
8. Do you have special religious leaders? How do you view them?
9. What would help you maintain your spirituality?
10. Does prayer provide comfort for you? If you pray, about what do you pray? When do you pray?
11. What happens when you pray or meditate?

- Expresses bitterness or anger over perceived abandonment by God or belief that God is causing the suffering
- Appears depressed
- Expresses feelings of helplessness or hopelessness
- Does not derive enjoyment and satisfaction from formerly pleasurable activities

Thoughts, Beliefs, and Perceptions

- Believes that nothing can help
- Exhibits global, all-or-nothing thinking

- Believes that life is overwhelming and that he or she cannot continue living
- Questions long-held beliefs and may doubt his or her faith
- Believes that he or she has committed sins that cannot be forgiven
- Believes they may be separated from God or a higher power
- Is self-absorbed in own belief system
- Views self as guilty and in need of punishment
- Views self as spiritually superior to others
- Believes that a higher power requires suffering and pain and therefore refuses pain control measures
- Views self as having a great mission to accomplish
- Claims to hear voices of God, Moses, or other religious figures
- Holds omnipotent view of self—a specialness that rests in the inability to be forgiven by God or higher power

Relationships and Interactions

- Feels isolated and alone even in the presence of others
- May be so preoccupied that they are unable to interact with others
- Withdraws from others who do not share similar beliefs
- May experience change in relationship with family or friends who are involved with religious beliefs
- May seek out members of similar religious group for support, caregiving

Physical Responses

- Reports increased discomforts
- Change in eating or sleeping patterns
- May have increase of somatic symptoms and medication-seeking behaviors

Pertinent History

- Involved in specific religious groups, cults, or a variety of different religious groups
- History of emotional disorders or emotionally charged previous situations, such as abortion or catastrophic events

COLLABORATIVE MANAGEMENT

Chaplaincy/Clergy

Some health-care agencies have full-time chaplains on staff. Others may have volunteer chaplains or links to clergy in the community. Chaplains provide spiritual counseling and are often knowledgeable about community support resources that may be useful for the patient. Working with the social workers, they can help in making funeral arrangements or locating needed services or volunteers.

Chaplains can help both patients and staff members to find ways to cope with the problem situation. However, not all patients hold clergy in high regard. Some can talk about spiritual concerns more effectively to a nurse. Others may view clergy negatively or with suspicion or fear that they are associated only with bad news, depending on previous life experiences. Also, depending on the situation, the patient may prefer to share concerns with a chaplain other than the one associated with the place where he or she worships.

Clergy are restricted as to what information they can share with nursing staff and others. Like mental health professionals and lawyers, clergy are bound by professional ethics and law regarding what they may reveal of anything told to them in confidence.

Pharmacological

Psychoactive substances can influence mood and consequently the way in which the individual perceives the situation and how well he or she functions in responding to it. This can contribute to spiritual distress. Nurses need to be aware of the many prescription drugs that have such effects, such as beta-blockers, steroids, antihypertensives, immunosuppressants, and chemotherapy. Patient's spiritual or religious beliefs may also influence their acceptance of some medications such as analgesics and psychotropics. Individuals may believe that these medications could block their access to their higher power.

NURSING MANAGEMENT

SPIRITUAL DISTRESS evidenced by questioning beliefs, despair, hopelessness, or inability to practice beliefs related to suffering, illness, or hospitalization.

Patient Outcomes

- Verbalizes "I feel better," "I feel relieved," "I feel at peace," or similar statements
- Demonstrates increased social interaction
- Reports feeling rested and comfortable
- Demonstrates reduced crying or other signs of distress

Interventions

- Empathize with patient's degree of pain or despair.
- Recognize that your own personal values and beliefs may not be effective for others. Be willing to set aside your own beliefs when analyzing the patient's spiritual needs.
- Become familiar with the patient's beliefs and practices.
- Use self-disclosure of own spiritual beliefs *only* to foster patient's therapeutic goals.

- Use questions to determine the role that religion and spirituality play in the patient's life. For example, "The chart says you are Catholic. What religious practices are important to you during your illness?"
- Seek assistance of or referrals to hospital chaplain or other resources when you feel uncomfortable or unable to meet the patient's spiritual needs. Recognize the role that members of the patient's church or temple can play in providing support.
- Involve chaplains in team meetings and patient care conferences to collaborate on treatment plan.
- Promote use of prayer and scripture when appropriate if within patient's belief system (Box 18–3).
- Become familiar with agency policy regarding praying with patients.
- Provide supportive, private environment to meet spiritual needs.
- Be honest with the patient. If you are not comfortable praying, it is appropriate to disclose this, but offer to be present while the patient says a prayer.
- Substitute supportive response for prayer when the setting or timing is inappropriate.

BOX 18–3
Guidelines for Use of Prayer and Religious Literature

1. Prayer combined with therapeutic use of self can be used to meet the patient's spiritual needs and show empathy. A therapeutic relationship must already be established with the patient before engaging in prayer, a more intimate form of communication.

2. Prayer can consist of simply sharing a few brief sentences to express an immediate need or can be taken from a formally written source.

3. The request for prayer and religious literature should be initiated by the patient. If you are not comfortable, discuss with colleagues other alternatives.

4. Ask the patient to define the specific needs for which he or she is requesting prayer.

5. Ask what passages the patient wants to read and how they are significant.

6. Validate expressed feelings such as pain, fear, anxiety, stress, helplessness, or anger at God.

7. Know that prayer can be an affirmation of God's presence and hope for the patient.

8. If reading from religious literature, select passages carefully. Consult with chaplain or other staff if in doubt. Some passages may be misinterpreted, be interpreted literally, or be beyond the level of this patient.

- Work with patient and staff to adapt patient's schedule or activities to incorporate religious rituals whenever possible.
- Allow patient to ventilate thoughts and feelings. Explore what precipitated the feeling of loss. Help patient clarify any underlying feelings of guilt. Help the patient explore and evaluate whether the source is rational or distorted.
- Help patient explore previously held false assumptions and, as indicated, refer to spiritual passages affirming hope, if within the nurse's comfort and knowledge.
- Allow family to participate in religious rituals such as ritual body care after death or baptism of a critically ill child.
- Be open to patient's expression of spiritual concerns. Avoid dismissing practices as inappropriate or pathologic.
- If the patient shares fears, remember that acceptance and listening are more important than having the answers.

SPIRITUAL DISTRESS evidenced by religious delusions or obsessions related to impaired thought process.

Patient Outcomes

- Demonstrates improved reality orientation
- Verbalizes concerns and conflicts
- Verbalizes improved sense of peace and well-being
- Demonstrates appropriate social interactions

Interventions

- Become familiar with the norms of the patient's particular religious group to assess the patient's deviation from standard practice.
- Be aware that delusions may represent areas of personal conflict or concerns. For example, the Messiah complex may reveal that patient has a need to feel special, and dwelling on past sins may show that patient feels badly about self. Focus on feelings the patient is having rather than on content of delusion.
- Use great caution in reinforcing religious beliefs with psychotic patients because this may perpetuate reality distortions. Seek assistance from available mental health resources as well as chaplain or clergy.
- Set limits on time spent talking about obsessions and performing ritualistic behavior with the patient. Make a contract regarding time when you will listen. Be consistent.
- Encourage patient to discuss concerns other than religious issues. Bring patient back to recent specific experiences or events.
- Avoid arguing with the patient about the validity of his or her beliefs. Rather, acknowledge the feelings these beliefs may evoke, such as fear or sadness.

- Recognize that reducing obsessional thoughts or compulsive behavior may result in increased anxiety or possibly even a panic reaction (see Chapter 7, Problems with Anxiety, for interventions). Discuss with the physician the need for evaluation by a mental health professional and appropriate medication.

HOPELESSNESS evidenced by depression, apathy, withdrawal, rejection of spiritual beliefs related to loss, impending death, incurable disease, lack of meaning; spiritual crisis.

Patient Outcomes

- Verbalizes phrases like "I hadn't thought of it that way" or "I feel better"
- Demonstrates increased social interactions
- Able to identify one or more future goals

Interventions

- Encourage patient to share feelings and concerns and talk about what has triggered the sense of hopelessness.
- Maintain a concerned yet positive attitude around patient, but avoid an overly cheerful approach that may inhibit communication.
- Focus on short-term, concrete goals; identify specific things the patient can do now. For instance, focus on the pleasure of visiting with granddaughter today rather than the hope to be playing tennis next year. Make a plan with patient for achievable goals, such as sitting up in chair for 5 minutes longer today than yesterday. Often a patient may feel less hopeless and depressed if progress in one area can be achieved.
- Recognize that pain, fatigue, and other stressors will affect ability to maintain hope. Use interventions to deal with these stressors.
- Seek out chaplain to discuss patient's beliefs to help challenge hopelessness and support a more hopeful view.
- Recognize that, with time to work through a loss or crisis, the patient may be able to focus on the future. Allow the patient time to work through the grieving process.
- Be aware of your own anxiety around patient. Patient could sense your tension and think that his or her issues are unacceptable.

ALTERNATE NURSING DIAGNOSES

Anxiety

Grieving, Dysfunctional

Spiritual Well-Being, Readiness for Enhanced

Thought Processes, Disturbed

WHEN TO CALL FOR HELP

- Patient is suicidal or homicidal.
- Religious practices interfere severely with healthcare regimen.
- Patient becomes psychotic.

WHO TO CALL FOR HELP

- Chaplain
- Patient's personal spiritual leader
- Family members
- Social Worker
- Psychiatric Team

PATIENT AND FAMILY EDUCATION

- Educate patient and family on ways to incorporate religious practices into the treatment plan for the specific illness. For instance, the patient can adapt dietary restrictions and fasting requirements around specific beliefs.
- Educate the family on the importance of patient's spiritual beliefs if the family is not supportive of them.
- Encourage family to not impose their beliefs on the patient if they are different.
- Encourage family to bring in Bibles or religious articles, as appropriate.

CHARTING TIPS

- Document patient's beliefs, especially as they relate to patient's illness.
- Document conflicts between patient and family.
- Document patient's response to visit with clergy.
- Document nursing interventions and patient responses to spiritual interventions such as prayer, scripture reading, or meditation.
- For patient's at the end of life, document any prayers or rituals done in preparation for death, e.g., Sacrament of the Sick.

COMMUNITY-BASED CARE

- Refer to clergy or agency chaplain, as appropriate.
- Encourage attendance at religious or health-related support groups, such as Reach for Recovery.
- Encourage participation in patient's own house of worship as indicated.
- Use members of patient's religious community to assist with home care when appropriate.

19

Nursing Management of Special Populations

The Patient with Sleep Disturbances

Learning Objectives

- Differentiate between mild, moderate, and severe sleep pattern disturbances.
- Identify factors leading to poor sleep and fatigue.
- Select appropriate interventions for dealing with sleep pattern disturbances.

Glossary

Fatigue – *An overwhelming, sustained sense of exhaustion or lack of energy and decreased capacity for physical or mental work.*

Insomnia – *Abnormal wakefulness or an inability to fall asleep easily or to remain asleep during the night.*

Narcolepsy – *An infrequent but serious disorder consisting of recurrent episodes of uncontrollable sleep.*

Nocturnal enuresis – *Involuntary loss of urine at night in absence of physical disease when a child is of the age when he or she would be expected to remain dry.*

Obstructive sleep apnea – *A serious sleep-related breathing disorder mani-fested by daytime sleepiness or excessive loud snoring. Frequently associ-ated with cardiac dysrhythmias.*

Sleep apnea – *Cessation of breathing for at least 30 episodes during sleep.*

Sleep deprivation – *Periods without normal sleep pattern, resulting in irri-tability, fatigue, difficulty concentrating and memory, poor muscle coordi-nation, and sometimes hallucinations and illusions with delirium.*

Sleep disorders – *Chronic disturbance of sleep patterns affecting the amount, quality, or timing of sleep or events occurring during sleep includ-ing dysomnias (insomnia), hypersomnias (excessive sleeping), and para-somnias (abnormal behavior during sleep as in sleepwalking).*

Sleep is unconsciousness from which a person can be awakened by sensory stimuli such as sound, light, and touch. Sleep disorders put an individual at risk for experiencing a change in the quantity or quality of rest and sleep as related to biological and emotional needs. Adverse physical, mental, and emo-tional changes may occur if normal rest and sleep patterns are interrupted. Most people have suffered from at least transient sleep disturbances. Many factors lead to poor sleep, such as the environment of the sleeping area (levels of sound, light, and temperature), the age and general physical and psychological condition of the patient, and recent stressful events.

Sleep was considered a homogeneous quiet period with minimal brain activity until the discovery of the electroencephalographic (EEG) record. With this technology, the description of rapid eye movement (REM) and nonrapid eye movement (NREM) periods during sleep and their association with dreaming has provided better understanding of sleep physiology and sleep disorders.

Sleep research has shown that there are two types of sleep during a sleep period: sleep when the brain is very active (REM) and sleep with slow brain waves (NREM). The reason why these two types of sleep exist is unknown. The sleep center is located in the pons and the medulla. Most sleep at night is NREM sleep; it occurs when a person first falls asleep and is a deep and rest-ful sleep.

On the basis of EEG studies, sleep is divided into five distinct stages: REM sleep and four stages of NREM sleep.

Stage 1 NREM: Transition from wakefulness to sleep; about 5% of time spent asleep in adults; person feels very drowsy; musculature relaxes.

Stage 2 NREM: Characterized by specific EEG waveforms; occupies about 50% of sleep time; muscles relax further; cerebral activity decreases.

Stage 3 NREM: Physiological changes evident; vital signs decrease; gastroin-testinal functions and venous dilation increase to facilitate cellular metabo-lism and exchange.

Stage 4 NREM: Known as slowwave, deepest level of sleep with lowest level of body function. Stages three and four together occupy about 10% to 20% of sleep.

During NREM sleep, pulse and respirations drop 20% to 30%, blood pressure decreases, muscles relax, skin vessels dilate (increasing heat loss), metabolic rate decreases by 10% to 30%, and body temperature decreases. NREM stages three and four tend to occur in the first half of the night and increase in duration in response to sleep deprivation.

REM sleep occurs cyclically throughout the night, alternating with NREM sleep about every 80 to 100 minutes, lasts about 5 to 30 minutes, and is associated with dreaming that is remembered. REM sleep increases in duration toward the morning. During REM sleep, heart rate and respirations often become irregular and metabolism and temperature increase.

The need for sleep decreases with age: Newborns should sleep 18 hours or more a day, school-age children and teenagers about 10 to 12 hours, adults 7 to 8 hours (National Institute of Neurological Disorders and Stroke, 2007). Sleep needs increase during illness. Lack of sleep results in progressive deterioration of mental functioning, physical fatigue, discomfort, and emotional instability. Ten percent of the population has chronic insomnia that is associated with daytime functional impairment and 30% to 40% have problems with some insomnia in any given year (National Center on Sleep Disorders Research, 2006).

Sleep deprivation is a major concern for safety. Driving while drowsy creates similar reactions as if driving while intoxicated. The National Sleep Foundation (2007) reports that a person is too drowsy to drive if they are having problems focusing their eyes, can't stop yawning and cannot remember driving the last few miles. Those at highest risk include shift workers driving home from work, people with a history of sleep disorders, and business travelers suffering from jet lag.

Chronic insomnia can lead to the following daytime impairments: poor attention, concentration or memory; anxieties about sleep; making errors or mishaps at work or driving; irritability; and tension headaches (Ramakrishnan & Scheid, 2007).

Eighty percent of patients with psychiatric disorders describe sleep complaints (Czeisler, Winkelman, & Richardson, 2005). Depression is associated with reduced total sleep time, a shift in REM activity, and early morning awakening. Manic phase of bipolar disorder is associated with insomnia, shortened REM latency, and increased REM activity. Schizophrenia is associated with frequent awakenings and reduced slow wave sleep.

More than 100 different disorders of sleeping and waking have been identified. Both the American Psychiatric Association (2000) and the Association of Sleep Disorders have developed a system for classifying sleep disorders into four main categories (Box 19–1).

The term sleep hygiene is used to describe a holistic approach to sleeping that encompasses many behaviors. Everyone should practice good sleep hygiene to prevent or relieve insomnia, or simply to safeguard sleep, making it more restful and pleasurable (Box 19–2).

BOX 19–1
Classifying Sleep Disorders

DSM-IV-TR Classification

- Dyssomnias—primary insomnia, primary hypersomnia, narcolepsy, breathing-related sleep disorder, circadian-rhythm sleep disorder (jet lag, shift work)
- Parasomnias—nightmares, sleep terror, sleepwalking
- Sleep disorder related to another mental disorder such as anxiety, grief, depression, psychosis
- Sleep disorders caused by a medical condition and substance-induced sleep disorder

Association of Sleep Disorders Centers Classification

- Problems with falling and staying asleep
- Problems with staying awake (excessive sleepiness)
- Problems with adhering to a regular sleep-wake schedule
- Sleep-disruptive behaviors (parasomnias) such as sleepwalking

BOX 19–2
Sleep Hygiene

Suggestions for Increasing Adequate, Restful Sleep

- Establish a regular time for going to bed and getting up in the morning, and stick to it, even on weekends and during vacations.
- Use the bed for sleep and sexual relations only, not for reading, watching television, or working; excessive time in bed seems to fragment sleep.
- Avoid naps, especially in the evening.
- Exercise before dinner. A low point in energy occurs a few hours after exercise; sleep will then come more easily. Exercising close to bedtime, however, may increase alertness.
- Take a hot bath about an hour and a half before bedtime. The body temperature then begins dropping rapidly, which may help sleep after that time. (Taking a bath shortly before bed increases alertness.)
- Do something relaxing in the half hour before bedtime. Reading, meditation, and a leisurely walk are all appropriate activities.
- Keep the bedroom relatively cool and well ventilated.
- Do not look at the clock. Obsessing over time will just make it more difficult to sleep.

- A light snack before bedtime can help sleep, but a large meal may have the opposite effect.
- Avoid fluids just before bedtime so that sleep is not disturbed by the need to urinate.
- Avoid caffeine in the hours before sleep.
- Quitting smoking not only brings many health benefits to any smoker, it also eliminates the effects of nicotine that contribute to sleep loss.
- When unable to sleep after 15 or 20 minutes, one should get up, go into another room, and read or do a quiet activity using dim lighting until they are sleepy again. (Do not watch television, which emits too bright a light.)
- Sleeping alone may be more restful than sleeping with another person. If a person with insomnia is distracted by a sleeping bed partner, moving to the couch for a couple of nights might be useful.
- Take a nap in the early afternoon if needed to stave off drowsiness. But remember that naps can disrupt nighttime sleep. If you must nap, do so for no longer than 30 minutes in the late afternoon.

ETIOLOGY

Sleep disorders are often caused by a variety of medical and psychiatric disorders. Short-term insomnia is often due to stress and acute grief. Some chronic sleep disorders may be due to dysfunction with the sleep/wake cycle.

Before a sleep disorder diagnosis can be made, the patient should have a thorough physical examination; review of all medications (prescribed, illicit, and over-the-counter); and the person's spouse or bed partner should be asked about the person's sleeping habits. Evaluating a sleep-wakefulness complaint requires a thorough history that considers medical, toxic, and environmental conditions, as well as drug and alcohol use. If tolerance to or excessive use of drugs or alcohol is the likely cause of the insomnia, the patient must undergo withdrawal under careful supervision. Sleep problems are associated with a long list of drugs, including stimulants and alcohol. Hypnotics used over a long period of time can also cause insomnia because of the development of tolerance and suppression of REM sleep.

Insomnia is the most common sleep disorder across all ages (NIH, 2005). Anxiety and stress are the most common causes of intermittent, short-term insomnia. Other common causes of short-term insomnia include medication side effects and jet lag. Initial treatment for short-term insomnia includes behavioral approaches and use of hypnotics for the short-term. In the absence of comorbidities, chronic insomnia is now considered to be a primary disorder unto itself. Chronic insomnia is identified as symptoms of insomnia that last more than 30 days.

Sleep lab studies reveal that some patients with obstructive sleep apnea have about 30 episodes of upper airway obstruction each night, resulting in an inability to achieve a deep sleep state because of hyperventilation, carbon dioxide retention, and severe hypoxemia. Treatment possibilities include weight loss for obese patients and positive-pressure respiratory treatments (CPAP) to keep the airway open. Surgical intervention (a procedure to remove excess tissue in the pharynx or a tracheotomy) may be required for more serious cases. Sleep apnea is usually caused by obesity and history of cardiovascular disease is another risk factor.

Narcolepsy is caused by an abnormality in REM sleep. It is sometimes accompanied by cataplexy (partial or complete loss of muscle tone), presleep hallucinations, and sleep paralysis. These symptoms are more debilitating than the sleepiness. Specific treatment includes short daytime napping and prescription of a central nervous system stimulant.

Parasomnias including sleepwalking and nightmares are considered REM sleep disorders. Treatment usually includes use of benzodiazepines.

Conditions most frequently associated with excessive daytime sleepiness include the following:

- Regularly sleeping 10 to 14 hours
- Psychophysiological causes: Transient and situational sleepiness caused by stress, boredom, or depression
- Nocturnal myoclonus, also known as "restless legs" or leg jerking
- Idiopathic central nervous system hypersomnolence not caused by head trauma
- Menstrual cycle–associated syndrome: Increased daytime sleepiness around time of period
- Self-induced insufficient sleep: Related to increased work hours, pressured deadlines, or other self-imposed behavior.

Risk factors for sleep disorders include the following:

- Older age associated with more comorbidities
- Female gender
- Psychiatric disorder
- Medical condition
- Shift work

RELATED CLINICAL CONCERNS

Many medical and psychiatric conditions affect the patient's ability to maintain a normal sleep pattern. Patients with respiratory conditions, Alzheimer's disease, and chronic pain frequently complain of sleep problems. Anxiety, depression, mania, and delirium are also often accompanied by inability to sleep satisfactorily.

For hospitalized patients, institutional routines and policies, such as how late sleeping medication may be given or giving baths on the night shift, can actually restrict nurses in effectively intervening with the more common sleep disturbance problems. Patients often complain that hospital rules and routines are disturbing to their normal sleep patterns. After just a few days in an unfamiliar environment with multiple sleep interruptions, a patient's usual sleep routine can be almost totally reversed, with the patient sleeping most of the day and awake most of the night (Redeker, 2000).

If the patient's physical condition requires intense nursing care, sleep needs will be secondary until physical stability is achieved. However, the need for sleep and its role in a patient's care plan must not be overlooked, even during acute care periods. Sleep deprivation is a major contributor to intensive care unit psychosis. Nocturnal sleep is severely disturbed in the critical care area even with sleep medications owing to psychological stress, physical stress, the stressful environment, and frequent interruptions. Patients with sleep deprivation may become more irritable and display other behavior changes. Efforts should be directed to incorporate the patient's normal routine for sleep, as soon as feasible in the hospital setting (Kahn et al., 1998; Freedman, Kotzer, & Schwab, 1999).

Cancer patients commonly complain of increasing fatigue in their treatment. Evaluation of sleep disorders should be made to determine if they are contributing to fatigue rather than assuming fatigue is just related to cancer treatment (Roscoe et al, 2007). Biochemical changes associated with neoplastic growth can contribute to the development of sleep disorders.

LIFE SPAN ISSUES

Children

Sleep terrors, nocturnal enuresis, and bedtime fears are more common in toddlers and in children 7 to 12 years of age. Sleepwalking and tooth grinding (bruxism) are considered childhood sleep disorders because they are probably developmentally related and usually disappear before or during adolescence.

Children can develop distress at bedtime because of fears of separation and other anxieties. Providing a calm, reassuring routine is important.

Older Adults

Age is the single most powerful determinant of a person's sleep physiology. As a person ages, sleep becomes more fragmented: a 60-year-old awakens on average 22 times each night compared with about 10 times for a younger person. The cause of this sleep disturbance is usually health related as in the frequent need to urinate, restlessness from medications, shortness of breath from heart failure. Sleep disturbances increase with age and change in type during the aging process. Elderly people typically have more trouble falling asleep and awaken frequently throughout the night and early in the morning. They are more easily awakened by noise or other stimuli and are especially prone to drug toxicity with hypnotics because of reduced renal function. Antihistamines are frequently used as treatment for insomnia, however potential side effects of delirium and anti-cholinergic symptoms can put the patient at risk for other problems including falls and urinary retention. Insomnia is more common in women than men, although older men have more disrupted sleep than older women (Schnelle, Alessi, Al-Samarrai, Fricker, & Ouslander, 1999).

Risk of falls is a concern for the elderly with sleep pattern disruption. These patients may be getting out of bed frequently during the night in the dark. It is important to maintain a safe pathway to the bathroom.

POSSIBLE NURSES' REACTIONS

- May experience patient-staff conflict because patient states that he or she was awake all night and the nurses reported that the patient had slept.
- May be unwilling to or feel incapable of doing anything about patients' sleep problems.
- May feel that hospital rules cannot be changed and patients will just have to tolerate frequent interruptions.
- May become frustrated because patients who are awake all night require more care.
- Nurses on the night shift or on rotating shifts may be experiencing sleep deprivation and be less tolerant of patients sleep concerns

ASSESSMENT

Behavior and Appearance

- Tired, lethargic, depressed, agitated, even delirious, depending on cause and duration of sleep disturbance
- Drawn and pale, with puffy dark circles under eyes
- Frequent yawning, dozing during the day
- Forgetting appointments or responsibilities
- Minor accidents, such as dropping things, hitting self on cupboard or table corners, not being able to complete or misdoing routine tasks

Mood and Emotions

- Changes in mood
- Less tolerance for even minor problems
- More frustrated at difficult tasks
- Severe anxiety
- Irritable
- Angry and hostile
- Depressed

Thoughts, Beliefs, and Perceptions

- Minor errors in memory or ability to calculate
- Confusion
- Inability to retain information
- Inattention and lack of concentration
- Hallucinations, paranoia, or psychotic thinking

Relationships and Interactions

- Spouse or partner complaints about patient's sleep problems
- Changes in sexual relationships
- Change in relationship caused by patient's irritability and fatigue

Physical Responses

- Decreased energy for usual activities
- Daytime sleepiness and napping
- Increased fatigue
- Sleep apnea
- Cardiac dysrhythmias
- Low arterial oxygen levels
- Morning headache
- Less pain tolerance
- Injuries as a result of sleepwalking, narcolepsy, or sleep deprivation

Pertinent History

- History of sleep disturbance
- Medical diagnosis associated with sleep disturbances
- Situation or lifestyle events that affect sleep pattern
- Immobility as a result of casts or traction
- Pain, illness
- Pregnancy
- Anxiety
- Depression
- Lifestyle disruptions, such as changes in occupation, finances, or relationships
- Environmental changes, such as hospitalization or travel
- Use of medication or other chemical substances, such as alcohol, caffeine, tranquilizers, sedatives, hypnotics, antidepressants, antihypertensives, amphetamines, anesthetics, barbiturates, or steroids
- Alternative work schedules such as evening or night shift work
- History of motor vehicle accidents, accidents in the work setting

COLLABORATIVE MANAGEMENT

Pharmacological

Pharmacological treatment of insomnia generally includes hypnotics and sedatives used for short periods of time. Effective management of pain and other symptoms will enhance sleep as well. Using sedatives to induce sleep confounds the sleep stages and may actually lead to worsening of the sleep disturbance and to depression if used for more than a few days or weeks. They inhibit other mental and physical activities, such as respiration, cognition, circulation, digestion, and elimination. However an occasional sleeping pill may be beneficial to patients with a short-term sleeping problem (Beck-Little & Weinrich, 1998; Ford & Kamerow, 1989).

Tricyclic antidepressants, monoamine oxidase (MAO) inhibitors, and benzodiazepines are sometimes used to help with sleep due to their side effect of drowsiness. These may cause sleep disturbances when discontinued or reduced. With antidepressants and some hypnotics, REM sleep is actually suppressed and, when these medications are discontinued, the REM rebound can cause agitation and frightening dreams.

Some of the newer sleep medications are now approved for longer term use for patients with chronic insomnia. These includes eszopiclone (Lunesta) and ramelteon (Rozerem). These newer sleep agents work to modify the disruption in the sleep cycle. Other newer hypnotics have long-acting formulations such as zolpidem-CR (Ambien CR) that are more effective for patients who have frequent awakenings throughout the night.

Herbal remedies include chamomile, kava kava, and St. John's wort. Natural products such as melatonin and L-tryptophan are also useful. Some herbal products, such as ephedra and ginseng, can contribute to insomnia.

Many medications used to treat medical conditions can contribute to sleep problems, including many asthma medications, levodopa, thyroxine, steroids, SSRIs, and some chemotherapies.

Nonpharmacological

Cognitive-behavioral therapies, such as relaxation techniques, hypnosis, massage, guided imagery, and even aromatherapy, can break the self-perpetuating nature of some insomnias—"the less you sleep, the more you worry about losing sleep."

Exercise is one of the best ways for persons of all ages to achieve healthy sleep. Light therapy has proven effective for delayed sleep syndrome and jet lag. Shift workers can adjust well by working in bright light and sleeping in a completely darkened room.

Sleep clinics may provide a multidisciplinary approach to chronic sleep disorders. These programs generally provide a thorough diagnostic work-up with the patient actually sleeping at the clinical setting while closely monitored. Sleep specialists may use multichannel polysomnography at home or in the laboratory to evaluate the patient's sleep pattern.

Psychotherapy

Many people are reluctant to seek nonmedical therapy for sleep-related problems. Yet insomnia is commonly caused by emotional stress and mental disorders that can be successfully treated. For those who follow through with treatment, about three fourths benefit from psychotherapy (DSM-IV-TR, 2000).

NURSING MANAGEMENT

DISTURBED SLEEP PATTERN evidenced by difficulty falling asleep, frequent awakenings, and early morning rising related to sleeping in unfamiliar environment, postoperative or ICU care, or hospital care routines that interrupt sleep pattern.

Patient Outcomes

- Able to sleep a satisfactory amount of time and awaken feeling rested
- Able to rest between disturbances for required care
- Has enough rest to participate in activities ordered, including pre- and postoperative care and rehabilitation

Interventions

- Assess the patient's sleep for quantity and quality. Ask about patient's normal sleep habits. Determine what is promoting or inhibiting patient's sleep in the new environment.
- To help establish a sense of security, familiarize patient with environment; walk around unit, and describe building.
- Establish a sleep routine for the patient using familiar sleep habits if possible, such as special activities in preparation for sleep, fixing the bedding, or playing music.
- Allow the patient some personal comfortable bedding and pajamas and other personal possessions, if available.
- Encourage the use of presleep relaxation measures including back rub, meditation, prayer, soft music, reading, or bedtime snack if patient desires.
- Position patient comfortably; assist in turning and using bathroom as needed.
- Minimize use of caffeine or other stimulants in afternoon and evening.
- Provide a quiet, undisturbed period of sleep with comfortable room temperature and nonglaring, dim lighting if needed. Adjust schedule of treatments where possible to allow for uninterrupted sleep.
- Use hypnotics or sedatives only as a last resort or if patient is experiencing unusually stressful events.
- Teach the causes and interventions for sleep disturbance provoked by new environment. If sleep-rest pattern continues to be disturbed after a

reasonable amount of time for adjustment, reassess for other possible problems, such as depression or anxiety.

- If possible, assess patient's sleep habits before and after surgery and observe for behavior changes that may indicate sleep deprivation, such as confusion or agitation. Plan nursing care activities with patient to limit number of disturbances and to increase sleep periods within patient safety and postoperative care requirements
- Have staff members on night shift provide the patient with feedback on his or her sleep pattern and emotional support to address anxieties.

SLEEP DEPRIVATION evidenced by pacing, agitation, inability to regulate one's own behavior related to hyperactivity, hallucinations, and other psychotic symptoms.

Patient Outcomes

- Remains awake during the day
- Sleeps at least 4 hours every night
- Demonstrates appropriate nighttime behavior

Interventions

- Identify factors that increase stimulation to patient and attempt to reduce or eliminate these factors.
- Provide a calming environment.
- Monitor patient safety from falls
- Limit coffee and other caffeine-containing foods and drinks such as tea, cola, or chocolate, especially after 4:00 p.m. Encourage use of decaffeinated products.
- Establish a contract with the patient to lie down and remain quiet for a specified period of time at night.
- Discourage daytime naps. During the day, encourage patient to keep drapes open and remain active. Provide structured activities during the day if needed.
- Avoid reinforcing behaviors that encourage being awake at night such as not allowing eating, watching television, or socializing.
- Administer ordered medications as indicated. Discuss with physician and pharmacist the changing of doses or timing of medications.
- Move patient to a private room if needed.

ALTERNATE NURSING DIAGNOSES

Anxiety
Breathing Pattern, Ineffective
Coping, Ineffective

Fear

Gas Exchange, Impaired

Hopelessness

WHEN TO CALL FOR HELP

- Increased complaints of inability to rest or sleep to the point of physical or mental fatigue affecting patient's ability to participate in treatment or rehabilitation or safely perform daily activities
- Onset of delirium, paranoid thinking, or hallucinations related to sleep deprivation
- Long-term or episodic misuse or abuse of sedatives or hypnotics
- Idiosyncratic response to sleep medication
- Evidence of serious complications of sleep apnea, such as chest pain, shortness of breath, cardiac dysrhythmias, or dyspnea
- Presence of parasomnias such as sleep walking

WHO TO CALL FOR HELP

- Social Worker
- Sleep specialist
- Chaplain
- Pharmacist
- Attending Physician
- Psychiatric Team

PATIENT AND FAMILY EDUCATION

- Teach patient and family about improving sleep hygiene.
- If the patient is using sleep medications, review the potential adverse effects and potential problems with long-term use with some of them. Instructions should include to avoid alcohol. Also patients should be prepared for side effect of memory problems with some sleep medications.
- Review negative effects of poor sleep habits, especially irregular bedtimes and use of stimulants including caffeine and nicotine before bedtime.
- Review the role of diet and exercise in helping enhance sleep.
- Educate patient that sometimes short-term insomnia during times of grief or stress is normal and will usually resolve.
- Promote the use of sleep diary to document symptoms and quality of sleep.
- Provide information on therapies such as CPAP and safety for patients with narcolepsy and sleepwalking.

- Instruct on avoiding driving when unable to get enough sleep.
- Provide information on effective sleep hygiene including websites for the National Sleep Foundation.

CHARTING TIPS

- Document the patient's reports of poor sleep, increased tiredness, or fatigue.
- Make note of the patient's sleep history and bedtime routines to enhance continuity of care.
- Document the patient's response to sleep interventions.
- Document the use of and response to sleep medications.
- Document time patient is observed sleeping.

COMMUNITY-BASED CARE

- Educate the patient and family about general benefits of a regular sleep schedule and offer suggestions for better sleep.
- Provide referrals, as indicated, to sleep disorder centers for patients with obstructive sleep apnea, narcolepsy, or other serious disorders.
- Encourage the patient to minimize use of sedatives and/or hypnotics.
- Provide information about sleep problems to other staff members if patient is transferred to another unit or facility.

The Chronically Ill Patient

Learning Objectives

- Describe some important tasks that a person needs to accomplish to adapt to chronic illness.
- List common nurses' reactions to the chronically ill.
- Describe appropriate interventions for chronically ill patients with self-care deficit, alteration in self-concept, and impaired social interactions.

Glossary

Acute illness – *A condition caused by a disease that produces symptoms and signs soon after exposure to the cause, that runs a short course, and from which there is usually a recovery or an abrupt termination in death.*

Chronic illness – *A medical condition or disability that required long term (greater than 3 months) management.*
Disability – *Any long- or short-term reduction of activity that results from an acute or chronic condition.*
Exacerbation – *Resumption of pronounced symptoms from an illness.*
Remission – *Period during which the disease is controlled and symptoms are not obvious.*

Even though more Americans are affected by chronic illness than acute illness, the U.S. health-care system focuses more money and research on treating acute illness. In 1995, there were 99 million Americans living with one or more chronic illnesses including arthritis, hypertension, diabetes mellitus, respiratory disease, visual impairments, and mental illness (Robert Wood Johnson, 1996). In 2005, the NCHS found 12% of the U.S. population were limited in their usual activities due to one or more chronic illness (National Center for Health Statistics, 2007). In addition, heart disease, cancer, and stroke, which are the leading causes of death in adults, can cause major disability and have significant impact on long-term care, caregiver burden, and symptom burden. Acute illness accounts for only 10% of deaths in the United States (Center for Advancement of Palliative Care, 2006). Death from chronic illness is much more likely. Although the highest incidence of chronic illness is in the population older than the age of 65, all ages are affected. One third of Americans older than the age of 75 report their health as fair to poor (NCHS, 2007). By 2010, it is estimated that the number of Americans with chronic illnesses will increase to 120 million (Robert Wood Johnson, 1996). The increase in the chronically ill population is a result of increased life expectancy, new technologies, pharmaceuticals that prolong life with chronic illness, and breakthroughs in treating acute illnesses such as myocardial infarctions and infections. Another change today is most chronic illnesses are managed at home now rather than in the hospital (Corbin, 2004).

Unlike acute illness, which is time limited, chronic illness is often permanent, with no definite timetable to give the person a frame of reference to plan for the future. Most chronic illnesses require major adjustments in the individual's lifestyle. The periods of uncertainty, remissions, and exacerbation, and in some cases, a slow, steady decline in health can significantly strain the coping mechanisms of the individual and his or her family. Whether the individual and family can continue to cope effectively with the anxiety this creates depends on how long the individual's normal routine can be maintained, how frequently medical crises require treatment, and how easily treatment can be incorporated into the individual's normal lifestyle. In addition, changes in family routines such as caregiver responsibilities, role changes, financial strain, and changes in socializing patterns and sexual relationships significantly influence the psychosocial response to chronic illness. Some chronic illnesses can remain fairly stable throughout one's lifetime and others will decline and eventually cause one's death. See Table 19–1 for common phases of chronic illness.

TABLE 19–1

Phases of Trajectory of Chronic Illness

Phase	Description
Pretrajectory	Individual at risk for chronic illness due to genetics or lifestyle
Trajectory onset	Appearance of symptoms, diagnostic work-up, diagnosis made
Stable	Symptoms under control
Unstable	Reactivation of illness or symptoms become more evident
Acute	Severe and unrelieved symptoms or complications
Crisis	Life-threatening complications
Comeback	Gradual return to acceptable way of life within limits imposed by illness
Downward	Rapid or gradual decline
Dying	Shutting down of body processes

Source: Adapted from Strauss, A. L. (1984). *Chronic illness and the quality of life* (2nd ed.). St. Louis: CV Mosby; Corbin J. (2004). Chronic illness. In S. C. Smeltzer & B. G. Bare (Eds.), *Brunner and Suddarth's textbook of medical-surgical nursing* (pp. 146–157). Philadelphia: Lippincott Williams & Wilkins.

ETIOLOGY

Chronic illness can be due to illness, injury, or genetics (Corbin, 2004). Chronic illness requires facing a number of losses and changes that affect the patient and family. Many psychological theories address the process of adapting to a chronic illness. *Grief* theory is one of the most significant. During the grieving process, the individual can experience denial, anger, depression, and finally, acceptance.

Denial can occur at the time of diagnosis or during remissions or exacerbations as a protective mechanism against the distress and fear created by the disease. Anger occurs as the individual struggles with giving up dreams and hopes because of the illness. Anger can energize the person to try to gain control over the illness. There may be a need to obsessively seek second or third opinions, call information hotlines, use the Internet, talk to others with the condition to gain information on new treatments, and go to extremes to implement lifestyle changes such as diet or giving up smoking. Depression occurs when the individual feels the pain of giving up his or her former healthy self. Experiencing fear, sadness, and discouragement and reminiscing about the past can occur as part of the grieving process. Acceptance occurs gradually and may come and go as the illness changes. If the individual is unable to come to some acceptance, each new limitation will feel like a fresh emotional injury and the person will experience ongoing demoralization.

Poor adaptation to chronic illness can cause noncompliance, dependency, loss of self-esteem, and depression. Noncompliance may be the result of denial, used to protect one's self from having to acknowledge the illness; anger, used to maintain control over the situation; or fear of dependency.

Most patients with chronic illness need to accept a dependent role at some point in their illness, even if it is for a short time with dependence on medication or equipment. However, people who view themselves as weak and vulnerable may become dependent for longer amounts of time, possibly for the rest of their lives.

Because our society values independence so much, adjusting to chronic illness can be a blow to self-esteem when the individual must face relying on others for help. For those individuals who have pre-existing low self-esteem, physical or lifestyle changes such as becoming dependent on medical equipment can negatively affect body image and, ultimately, lower self-esteem even further. These patients may reject others because they feel unlovable. As they become more isolated, they are at a higher risk for depression.

Miller (2000) identifies four factors that influence adjustment to chronic illness:

1. Knowledge of the illness and therapies
2. Coping resources
3. Problem-solving skills
4. Personal mastery as well as motivation

CLINICAL CONCERNS

Chronic illnesses can influence an individual's response to an acute illness and the potential for recovery. For example, persons with chronic pulmonary disease may have difficulty surviving major surgery. The presence of more than one chronic illness often adds to the demands made by even a relatively minor illness. The survey by Robert Wood Johnson (1996) identified the five most disabling chronic conditions:

1. Mental Retardation
2. Respiratory cancers
3. Multiple Sclerosis
4. Blindness
5. Paralysis of extremities

LIFE SPAN ISSUES

Children

Up to 20% of children have a chronic illness, with the most common being asthma (Copeland, 1993). In 2003, 6.9% of children had chronic illnesses that limited their daily activity (NCHS, 2006). How the child responds to the condition depends on the child's developmental stage and the parent's response. Under stress, the child may regress to a previous developmental stage. Denial, overprotectiveness, rejection, and overcompensating are examples of poor parental responses and can significantly influence the child's adaptation response. The child's illness can cause dysfunction within the family as frequent doctor's appointments, changing living arrangements, and financial stress cause disruption in family life and increase the child's anxiety. Siblings may experience jealousy and resentment for the increased attention to the ill child, embarrassment, shame, fear of becoming ill, guilt from believing they caused the illness, or an extreme sense of overprotectiveness. These feelings are influenced by the parent's response. The sibling may also regress to a previous developmental stage during times of stress.

Adults

Chronic illness can be a devastating blow in adulthood, a time when expectations are highest. Many illnesses can impede performance of an important role such as breadwinner or parent.

Older Adults

The most common chronic conditions in the group older than 75 years of age include arthritis, hypertension, heart disease, diabetes, and chronic joint symptoms (NCHS, 2006).

Adapting to chronic illness depends on the resources available to the person, including caregiver availability, financial resources, and living arrangements. Spouses or other supportive people may be chronically ill as well. Advancing chronic illnesses may force elderly persons to move out of the home into unfamiliar surroundings, such as to a retirement home or nursing home. Also, treatment for multiple chronic illnesses can drain one's coping reserves, and the symptoms of one chronic illness such as reduced vision from cataracts affects the management of another one such as being able to give insulin to one's self. Elderly spouses who must be the primary caregivers provide an additional stress and can contribute to poor compliance because of their inability to cope with the illness.

POSSIBLE NURSES' REACTIONS

- May view caring for the chronically ill as depressing because of deteriorating patient health.
- May have difficulty defining care goals as optimal maintenance rather than curative.
- May lack empathy and blame noncompliant patient as causing his or her own problems.
- May feel powerless to provide any hope to the patient for the future.

ASSESSMENT

Behavior and Appearance

- Obvious disability or change in appearance caused by illness
- Unkempt, poor hygiene because of depression and lack of energy
- May require obvious assistive devices such as oxygen or a wheelchair

Mood and Emotions

- Depressed
- Angry
- May lack emotional reaction as a result of denial
- Guilt over burden created by illness
- Fear and anxiety caused by uncertain future or physical discomfort

Thoughts, Beliefs, and Perceptions

- Powerless to control condition, complications, or side effects
- May generalize view of self as weak and ineffectual into all areas of life
- May think obsessively about his or her health or physical condition
- May view body as unattractive or damaged
- May be able to maintain self-esteem and sense of competence

Relationships and Interactions

- May need to become dependent on others for care, transportation, financial support
- May have difficulty in maintaining personal relationships because of lack of energy, physical discomfort, or embarrassment
- May need to change living arrangements to facilitate care, causing the individual to develop new or changed relationships with others
- May experience changes in sexual relationships because of physical discomfort, loss of energy, or poor self-image
- May experience a sense of social isolation or rejection because friends and family may avoid patient if they are uncomfortable being around someone with a disability

Physical Responses

- These vary depending on specific illness.
- Symptoms must be reassessed frequently because they may or may not be related to the chronic illness.
- Ability to perform activities of daily living can be affected.

Pertinent History

- Past history of chronic illness, other conditions, or disabilities
- History of psychiatric disorders, especially depression and substance abuse

COLLABORATIVE MANAGEMENT

Pharmacological

Because patients with chronic illnesses often take multiple medications, there is an increased risk of interactions between medications or between medications and food. Each new symptom needs to be assessed carefully to determine if the cause is the illness or the treatment. For example, confusion and lethargy could be a sign of a deteriorating medical condition or the result of overmedication.

Individuals may utilize a variety of complementary or alternative approaches to deal with symptoms and/or treat the illness.

NURSING MANAGEMENT

IMPAIRED SOCIAL INTERACTION evidenced by inability to establish and/or maintain stable, supportive relationships related to loss of body function because of chronic illness.

Patient and Family Outcomes

- Patient identifies behaviors that deter socialization.
- Patient demonstrates behaviors that encourage socialization.
- Family provides support to patient.

Interventions

- Assess the patient's support system, living arrangements, and care needs. Identify areas where patient needs assistance in his or her care routine.
- Identify types of behavior that may impede socialization, such as manipulative, dependent, hostile, depressed, or passive-aggressive behavior. As needed, help patient become aware of how these types of behaviors may discourage interactions with others. Explore ways to change these behaviors.
- Encourage patient to share worries and concerns with others, as appropriate. Also encourage patient to make an effort to provide support to family members as they learn to adjust. If the patient consistently focuses others' attention on his or her health problems, give the patient feedback on understanding others' responses.
- Encourage patient to accept help from others, as needed, while maintaining independence within the limitations of the illness.

- Address burden on caregivers and provide assistance as needed.
- Patient may need assistance to express feelings and wishes to his or her caregiver in a nonthreatening way. Role-play with patient. This promotes independence and self-esteem in patient and caregiver.
- Encourage patient and family to be aware of communication patterns when under stress, and explain how these may negatively affect their relationships.
- Allow family to share their concerns and frustrations about the patient with you. Explore with the patient ways to resolve issues. If both agree to participate, consider bringing patient and family together to discuss these issues.
- Encourage patient to participate in activities and interests that do not involve his or her illness.
- Encourage patient to maintain contact with supportive people through phone calls, letter writing, e-mail, and tapes.
- Assist patient in identifying ways to establish new relationships.

DISTURBED SELF-CONCEPT evidenced by self-destructive behaviors, unwillingness to face effects of illness, excessive dependency, depression related to alteration in body image from chronic illness.

Patient Outcomes

- Remains as independent as possible within limitations of illness
- Demonstrates acceptance of his or her body by such behaviors as talking positively about self, taking care of own physical needs
- Implements adaptive coping mechanisms

Interventions

- Develop a trusting relationship with patient to encourage sharing feelings with you. Providing privacy and respect for patient's feelings and body will enhance that trust.
- Encourage patient to express feelings and thought about the illness and the way the illness has changed self-image.
- Assess the effect of illness on the patient. Clarify misconceptions, myths about illness, treatment, and functional ability. For example, patient may believe the portable oxygen tank cannot be taken in the car, so he or she no longer goes out with friends.
- Help the patient begin to accept self with the new limitations. Involve the patient in own care, gradually increasing those areas for which the patient can take responsibility. Encourage expressing feelings about the illness and body image. As appropriate, involve the family.
- Be aware of what others' behavior communicates to patient. For example, if patient's wife puts on disposable gloves every time she is with patient,

she is nonverbally communicating her discomfort being around him. She needs to be encouraged to examine how this behavior affects him.

- Explore the patient's strengths and interests. Provide encouragement to focus on these, not just on the illness. Explore ways to develop former interests that are within his or her functional abilities.
- Encourage participation in rehabilitation and education programs, as appropriate.

POWERLESSNESS evidenced by not participating in activities of daily living, anger, and depressive behavior related to the impact from chronic illness.

Patient and Family Outcomes

- Demonstrates participation in care within limitations of illness
- Performs activities of daily living within limitations of illness
- Verbalizes one area in which he or she can have some control

Interventions

- Assess patient's ability to perform activities of daily living and to maintain medical regimen for chronic illness care.
- Identify some aspect of patient's care in which he or she can retain control. Then make sure all caregivers support this.
- Provide needed education and resources to enhance performing these activities to encourage independence.
- Involve family and caregivers in identifying ways to promote independence. Teach them ways to help patient without taking over completely.
- In areas in which patient must be dependent on others, promote patient participation in decision making and timing of care to promote some control.
- To successfully promote independence in an activity, you may need to break down each activity into small segments and then focus on one segment at a time.
- Explore the patient's feelings regarding activities that he or she is no longer able to perform. Encourage the grieving response to express feelings and encourage acceptance. Then explore activities of interest within the patient's functional abilities.

ALTERNATE NURSING DIAGNOSES

Coping, Family: Compromised
Coping, Ineffective
Grieving, Anticipatory or Dysfunctional

Hopelessness

Knowledge Deficit

Noncompliance

WHEN TO CALL FOR HELP

- There are indications that the patient is not being cared for adequately, such as poor hygiene, pressure ulcers, poor nutrition, or dehydration.
- Patient is not complying with treatment plan, which could lead to life-threatening complications—for example, the patient is not taking insulin or is refusing dialysis.
- Patient is demoralized by destructive behavior within his or her family, such as substance abuse.
- Severe depression, threat of suicide.

WHO TO CALL FOR HELP

- Attending Physician
- Social Worker
- Chaplain
- Psychiatric Team

PATIENT AND FAMILY EDUCATION

- Provide appropriate education for the individual's chronic illness and medical regimen.
- Encourage patient and caregivers to consolidate prescriptions with one pharmacy so interactions can be monitored.
- Provide information on prevention of complications or progression of the illness and side effects of treatment.
- Involve family and/or caregivers in this education.
- Teach assertive and problem-solving skills to patient who is dependent on others for much of his or her care to gain a sense of control over health care.
- Review with family ways to promote independence and self-esteem in the patient.
- Teach relaxation techniques as a way to reduce anxiety (see Box 3–2)
- Teach family the stages of grieving and ways to cope with these.
- For patients with advanced, progressive illness, promote completion of advance directive and discussion with caregivers about wishes if disease progresses

CHARTING TIPS

- Document patient and family response to health teaching.
- Note caregiver responses to patient. Use specific examples rather than a subjective opinion of the response.
- Document patient's reaction to illness, prognosis, and body image changes.
- Document patient's participation in treatment plan.
- Document side effects to medications/treatments
- Document patient expressed wishes regarding aggressiveness of treatment

COMMUNITY-BASED CARE

- Involve patient and family in the discharge plan early in treatment.
- Provide specific referrals for additional help in the home or alternative care options as needed.
- Identify equipment patient will need in the home, such as hospital bed or wheelchair, to enhance independence and caregiving.
- Refer patient and family to support programs and self-help groups specific to patient's illness, such as ostomy or stroke groups.
- Refer to counseling as needed.
- Consider home health referrals to assess caregiver's ability to provide care and patient's compliance in the home.
- Communicate with all referring agencies regarding identified problems.
- Encourage seeking out information on the illness from the Internet or library.
- Refer to adult protective services or child abuse services if evidence of patient does not appear to be receiving adequate care.
- Consider referral to palliative care and/or hospice with advanced illness

The Homeless Patient with Chronic Illness

William R. Whetstone, RN, CNS, PhD

Learning Objectives

- Describe the social origins of homelessness
- Describe common characteristics of homelessness

- Identify risk factors to health care for the homeless
- Describe effective patient-centered nursing interventions

Glossary

Community Mental Health Centers – *Funded agencies offering such core services as outpatient care, 24 hour-a-day emergency services, day treatment or partial hospitalization, and screening.*
Homeless – *A person without housing except the streets.*
Homeless Shelters – *Temporary residences in urban areas usually open during the night for sleeping. Some shelters do provide related services such as food, job training and skills.*
Marginalization – *To be excluded, ignored, relegated to the edge of a social system.*

Homelessness in America is an invisible and complex social problem. Marginalized by our society, the homeless include men, women and children of all races and socioeconomic backgrounds. According to the National Coalition for the Homeless (2006), the rate of our homeless population has tripled since 1981. Whereas people often think of men as the major homeless population, families–namely women with their children–are seen increasingly in this situation. Nurses are likely to come in contact with homeless patients in all settings including acute hospitals, emergency rooms or urgent care clinics, psychiatric settings, and long-term care institutions. These patients are often viewed in a negative way by health-care professionals who may be frustrated and alarmed by their behavior (Saarman, Daugherty, & Riegel, 2000; Chung-Park, Hatton, Robinson, & Kleffel, 2006).

The National Mental Health Association (2006) gives the following perspective on the homeless population:

- People who are homeless are the poorest of the poor. Unemployment, lack of job skills, and personal problems contribute to homelessness because the person is unable to make an adequate income. Decreases in the number of manufacturing and industrial jobs combined with a decline in the real value of the minimum wage, have left significant numbers of people without livable incomes.

- Cost of rental housing has increased in most urban areas. In 14 states and 69 metropolitan areas, the entire maximum Supplemental Security Income (SSI) benefits do not cover the Fair Market Rent for a one-bedroom apartment and no state in the nation offers SSI income equal to the federal minimum wage.

- The average adult man who is homeless is in his late 30s; the average adult woman is in her early 30s. Minorities, in particular, African Americans, are overrepresented among people who are homeless and have a mental illness.
- Approximately 40% of adult men who are homeless are veterans.
- An estimated one third of the approximately 600,000 Americans who are homeless on any given night have serious mental illnesses and more than one-half also have substance use disorders.
- Many people who are homeless and have addictive disorders want treatment, but the system is ill equipped to respond to their needs, leaving them with no access to treatment services and recovery support.
- The homeless population frequently suffers from concurrent severe mental illness and substance usage and/or dependency. The number of homeless with dual diagnosis or co-occurring disorders is difficult to estimate but the numbers have increased substantially over the past 2 decades.
- People who are homeless frequently depend on the highest cost public service systems—emergency rooms, hospital psychiatric beds, detoxification centers, residential treatment programs and, in some places, jail cells—which places a huge burden on health, mental health and correctional systems.
- Because men who are homeless are more likely to have substance abuse disorders than women who are homeless, men are more often excluded from emergency shelters because these facilities often require abstinence as a condition for admission. This partially explains why more men than women sleep on the streets.
- Lack of resources for transportation for the urban homeless is a major problem (U.S. Conference of Mayors, 2005). Not following through with medical appointments or referrals to shelters or employment programs can often be tracked back to lack of transportation.

ETIOLOGY

There are many reasons for being homeless today. The causes are complex and diverse. The causes interrelate with socioeconomic issues prevalent in our society: poverty, low-paying jobs, unemployment, alcohol and drug usage, or just temporarily being down on your luck. The lack of affordable housing, whether it is Section 8, single room occupancy hotels (SRO), or low rent apartments are at a premium in our urban areas. More and more urban areas are undergoing gentrification as the demand for trendy lofts and condo living is bringing suburbanites back to the inner core of cities that previously were on the decline. An individual may not have the financial resources to provide first and last month rent, credit card references, etc. to obtain a suitable living situation.

Mental illness and substance abuse are major contributors to homelessness. In the late 1970s and early 1980s, the advent of deinstitutionalization (Lamb,

2006) dramatically increased the number of mentally ill on the streets. Many institutionalized mentally ill (primarily schizophrenics) were returned to the community. Our communities were not well prepared to either receive them or accept them. Community mental health services that were supposed to be providing assistance with social skills, rehabilitation or retraining, health care, counseling and psychotherapy, were not well planned (Treatment Advocacy Center, 2006).

Instead of these services being seamless, such services were often fragmented, caught up in bureaucratic red tape, and inadequate in meeting the immediate and long-term needs of the mentally ill. The trend to keep the mentally ill out of institutions has continued today. Many mental health professionals, including nurses, are ill prepared to provide meaningful assistance in meeting the psychosocial needs of this population. So many of the severely mentally ill find their way onto the streets. The streets provide them the least restrictive environment, an escape from the confines of both board and care and nursing homes. However neither of these latter environments provide them with the necessary requisites for activities of daily living, health promotion or wellness, consistency, medication management, and reintegration into their own community.

Another large group of homeless are the many substance abusers caught up in the era of readily available street drugs–most commonly crack cocaine, heroin, and crystal meth (methamphetamine). Again, like the mentally ill, these homeless lack much needed social, rehabilitation, and welfare services. Service providers continue to offer fragmented care. Somehow, like the mentally ill, they survive; but survival is at a great cost of developing life threatening and chronic debilitating illnesses such as chronic obstructive pulmonary disease, uncontrolled diabetes, high blood pressure, cardiac problems, respiratory disorders, skin lesions, leg ulcers, sexually transmitted diseases, and HIV. The continual dangers of living on the streets without access to adequate healthcare and follow up predisposes them to a variety of chronic and serious health problems. Many of the homeless have a dual diagnosis of a psychiatric disorder and a substance abuse problem. These individuals may be using drugs or alcohol to self-medicate the uncomfortable symptoms from their psychiatric problem.

Homeless families—usually women with young children—are a more recent phenomenon that may be related to mental illness and substance abuse. Women may also be victims of domestic violence and are seeking a way to escape an intolerable living situation. With no financial assets and limited skills, these women may find their way to shelters with their children. Access to services may be limited by things we all take for granted like a phone number and mailing address.

RELATED CLINICAL CONCERNS

Because of self-care neglect and lack of resources, many of the homeless suffer from hypertension, arthritis, tuberculosis, coronary artery disease, sexually transmitted diseases, hepatitis, and HIV (Lewis, Andersen, & Gelberg, 2004). Other common conditions include anemia from malnutrition and orthopedic conditions from repeated injuries. Lack of good footwear may lead to feet problems, poor vision due to no resources to obtain glasses, and no access to preventative dental care are just a few of the common problems seen in this population. The homeless may have little way to obtain refills on prescriptions so routine medications for chronic conditions as well as psychotropic medications may be unavailable. Without psychotropic medications, the mentally ill homeless can become more of a problem contributing to this group being marginalized by society.

LIFE SPAN ISSUES

Children

Children and their mothers represent an increasingly frequent form of homelessness (National Coalition for the Homeless, 2006). Children in this situation must endure insecurity, fear, disruption of routine and education, and poor preventative healthcare. Family life is disrupted and physical and emotional health of family members is affected. Children may be exposed to unhygienic living conditions, violent and inappropriate behavior, and lack of age appropriate resources that will impact their mental, physical, and psychological development. Children may also have been exposed to domestic violence and child abuse. At times, women with little resources need to escape an abusive situation and end up living in their car or on the streets with their children.

Because these mothers are at increased risk for illness and death at an earlier age than in comparison to the rest of the population, children also face the chance of being alone on the streets or moved into foster care (Lewis et al., 2004).

Adolescents

The Center for Law and Social Policy (2003) estimates the homeless adolescent population can range from 500,000 to 1.3 million per year. The U.S. Conference of Mayors (2005) indicated that 3% of urban homeless are classified as "unaccompanied" youths.

Unlike homeless adults, adolescents become homeless due to failure of parental support or due to a problem with foster or institutional care. Once they reach 18 years of age, their chances for assistance may be reduced even further as they no longer qualify for programs for adolescents. These teenagers find themselves with little resources and often stigmatized by society. Many come from dysfunctional families where physical and sexual abuse as well as illicit drug abuse were the prevailing family dynamic. When family relationships are strained, parental neglect can follow (U.S. Department of Health and Human

Services, 1995). Other precipitating factors can include adolescent behavioral problems, family financial difficulties, lack of affordable family housing, low paying service jobs, uninsured parents and lack of welfare benefits (Shinn & Weitzman, 1996).

Young girls and boys often resort to prostitution to make a living on the streets. Referred to as "survival sex," young people may see this as their only way to obtain food and shelter. This leads to sexually transmitted diseases, HIV, victimization, substance abuse, and unwanted pregnancy. Other problems include criminal behavior and suicide attempts (Greene, Ennett, & Ringwalt, 1999). Because they lack health insurance, there is limited access to prenatal care or drug rehabilitation.

Homeless adolescents are also generally absent from the public school system. Even though a permanent address is no longer required, problems with accessing immunization and school records as well as grade placement make acceptance in a school problematic. Because basic needs of survival for food and shelter will take priority, education becomes a low priority.

Slesnick and Prestopnik (2005) found that the majority of adolescents in their study suffer from dual diagnosis. Also multiple street drugs may also be used. This problem demonstrates the need for better comprehensive treatment services.

Older Adults

With the expected increase in the geriatric population, the number of homeless elderly is expected to increase. Statistics on the scope of this problem are sparse as the elderly may not be included in surveys and studies. The U.S. Census Bureau (2005) roughly estimates that 9.6% of seniors live below the poverty level. Of this group, a smaller percentage are permanently homeless, living primarily on the streets. Permanent residency on the streets for the elderly may be caused by the lack of available, affordable housing along with poverty as well as problems of mental illness and substance abuse (National Coalition for the Homeless, 2006).

These individuals remain at high risk for complications from chronic illness, lack of access to prescriptions and poor nutrition. Access to health care may be impacted by lack of transportation, isolation, lack of knowledge about services, lack of a way to be contacted for follow up, and needed social services. According to O'Connell et al (2004), the elderly homeless may have anywhere from five to nine chronic health conditions placing them at continued risk for illness and death. These continued, untreated health risks forecast continual physical and mental decline beyond the limitations of just aging. As the elderly become more frail or suffer from advancing dementia, they may be moved to nursing homes for the remainder of their lives.

Bottomley (2001) has pointed out that many of our current policies and programs for the elderly are inadequate, fragmented, and provide a limited array of much needed services.

POSSIBLE NURSES' REACTIONS

- May view the homeless as disgusting, dirty, difficult, or ungrateful
- May be frightened by their behavior
- May feel overwhelmed with the patient's problems and then avoid dealing with the patient
- May view patient as being unmotivated to change
- May feel conflicted when patient wishes to return to the streets rather than accept offer of social services or a shelter
- Difficulty relating to patient's lifestyle
- Want to avoid caring for patient owing to negative feelings

ASSESSMENT

Behavior and Appearance

- Disheveled, torn, ill-fitting clothing
- Unkempt appearance
- Unshaven, dirty
- Unpredictable
- Demands to keep all belongings with him/herself

Mood and Emotions

- Mood swings
- Angry outbursts
- Low tolerance for frustration
- Anxiety when controlled

Thoughts, Beliefs, and Perceptions

- Poor concentration
- Paranoid and suspicious
- Delusional
- Hallucinations
- Loose associations

Relationships and Interactions

- Distrust of others
- Lack of social skills
- Poor eye contact
- No evidence of close relationships

Physical Responses

- Unusual or bizarre symptoms
- May deny complaints
- Fatigue due to poor nutrition, physical problems
- Sleep disturbances
- Chronic illness
- Substance abuse/withdrawal syndrome
- Chronic pain due to back and feet problems

Pertinent History

- Psychiatric disorder
- Substance abuse
- Domestic violence, child abuse
- Minor infractions of the law

COLLABORATIVE INTERVENTIONS

Social Services

When working with the homeless population, it is essential to involve social services to access appropriate community agencies (HELP, 2006). These services can include:

- Case management
- Legal aid
- Assistance obtaining benefits include veteran benefits
- Employment services or retraining
- Day care
- Mental health services
- Housing placement and temporary shelters
- Substance abuse treatment
- Financial aid
- Adult education
- Follow-up health care
- Obtaining prescriptions

Psychiatric and Addiction Services

Because of the frequency of dual diagnoses of psychiatric disorders and substance abuse, the homeless population is at particular risk for many complications from these two disorders. Denkins (2005) recommends prioritizing treatment based on the individual's most pressing need rather than try to treat what the healthcare professional thinks is the most pressing problem. When homeless patients are identified as having a substance abuse problem and a psychiatric diagnosis, an integrated approach of addiction specialists and mental health professionals is needed.

NURSING MANAGEMENT

INEFFECTIVE THERAPEUTIC REGIMEN MANAGEMENT evidenced by poor management of chronic illness related to impaired mental status and/or substance abuse in the homeless

Patient Outcomes

- The patient will keep medical appointments.
- The patient will be able to describe his/her healthcare needs.
- The patient will be able to identify symptoms that indicate immediate need for health-care.
- The patient will accept treatment for ongoing health problems including psychiatric disorders and substance abuse

Interventions

- Provide small amounts of information at one time; do not overwhelm patient with rules, instructions.
- Focus on realistic interventions that would work in the patient's environment
- Encourage the patient to participate in self-care as soon as possible
- Provide written instructions in language and reading level the patient is able to understand.
- Promote trust by communicating in a non-judgmental way, listening to patient's concerns
- Focus interventions on here and now rather than future orientation
- Encourage patient to verbalize concerns about health issues and lifestyle
- Be flexible; remember that this patient may be very uncomfortable, distrusting, and fearful in the healthcare setting
- Make sure social worker is involved early to provide practice information on shelters, clinics, financial services, and taxi vouchers.
- Be alert for increasing frustrations with rules and restrictions that could trigger violent outbursts
- Reassure patient about safety of his/her belongings. What may look like trash to the nurse may be a meaningful item to the patient. Patient may be very protective of them and want to keep them in view at all times.
- For patients with psychiatric disorders address the use of long-acting psychotropic injections that may last a few weeks
- Explain how best to access required health-care services within the community

- Assess for psychiatric diagnoses and substance abuse. Observe for signs of drug withdrawal. Promote continued psychiatric treatment and/or substance abuse treatment where appropriate.
- Assess response to psychotropic medications and discuss with patient need to follow through on obtaining prescriptions.
- Provide specific information on follow-up appointments including directions, transportation, taxi vouchers.

DISABLED FAMILY COPING evidenced by parent and children living on the streets related to alcohol/substance abuse, psychiatric disorders, and abuse

Patient/Family Outcomes

- The homeless family will be able to identify ways to maintain a safe and consistent environment.
- Parent will be able to identify healthcare needs and concerns of the family
- Family will accept assistance to provide a safe and stable environment for the children

Interventions

- Reassure parent about the care of the child and reinforce good parenting practices. Provide concrete interventions to ensure good health care.
- Promote resources for preventative care including vaccines for children.
- Encourage family to talk about their life and share concerns.
- List community resources specific for homeless families
- Identify agency resources that would have information on child care services.
- Observe for any signs of child abuse and/or domestic violence. Seek out social work input to address these concerns and promote safety for the family including appropriate shelters.
- Seek input from pediatric team to address healthcare issues and schooling for the children
- Observe for signs of substance abuse in all members of the family and address as appropriate

ALTERNATE NURSING DIAGNOSES

Coping, Ineffective
Home Maintenance, Impaired
Knowledge, Deficient
Social Isolation, Impaired
Violence, Risk for

WHEN TO CALL FOR HELP

- Escalation of anger and frustration to threats of violence
- Evidence of illegal substance abuse
- Evidence of extreme noncompliance with rules and procedures
- Evidence of child abuse/neglect, domestic violence, or elder abuse

WHO TO CALL FOR HELP

- Security
- Social Worker
- Psychiatric Team
- Addiction specialists
- Pediatric Team

CHARTING TIPS

- Document any information the patient provides about lifestyle, resources used, future plans, health problems and concerns
- Document response to education
- Describe any indication of inappropriate drug use
- Document any information from patient on services he/she has used in the past

PATIENT AND FAMILY EDUCATION

- Discuss ways to maintain personal hygiene in patient's living environment
- Provide information on ways to incorporate quality nutrition into the daily diet
- Give written information that patient can understand on the illness
- Give parent written information on normal growth and development of children, vaccine needs, preventative healthcare
- Review effective parenting techniques
- Teach all involved signs of abuse
- For patients with substance abuse problems, educate them on ways to avoid situations where drugs are readily available
- Provide information on risks of hepatitis, HIV, sexually transmitted diseases
- Educate women on effects of drugs and alcohol on pregnancy.
- Provide birth control information as appropriate to women
- Discuss need for consistent school attendance for children

COMMUNITY-BASED CARE

- Refer to social worker as soon as it is identified that patient is homeless so resources for health-care, shelter, financial aid, and nutrition can be developed
- Provide transportation information on public transportation, taxi vouchers for medical appointments, shelters, employment/educational opportunities
- Identify resources for obtaining prescription refills
- Arrange follow-up for administration of long-acting psychotropic medications where appropriate to ensure that the patient is getting needed medication
- Make referrals for substance abuse programs and psychiatric treatment as needed
- Identify resources through the VA (Veterans Administration) for support and health-care where appropriate
- Work with patient to identify contact information–post office box, phone at local shelter, family member so patient can be reached
- When appropriate, encourage patient to accept short-term placement in facilities like nursing home or home health care in a shelter for continued treatment/observation of a condition.
- When patient is discharged from in-patient care, ensure that follow-up care is attempted
- Make every effort to provide a realistic discharge plan that gives the patient some resources if he/she chooses to use them.

The Dying Patient

Learning Objectives

- Describe common fears faced by the dying patient.
- Describe common nursing staff reactions when caring for the dying patient.
- Discuss the role of palliative care and hospice in the caring for the dying patient and family.
- Describe effective nursing interventions to help the dying patient and family.

Glossary

Advance directive – *A document prepared by an individual to provide guidance to the healthcare team in the event that the person is no longer capable of making decisions.*

Euthanasia – *The act by a physician or another person of administering a treatment with the specific intent to end a person's life.*

Hospice – *A philosophy of care and a program for the terminally ill that focuses on providing dignity, comfort, control, and choices at the end of life. At home or in a facility, hospice care is provided by an interdisciplinary team of specially trained professionals who coordinate services for the patient and family to enhance the quality of life for the time remaining.*

Palliative care – *Management of patients with active, progressive, far-advanced disease for whom the prognosis is limited and the focus is on care to enhance quality of life. Goals for interventions are generally focused on symptom management.*

Physician-assisted suicide – *Means provided by a physician to be used by the patient to end his or her life. Also may be called Aid in Dying.*

Facing the end of life, whether from a prolonged terminal illness, advanced age, or injuries remains the greatest and final challenge. For some people, facing this challenge may be a gradual process as a disease advances; for others, it may come suddenly and unexpectedly. With advanced disease, some individuals may be preparing themselves all the way through the course of the illness, whereas others maintain strong optimism or denial.

The National Hospice and Palliative Care Organization reports that in 2005 75% of deaths in the United States occurred in institutions (50% in acute hospitals) and 25% at home. Home deaths are most associated with hospice care. It is predicted that nursing homes will be increasingly common as the site of death in the United States. Although most people report that they wish to die at home, the acute hospital remains the most common location at the end of life because some people still pursue aggressive treatment, their wishes about resuscitation are unknown, or the family is uncertain about what to do when a crisis occurs. Unfortunately, the hospital may not always be the best prepared for providing a peaceful, comfortable setting for patient and family because of the focus on aggressive interventions (Teno et al, 2004). More hospitals are now developing palliative care programs to address these issues. CAPC (Center for Advancement of Palliative Care) reports that 75% of hospitals with bed capacity over 250 have a palliative care program in 2006.

Policies need to be in place to address comfort care and provide adequate medications. Families and staff members need to be clear on the appropriate use of analgesics and sedatives at the end of life and that the use of these is different from physician-assisted suicide and euthanasia. Wherever the patient is, however, the nurse remains the key person to advocate for the patient's care and provide care and support at the end of life.

The National Hospice and Palliative Care Organization has developed three outcomes that embody quality end-of-life care and can be adapted to any setting:

1. Safe, comfortable dying—providing appropriate symptom management to achieve comfort
2. Self-determined life closure—patient autonomy and participation throughout the process
3. Effective grieving for survivors

These outcomes provide an effective model for healthcare professionals to use when providing care to dying patients.

ETIOLOGY

As a person faces the end of life, coping takes many forms. There are no consistent expected behaviors, although generally the person copes in the same way as he or she has at other times of crisis. For example, if a person has tended to be angry and isolated, it is common to see the same reactions during the dying process. The following are some of the common fears faced by the dying patient and family that influence how they will cope.

Fear of Pain and Suffering

This is often listed as the greatest fear of the dying. Images of loved ones who died in severe pain are particularly associated with cancer. These memories may cloud the perceptions of what the end of life will be like. Fear of pain and suffering has received more attention in the last few years because pain and hospice professionals are attempting to educate the public and health-care professionals that the vast majority of pain can be treated by relatively simple means (Agency for Healthcare Policy and Research, 1994; Paice & Fine, 2006). Nearly all pain and suffering from end-stage disease can be effectively controlled with the knowledge and technology available today. The experience of pain and suffering can create isolation and depression for the patient and guilt for the family, so addressing this fear is essential to enhance physical and emotional comfort.

Fear of Abandonment

Increasing weakness and loss of control can increase anxiety and a sense of vulnerability in being left alone. This fear can be experienced in relation to the patient's physician, who may be less involved once aggressive treatment has stopped. This can even be reinforced if a physician communicates, "There is nothing more to do." It is important for the physician to remain involved throughout the course of the terminal illness. Family members and physicians who feel helpless and anxious may inadvertently avoid the patient to escape distress or because they do not know what to say. It is important to realize how this affects the dying patient.

Loss of Control

Because our society values self-reliance and independence, loss of control is particularly frustrating. Weakness, fatigue, confusion, incontinence and distressing symptoms can all contribute to this fear. Individuals who value their independence may try to retain it as much as possible, even to their detriment. For example, a patient who lives alone may refuse to hire a live-in caregiver, even though he or she is no longer able to care for basic needs. Families often struggle to try to help their loved one maintain valued independence, yet provide for their safety. Loss of control can induce feelings of guilt as the patient needs to rely on others. Making the decision to stop aggressive treatment in the face of advanced disease can represent a major loss of control because the patient may feel that he or she is "giving in" to the disease.

Loss of Hope

Hope is a natural part of human existence, and as death approaches, it may be more and more difficult to retain. This can contribute to depression and loss of control. Hoping for a peaceful death and hoping to achieve a specific goal before death are examples of reframing hope at the end of life.

Fear of the Unknown

Death presents the greatest unknown to many people. Questions such as "What will happen to my family, my life plans, my body?" are difficult to face. They are also very difficult for others such as family members and even caregivers. Yet the patient may need to express them. Even though we may not have answers to these questions, providing an environment in which fears can be expressed is a great support. Spiritual support may also provide more comfort at these times.

The dying person also faces grief in facing the loss of his or her self, body, and loved ones. Family members may experience many of these same fears.

RELATED CLINICAL CONCERNS

The three leading causes of death today in the U.S. (National Center for Health Statistics, 2003) are

1. Heart disease
2. Cancer
3. Stroke

All of these causes of death are most often associated with chronic, long-term illness characterized by exacerbations and progressive symptoms. Pain, suffering, and distressing symptoms are all associated with long-term illnesses. Uncontrolled pain is by far the greatest fear and a major contributor to patient wishes for hastening death.

Patients in the final weeks of life report fatigue and weakness as the most disturbing symptoms, contributing to emotional distress.

LIFE SPAN ISSUES

Children

Addressing the needs of dying children takes a dedicated team experienced in working with children and their families. Because of their young age, children are often medically treated very aggressively until the end, making preparation for death more difficult. Professionals may be ambivalent about when to bring up these issues. Parents, especially younger ones, may have little experience with death and will need special assistance in preparing for it. Accidents remain the most common cause of death of children but congenital conditions and cancer remain as frequent causes (NCHS, 2006).

Parents and professionals often struggle with how to prepare the child. Adults who do not want to face this may expend most of their energies denying the possibility of the child's death. Children are very sensitive to their parents' reactions and may very well realize what is happening without being told directly. The sick child needs to be approached according to developmental level as to how much he or she can understand. Adults need to stress a sense of comfort, security, and family closeness. A pediatric hospice can provide parental support and education in this area. Pediatric hospice remains underused in many settings though because treating physicians and parents continue to maintain hope (Levetown et al, 2001). The growth in recent years of Pediatric Palliative Care Programs provides a family-centered approach for children with life-threatening conditions to address suffering, goals, coordination of care amongst other services (Himelstein, 2006) even if the family continues to pursue aggressive treatment.

Siblings often need special attention at these times, yet their needs may be overlooked because of the crisis with the sick child. Siblings often struggle with many anxieties about their own health, jealousy for the sick child who gets special attention, and even feeling responsible for the illness. As with the sick child, the use of play and drawings can be used to help them express feelings that they are too young to verbalize. Siblings should also be included in the care of the ill child, but still be given permission to live a normal life. Seeking help from pediatric professionals is essential.

Older Adults

The major developmental task of old age is to prepare for death. Life review, letting go of responsibilities and possessions, and adjusting to health changes are normal parts of the life cycle that elderly people must face. The death of close friends may occur much more frequently as one ages. Women in particular have a greater likelihood of losing their spouse and living alone. Death is not as feared in this age group. For many, a gradual giving up of plans, hopes, and dreams may provide preparation. Maintaining independence for as long as possible, along with respect, support, and good symptom management, are important contributions to good end-of-life care in this population.

As more older adults spend more time in nursing homes, this will become a more common place to provide end-of-life care (Teno et al., 2004). Hospice care can be provided in a nursing home.

POSSIBLE NURSES' REACTIONS

- May become detached from the dying patient to avoid the pain of losing him or her
- May have unrealistic expectations of how the patient should die (e.g., that family members will all get along)
- May fear losing control of own emotions around the patient and family, as well as coworkers
- May fear participating in hastening the patient's death when aggressive symptom management is ordered or when a patient requests that life-prolonging measures such as tube feedings be stopped
- May identify with a patient of similar age or circumstances, leading to more anxiety
- Facing the death of a patient may stir up past unresolved losses for the nurse, leading to feelings of sadness or anger
- May experience intense anger with family of a dying patient who are not providing the type of support the nurse thinks is appropriate

ASSESSMENT

Behavior and Appearance

- Crying, agitation
- Unable to concentrate
- No apparent reaction
- Extreme change in usual behavior patterns
- Life review
- Completing efforts for estate planning, mortuary arrangements, distribution of personal belongings

Mood and Emotions

- Shock, numbness
- Depression

- Anxiety, panic
- Mood swings
- No obvious emotional reaction
- Anger
- Guilt, remorse

Thoughts, Beliefs, and Perceptions

- Maintaining hope for a variety of things, including cure, more time, completion of goals
- Difficulty making decisions
- Denial, avoidance of preparation
- Reviewing one's life work and seeking validation for one's contribution
- Seeking the meaning of one's life
- Pursuing spiritual beliefs, especially regarding the afterlife

Relationships and Interactions

- Seeks support from others
- Fears being alone
- Withdrawal
- Projection of anger onto others
- Need to see loved ones to say good bye
- Wish to resolve past conflicts
- Wish to pass on thoughts, memories, stories to others

Physical Responses

- Disrupted sleep
- Confusion, agitation
- Pain, other symptoms that can be exacerbated by emotions
- Possibility that family may develop symptoms similar to those of patient

Pertinent History

- Unresolved or multiple past losses
- Ambivalent relationship with loved ones
- Tendency to isolate self
- History of psychiatric disorder or substance abuse
- Experiencing traumatic, painful death of a loved one

COLLABORATIVE INTERVENTIONS

Pharmacological

Adequate pain and symptom management must be achieved before any psychosocial issues can be addressed. The vast majority of pain and other symptoms of end-stage disease can be controlled with analgesics, anxiolytics, antiemetics, and other drugs as needed. Fears about addiction by patients, families and as health-care providers need to be addressed to ensure that no one is allowing needless suffering to occur. Side effects of medications used must also be anticipated and measures used to treat them must be provided.

Because depression and hopelessness can affect the quality of life, antidepressants can be useful at the end of life, even in a patient with only weeks to live. The side effect profile needs to be carefully reviewed before selecting any medications. Antidepressants with shorter time to onset of effect should be considered in this population. Consultation with a pharmacist and/or psychiatrist might be helpful.

Patient and family may use a variety of complementary and alternative approaches to treat the symptoms of advanced disease or even to retain hope for a cure. Shark cartilage, Laetrile, and other unproven methods are sometimes continued at the end of life. The nurse needs to become familiar with possible side effects to help patients and families weigh the risks and benefits of using these products. For example, inserting a nasogastric tube just to administer shark cartilage may be too great a burden given the poor prognosis. Other approaches for relief of pain and other symptoms may include magnet therapy, acupuncture, biofeedback, and hypnosis.

Palliative and Hospice Care

Palliative care provides symptom management and support for patients with life-limiting illnesses when the goal may be to try to prolong life but still focus on comfort. Patients may still be receiving aggressive treatments such as chemotherapy to control symptoms. Palliative care is most associated with end-of-life care (Gorman, 2006) but in fact can be appropriate early in the disease trajectory of a life limiting illness. Increasingly available in acute hospitals, Palliative care programs provide an important link to quality end-of-life care. National standards entitled the National Consensus Project (2004) for Quality Palliative Care are now in place to establish guidelines for programs.

Hospice care provides an interdisciplinary approach to care of the dying patient and his or her family when the goal is comfort. Medicare has provided a model for hospice services for patients with less than 6 months to live that has also been adopted by Medicaid in most states as well as by most private insurance companies. The hospice benefit will provide multiple services to patients and families under the direction of a hospice-trained physician and nurse to enhance comfort and support of the patient, family preparation, education, support and bereavement follow-up, along with the chaplain, social worker, and volunteers. See Table 19–2 for Comparison of Palliative Care and Hospice. Hospice cares for patients with any type of terminal illness. In recent years there has been an

TABLE 19–2

Comparison of Palliative Care and Hospice

Palliative Care	Hospice
Generally acute hospital based	Care provided in home or nursing home generally
Patient criteria: Advanced life limiting illness with patient in need of symptom management, addressing goals of care or future planning. Aggressive treatment can be continued.	Patient criteria: Patient with terminal illness with prognosis of less than 6 months; aggressive, curative treatment is completed or stopped
Multiple models including interdisciplinary consultation team, unit, clinic. Make up of team varies.	Interdisciplinary team defined by Medicare to include physician, registered nurse, social worker, spiritual care and volunteers amongst others
National Consensus Project has established standards	Medicare establishes regulations
Palliative care can provide a bridge to hospice care by identifying appropriate patients earlier	Hospice uses the acute hospital setting for short-term admissions if symptoms cannot be controlled at home

increase in patients with non-cancer diagnoses such as dementia and heart failure (NHPCO, 2007).

Spiritual Care

Some people seek out spiritual support when facing the end of life. They may wish to renew past religious ties, address personal suffering, and seek to find meaning to their life and perhaps their suffering. The role of religious leaders and particularly chaplains at the end of life can be an important intervention. Most hospitals, as well as hospices, offer these services.

NURSING MANAGEMENT

ANTICIPATORY GRIEVING evidenced by distress at facing own death, including depression, anger, and guilt related to the terminal illness.

Patient Outcomes

- Acknowledges terminal illness
- Expresses concerns, feelings of grief

- Verbalizes feelings of being supported in the grieving process
- Identifies potential coping mechanisms, support systems

Interventions

- Accept grieving behavior. Recognize that responses to grief are highly individual.
- Use open-ended questions and reflection to give the patient the opportunity to share feelings and concerns. Listen for patient readiness to discuss issues concerning death. For example, a patient may say, "I don't think I'll be around much longer." The nurse can respond by saying, "Tell me what you're worried about."
- Recognize that your role may be that of listener if patient needs to vent feelings. Providing an accepting environment to share these feelings is extremely important. Let the patient determine what issues he or she needs to explore. The patient may feel more comfortable discussing his or her grief with a nurse because of not wanting to upset family and friends.
- Facilitate communication between family and patient, if appropriate. Ask patient if he or she would like you to share personal concerns with the family if communication has been blocked. Prepare family for some of patient's concerns if patient agrees to this.
- Be aware of the need to preserve hope. Recognize that hope may take on many faces in the dying process. It could move from hope for a miracle to hope for less pain to hope to live until a grandchild's wedding. Caution yourself and others not to promote inappropriate hopefulness based on your own needs or discomforts.
- Recognize that behaviors such as frequent demands, criticisms, and frequent questioning may be indicative of patient or family sense of loss of control. Provide those involved with a role in decisions and allow some control where possible. Acknowledge the family's important role as patient advocate.

KNOWLEDGE DEFICIENT evidenced by frequent questioning, lack of knowledge of the dying process related to facing the death of a loved one.

Patient Outcomes

- Demonstrates increased awareness of what to expect in the dying process
- Able to identify resources available for assistance
- Expresses questions and concerns

Interventions

- Keep the family informed about the patient's condition. Provide information on what they can do for the patient and what the staff is doing.

Discuss with family how they want to be informed about the patient's death. For example, some families want to be called at any sign of deterioration; others want to be notified only of the death.

- Assess family members' understanding of patient's prognosis and awareness that patient will die soon. Then tailor education based on their level of awareness and readiness to accept more information.
- Reassure patient and family about options available to maintain comfort without euthanasia or physician-assisted suicide.
- Support cultural and religious beliefs during the dying process. Recognize that mourners may have rituals that need to be carried out at a death such as chanting or lighting candles.
- Determine patient and family readiness to discuss issues around goals of care. Code status, hospice care, degree of sedation wished, and continuing life-prolonging measures such as TPN or dialysis need to be addressed. Families and patients may need more information on the risks and benefits of all decisions made. Identify if patient has advance directive or has expressed his/her wishes for end-of-life care.
- Talk to family members about what to expect throughout the dying process. Review the symptoms the family may be seeing. When the patient is very close to death, provide information to help them prepare for when death is likely to occur.
- If children are present, ensure that they are included in general discussion to prepare them for what will happen. Speak with the adults away from the children when reviewing some information. Assist them on how to prepare the child. Adults should be encouraged to inform the child's teachers of what is happening.
- Provide information on local hospice programs, if appropriate. Give information on bereavement support programs available in the area.
- Remember that family members have other responsibilities such as child care and jobs. Talk with them about how they are managing and support their decisions about when to stay with the patient and when to leave. Assess whether they are getting adequate sleep and nutrition. They may need permission to take care of themselves.
- Once the patient has died, inform family members in private. Give them the opportunity to have some private time with the patient. Assist them in getting other family members to the bedside if possible to provide support. Provide information as appropriate on procedures regarding mortuary arrangements, organ donation, autopsy, and so forth.

ALTERNATE NURSING DIAGNOSES

Anxiety

Body Image, Disturbed

Coping, Family: Compromised
Coping, Ineffective
Powerlessness
Self-Esteem, Disturbed
Sleep Pattern, Disturbed
Pain
Spiritual Distress (Distress of the Human Spirit)

WHEN TO CALL FOR HELP

- Long periods of depression
- Patient and family avoiding dealing with important issues around end-of-life planning, code status
- Family behavior that affects patient's comfort (e.g., withholding analgesics)
- Patient with suicidal thoughts, requests for physician-assisted suicide or euthanasia
- No emotional reaction to impending death
- Patients' symptoms not managed

WHO TO CALL FOR HELP

- Palliative care
- Hospice
- Chaplain
- Pain Team
- Attending Physician
- Social Worker
- Psychiatric Team
- Pharmacist

PATIENT AND FAMILY EDUCATION

- Prepare patient and family for normal stages of grieving.
- Review the role of hospice in end-of-life care.
- Provide information on issues around care such as code status, need for analgesics, side effect management, and so forth.
- Provide information on advance directives. Encourage patient to clarify his or her wishes and share these with loved ones.

- If appropriate, encourage the dying patient to make a videotape, audiotape, memory book, or other form of legacy for the family, especially for young children who might not remember the patient.
- Review the signs and symptoms of death with loved ones throughout the dying process.
- Review information on organ donation, mortuary arrangements, and so forth as needed.
- Educate caregivers on patient care needs.
- Provide patient and family with education resources to prepare including Web sites for the Hospice and Palliative Nurses Association (hpna.org), National Hospice and Palliative Care Organization (NHPCO.org), and CAPC (getpalliativecare.org). Pamphlets on making difficult decisions such as *Hard Choices for Loving People* by Hank Dunn may be available through many hospice and palliative care programs.

CHARTING TIPS

- Document grieving behaviors.
- Document patient's pain and comfort level.
- Avoid documenting judgments about patient and family behaviors.
- Document patient and family awareness of prognosis, goals, and wishes.
- Document presence and content of an advance directive and patient's verbalizations of any change in wishes.

COMMUNITY-BASED CARE

- Refer to hospice care if patient is going home or to assisted living or a nursing home.
- Refer to support programs for patients with advanced disease as well as bereavement groups for the family.
- Refer to pain clinics, palliative care programs as appropriate.
- Provide legal referrals for completing wills, managing finances.
- Refer family to caregiver support group, education programs.

20

Disaster Planning and Response–Psychosocial Impact

The Disaster Victim/Patient
The Disaster Responder/Nurse

Carl Magnum, RN, MSN, PhD(c), CHS, FF

Learning Objectives

- List interventions a nurse could use in working with a patient/victim of disaster.
- Identify possible nursing staff reactions to disaster.
- Describe signs and symptoms of stress related of victims and responders in a disaster.
- Describe interventions to reduce the risk of post-traumatic stress disorder after a disaster.

Glossary

Critical incident stress debriefing – *An organized, structured approach to support emergency personnel and survivors who are exposed to extreme stress that revolves around discussion, feelings, and reactions to the event.*

Disaster – *Tragic events that disrupt normal functioning and safety of a community.*

Disaster Psychiatry – *Psychiatric specialists who address an epidemiological approach to understanding the treating of effects of mass casualty situations.*

Human-made disaster – *Occur through human actions (accidental or intentional).*

Natural Disaster – *Occur by acts of nature.*

Post-traumatic stress disorder (PTSD) – *Anxiety and stress symptoms that occur after a massive traumatic event; often includes the feeling that the event is recurring. PTSD can last for weeks, months, or years.*

The past 2 decades have been a learning curve for nurses related to disasters and their victims. The Oklahoma City Bombing, September 11 attacks, anthrax scares, and Hurricanes Katrina and Rita have set the standard for modern disasters. Local community disasters can include such events as school shootings and factory explosions. Disasters are usually grouped as natural and human-made. The effects on victims from each are the same. Some people are even affected before the actual event. Psychosocial problems occur throughout the phases of a disaster. Some people do not present with psychosocial difficulties until the recovery phase.

Citizens in the disaster area are always the first concern. The response community also has concerns for responders/nurses during and after the disaster. Responders are also affected by many of the responses that citizens have. There are a few differences in how to prepare for and operate during a disaster.

When a disaster occurs, there are three types of victims (Williams & Boyd, 2005). First are the victims who suffer trauma from the disaster itself. These people are vulnerable to physical injury, post-traumatic stress disorder (PTSD) and depression after the event. The second type of victims are the rescuers/responders who are likely to be exposed to trauma and PTSD at seeing others suffer, as well fear for their own well-being. The third victim is the community at large, who may suffer psychological effects from observing the events from afar. These victims may experience anxiety, sadness, helplessness, and fear that the disaster could have happened to them. For example, after the terrorist attacks on September 11, a study of Americans across the country demonstrated that 90% experienced at least one stress symptom immediately after the event (Schuster et al, 2001).

Because nurses may be among the first responders in a community disaster, preparation and knowledge about the impact of a disaster on oneself and others is essential. Nurses suffer from the same emotional trauma as others and need to take precautions to take care of themselves as well as others.

More information is now available on disaster preparation that includes psychological preparation. Health-care providers, law enforcement officials, and school officials are important areas to concentrate preparation (Norwood, Ursano, & Fullerton, 2006). Involving mental health professionals, including specialists in Disaster Psychiatry, is important to address potential fears and help responders identify emotionally "at-risk" individuals.

One consistency seen in a disaster is that some individuals step up and rise above their training and position to help. In many disasters, we hear inspiring stories of responders and victims who put themselves at risk to help strangers. After the initial shock, victims may try to do something to resolve the situation and help others. Nurses, as leaders in a helping profession, are often active in this role. For example after Hurricaine Katrina in 2005, many nurses sought out ways to help victims and local healthcare professionals. Many nurses went to the disaster area to help set up emergency medical care for the victims.

ETIOLOGY

There are many factors that influence emotional response to a disaster.

Biological: The stress response prepares the individual for "fight or flight." During the fight response, the individual is physiologically prepared to attack. The flight response involves efforts to conserve body resources. During a disaster, these physiological responses affect the initial response.

Psychological: Many psychological factors contribute to the emotional response to a disaster. Fear, anger, shock, sadness, and disbelief are all common and normal emotional responses. These responses may be based on the person's personality and normal coping patterns, coping reserves, and support system available. After a disaster, common responses can include sleep disturbances, and increased use of alcohol, tobacco, and illicit drugs to treat uncomfortable, residual symptoms,

Sociocultural: During a disaster, the community response as people rush to help can promote a sense of support and reassurance to victims. This social support from all levels of the community can expose victims to many strangers from other cultures and walks of life. This sense of support and community can be reassuring to victims, who realize that they are not alone. It is common that traumatic events can bring out some of the best in people (Deeny & McFetrige, 2005).

CLINICAL CONCERNS

The presence of chronic illnesses, required medical treatments, and dependency on medications may be factors on how individuals respond in a disaster. Victims and responders may also be dealing with physical injury, exposure to toxins, dehydration, lack of sleep, and no access to normal medications, which can create more complicated emotional responses. Patients who are being treated for serious illnesses like cancer may have many concerns when they are unable to access their health care providers (Tariman, 2007).

LIFE SPAN ISSUES

Children

Younger children may experience separation anxiety from parents. Older children may be mad, sad, or afraid the event may happen again. Difficulty concentrating and obsession with the event may be prevalent. Sleep disturbances, night terrors, and fear of the dark may be seen after the disaster. Regression to an earlier developmental stage, including bedwetting, clinging behaviors, and an inability to articulate, may be seen for short periods.

Children who are experiencing feelings of anxiety and helplessness can benefit from participating in altruistic activities like fundraising and volunteer activities such as food or clothing drives to help others (American Psychiatric Association, 2004).

Adolescents

They may respond similarly to adults (Norwood, Ursano, & Fullerton, 2007). Others may regress to a more childlike phase. They may be afraid to leave home and not want to spend time with their friends. Emotions may lead to increased friction, arguing, and even fighting with siblings, parents, and other adults. Teens may be put into adult roles for a short period to help others. This can lead to feelings of guilt and anxiety when faced with decisions that they are not prepared to handle. They may become preoccupied with decisions they made. An increase in high-risk behaviors after a traumatic event is sometimes seen.

Older Adults

Although older adults have many life experiences, a major disaster can have a tremendous impact. The unexpected, unfamiliar, and uncontrollable events bring fears for safety, loss of life-long treasures, and can affect chronic conditions. Lack of access to regular medications may contribute to additional emotional problems.

POSSIBLE NURSES' REACTIONS

- Fear for own safety and victim's safety
- Sympathy for victims
- Anxiety related to the situation
- May identify with victims' suffering and fears
- Guilt over leaving one's own family or focusing on personal fears/needs
- Resentment over victim's emotional reactions
- Overwhelmed with responsibilities and needs
- Feeling need to flee disaster

ASSESSMENT OF THE DISASTER VICTIM/PATIENT

Behavior and Appearance

- Suspicion
- Irritability
- Arguments with friends and loved ones
- Withdrawal
- Excessive silence
- Inappropriate humor

- Increased/decreased eating
- Change in sexual desire or functioning
- Increased smoking
- Increased substance use or abuse

Mood and Emotions

- Shock
- Numbness
- Feeling overwhelmed
- Depression
- Feeling lost
- Fear of harm to self and/or loved ones
- Feeling nothing
- Feeling abandoned
- Uncertainty of feelings

Thoughts, Beliefs, and Perceptions

- Poor concentration
- Confusion
- Disorientation
- Indecisiveness
- Shortened attention span
- Memory loss
- Unwanted memories
- Difficulty in making decisions

Relationships and Interactions

- Close attachment with other victims or responders
- Distant from family and friends
- Others avoiding victim due to volatile emotions

Physical Responses

- Nausea
- Lightheadedness
- Dizziness
- Gastrointestinal problems
- Rapid heart rate
- Tremors
- Headaches
- Grinding of teeth

- Fatigue
- Poor sleep
- Pain
- Hyperarousal
- Jumpiness

Pertinent History

- History of psychiatric disorders
- History of violent behavior
- Past experience in a disaster situation

ASSESSMENT OF THE DISASTER RESPONDER/NURSE

See Box 20–1 for Normal Responses to a Disaster and Box 20–2 for Signs of Stress after a Disaster.

Behavior and Appearance

- Intense anger
- Withdrawal
- Temporary loss or increase of appetite
- Emotional outbursts
- Excessive alcohol consumption
- Inability to rest, pacing

Mood and Emotions

- Anxiety
- Guilt
- Grief

BOX 20–1
Normal Reactions to a Disaster

- No one who responds to a mass casualty event is untouched by it.
- Profound sadness, grief, and anger are normal reactions to an abnormal event.
- You may not want to leave the scene until the work is finished.
- You will likely try to override stress and fatigue with dedication and commitment.
- You may deny the need for rest and recovery time.

BOX 20–2
Signs of Stress after a Disaster

- Difficulty remembering instructions
- Difficulty maintaining balance
- Uncharacteristically argumentative
- Difficulty making decisions
- Limited attention span
- Unnecessary risk-taking
- Tremors/headaches/nausea
- Tunnel vision/muffled hearing
- Colds or flu-like symptoms.
- Disorientation or confusion

- Difficulty concentrating
- Loss of objectivity
- Easily frustrated
- Unable to engage in problem-solving
- Unable to let down when off duty
- Refusal to follow orders
- Refusal to leave the scene
- Increased use of drugs or alcohol
- Unusual clumsiness

- Denial
- Severe panic (rare)
- Fear
- Irritability
- Loss of emotional control
- Depression
- Sense of failure
- Feeling overwhelmed
- Blaming others or self

Thoughts, Beliefs, and Perceptions

- Confusion
- Nightmares
- Disorientation
- Heightened or lowered alertness
- Poor concentration
- Memory problems
- Poor problem solving
- Difficulty identifying familiar objects or people

Relationships and Interactions

- Arguments with friends and loved ones
- Suspicion of others
- Change in sexual desire or functioning

Physical Responses

- Chest pain
- Difficulty breathing
- Shock symptoms
- Fatigue
- Nausea/vomiting
- Dizziness
- Profuse sweating
- Rapid heart rate
- Thirst
- Headaches
- Visual difficulties
- Clenching of jaw
- Nonspecific aches and pains

Pertinent History

- Type and amount of training the responder/nurse has had.
- Actual disaster experience.
- Has responder/nurse been personally affected by the event.
- Predisaster preparation.

COLLABORATIVE MANAGEMENT

Pharmacological

Antianxiety medications are used for relief of feelings of tension and anger. The choice of medications is dependent on the diagnosis and the availability of medications. During a large-scale disaster, medications become limited and it may be days or weeks for a medication of choice to be available. Many victims may try to self-medicate.

Mental Health Interventions

Mental health professionals are developing more strategies to address these issues. The American Psychiatric Association has developed principles for Disaster Psychiatry to provide training for mental health professionals on appropriate interventions to minimize exposure to traumatic stressors, education about normal responses to trauma and disasters, consultation with other health-care professionals and community leaders, and professional treatment for PTSD (Norwood, Ursano, & Fullerton, 2007).

Critical incident stress debriefing training can be completed by nurses, social workers, clergy, physicians among other professionals. People with this structured training can be helpful in assisting all types of victims or potential victims to prevent long-term emotional trauma. The American Psychiatric Association (2004) has cautioned that anxiety can be increased by the process of retelling about the event.

NURSING MANAGEMENT FOR THE DISASTER VICTIM/PATIENT

POST-TRAUMA SYNDROME (ACUTE), evidenced by anxiety, hypervigilance, anger, altered mood states, nightmares or flashbacks, headaches, loss of interest in normal activites, hopelessness, gastric irritability related to exposure to a disaster

Patient Outcomes

- Reports reduced anxiety when memories occur
- Demonstrates ability to deal with emotional reactions in an individually appropriate manner
- Demonstrates appropriate changes in behavior or lifestyle
- Reports absence of physical manifestations

Interventions

- Observe for and elicit information about physical or psychological injury and note associated stress-related symptoms such as numbness, headache, tightness in chest, nausea, pounding heart, and so forth.
- Identify psychological responses: anger, shock, acute anxiety, confusion, and denial.
- Provide crisis intervention techniques to assist with extreme reactions of panic, hysteria by remaining calm and providing consistent reassurance. See Chapter 5.
- Assess patient's knowledge of and anxiety related to the situation.
- Ascertain ethnic, background/cultural, and religious perceptions and beliefs about the occurrence.
- Determine degree of disorganization.
- Identify whether incident has reactivated pre-existing or coexisting situations.
- Determine disruptions in relationships.
- Note withdrawn behavior, use of denial, and use of chemical substances or impulsive behaviors.
- Be aware of signs of increasing anxiety.
- Note verbal or nonverbal expressions of guilt or self-blame when patient has survived in which others have died.

- Assess signs/stage of grieving for self and others. Recognize that traumatic bereavement can occur if the victim feels survivor guilt when others did not survive the disaster.
- See Box 20–3 for Communicating with Disaster Victims including suggestions on phrases to avoid that can increase the victims' anxiety, sense of loss, and powerlessness.

RELOCATION STRESS SYNDROME evidenced by feeling of powerlessness, lack of adequate support system, little or no preparation for the impending move, anxiety, depression, sleep disturbance, insecuirty, gastrointestinal disturbances, sad affect, withdrawal related to disruption of living arrangements after a disaster.

Patient Outcomes

- Verbalize understanding of reasons for change.
- Demonstrate appropriate range of feelings and lessened fear.
- Verbalize acceptance of situation.
- Demonstrates no escalation of emotions

Interventions

- Ascertain patient's perceptions about changes and expectations for the future.
- Monitor behavior, noting presence of suspiciousness or paranoia, irritability, defensiveness
- Note signs of increased stress, reports of new physical discomfort or pain, or presence of fatigue.

BOX 20–3
Communicating with Disaster Victims

Things to Avoid Saying:	More Helpful Phrases:
• "I understand."	• "There are people here to help you"
• "Don't feel bad."	• "We won't leave you alone"
• "You're strong/You'll get through this."	• "It's OK to let out your emotions"
• "Don't cry."	• "I know you are scared"
• "It's God's will."	• "We are in this together"
• "It could be worse" or "At least you still have…"	

- Determine the involvement of family and significant others.
- Encourage visiting new surroundings before transfer, when possible.
- Orient to surroundings and schedules. Introduce to staff members, roommate, and other residents. Provide clear, honest information about actions and events.
- Encourage free expression of feelings. Acknowledge the reality of the situation and maintain hopeful attitude regarding move or change.
- Identify strengths and successful coping behaviors the individual has used previously.
- Deal with aggressive behavior by imposing calm, firm limits. Control environment and protect others from patient's disruptive behavior.
- Involve patient in formulating goals and plan of care when possible.
- Discuss benefits of adequate nutrition, rest, and exercise to maintain physical well-being.
- Identify and provide concrete information on what happened to family and pets, condition of victim's home/belongings where possible. Recognize that victims may be fearful leaving the disaster site because of losing touch with family, friends, pets, belongings.
- Encourage participation in activities, hobbies, and personal interactions as appropriate.

INEFFECTIVE COMMUNITY COPING evidenced by deficits in social support services and resources, ineffective or nonexistent community systems, community powerlessness, high illness rates, increased social problems related to community response to a disaster

Patient Outcomes

- Recognize negative and positive factors affecting community's ability to meet its own needs.
- Identify alternatives to inappropriate activities for adaptation/problem solving.
- Report a measurable increase in necessary and desired activities to improve community functioning.

Interventions

- Provide support for victims who are frustrated with community response to the disaster. Recognize that community may be ill prepared for this event. Allow expression of anger
- Promote adaptive coping mechanisms that will not alienate others
- Seek out alternative resources available to the victims.
- Promote victims to participate in altruistic activities to help others if possible.

ALTERNATE NURSING DIAGNOSES FOR VICTIMS

Anxiety
Family Processes, Compromised
Fear
Hopelessness
Injury, Risk for
Powerlessness
Social Interaction, Impaired
Spiritual Distress, Risk for
Violence, Risk for

NURSING MANAGEMENT FOR THE DISASTER RESPONDER/NURSE

CAREGIVER ROLE STRAIN evidenced by caregiver health impairment, increasing care needs, unpredictability of care sitiuation, presence of violence, inadequate physical environment for providing care, caregiver isolation, insufficient information and finances or supplies, inadequate tranportation and equipment for providing care related to being present during or after a disaster.

Outcomes

- Identify resources within self to deal with situation.
- Identify outside resources to deal with the situation.
- Acknowledge limitations due to the extent of the disaster

Interventions

- Inquire about and observe physical condition of care provider and surroundings as appropriate.
- Assess caregiver's current state of functioning.
- Identify safety issues concerning caregiver and receiver.
- Determine availability of support systems and resources.
- Discuss caregiver's view and concerns about the situation.
- Acknowledge the difficulty of the situation for the caregiver.
- Discuss stress management techniques.
- Remove caregiver from situation, if needed.
- Contact other resources for assistance.
- Acknowledge feelings of being overwhelmed with situation
- Seek out assistance from others in the area who may want to help.

- Help caregivers and responders take breaks from the situation and encourage them to incorporate self-care where possible.

INEFFECTIVE COPING evidenced by situational crisis, high degree of threat, inadequate resources available, inadequate level of confidence in ability related to being called to help in a disaster.

Outcomes

- Assess the current situation accurately.
- Identify ineffective coping behaviors and consequences.
- Verbalize awareness of own coping abilities.
- Meet psychological needs as evidenced by appropriate expression of feelings, identification of options, and the use of resources.

Interventions

- Evaluate the ability to understand events, provide realistic appraisal of situation.
- Assess current functional capacity and note how it is affecting the individual's coping ability.
- Observe and describe behavior in objective terms.
- Actively listen and identify the nurse's perceptions of what is happening.
- Evaluate nurse's decision-making ability.
- Assist with relaxation techniques.
- See Box 20–4 for ways to manage stress after a disaster.

BOX 20–4
Ways to Help Manage Responder Stress in a Disaster

- Limit on-duty work hours to no more than 12 hours per day
- Make work rotations from high-stress to lower stress functions
- Make work rotations from the scene to routine assignments, as practicable
- Use counseling assistance programs available through your agency
- Drink plenty of water and eat healthy snacks like fresh fruit and whole grain breads and other energy foods at the scene
- Take frequent, brief breaks from the scene as practicable.
- Talk about your emotions to process what you have seen and done
- Stay in touch with your family and friends
- Participate in memorials, rituals, and use of symbols as a way to express feelings
- Pair up with a responder so that you may monitor one another's stress

ALTERNATE NURSING DIAGNOSES FOR RESPONDERS

Anxiety

Comfort, Impaired

Fear

Grieving

Hopelessness

Spiritual Distress, Risk for

WHEN TO CALL FOR HELP

- Threats against personal safety.
- Victims who become violent, threaten aggression
- Presence of firearms, other weapons
- Inability to handle patient load.
- Another event pending.
- Environmental hazards.
- Unable to continue response duties

WHO TO CALL FOR HELP

- Other team members on the scene.
- Command staff
- Local law enforcement
- Local medical providers
- State medical providers
- Federal medical providers
- Volunteers and bystanders

PATIENT AND FAMILY EDUCATION

- Planning and preparations by families is critical to getting through a disaster.
- Contact information for family, insurance, medical, and emergency personnel.
- Having current medication names and doses.
- Disaster kits for the home and the car.
- Promote the development of individual family disaster plans with a plan for how to contact each other in the event of being separated.

CHARTING TIPS

- Records are difficult to create and maintain during disaster situations.
- Basic information name and contact information.
- Include location of the treatment center; remember landmarks may not be available.
- Write down pertinent medical information.
- Identify if patients' medical records available electronically.

COMMUNITY-BASED CARE

- Planning and preparedness is the key.
- Be aware of disaster preparation in your work setting including information on where the command center would be, locate other communication resources, identify local radio stations that will have latest information.
- Seek out information in advance of a disaster in your community. The American Nurses Association has information on preparations for a disaster for nurses at www.nursingworld.org/news/disaster/. The Centers for Disease Control and Prevention (CDC) has a website on preparation of health professionals at www.bt.cdc.gov/masscasualties/copingpro.asp.
- Participate in a program on disaster preparation in schools and hospitals that includes psychological preparation.
- Be aware of humane resources for care of pets as it is well established that victims may not be willing to leave the disaster area if their pets would be left behind in potential danger.
- Participate in disaster exercises in your community that give potential responders and victims some preparation for the emotional reactions seen in a disaster.

21

Psychopharmacology: Database for Patient and Family Education on Psychiatric Medications

Yoshinao Arai, RN, MN, CNS

Learning Objectives

- Identify the indications and clinical uses for antianxiety, antidepressant, mood stabilizers, and antipsychotic medications.
- List safe administration practices for patients taking these drugs.
- Select the appropriate nursing interventions and patient education strategies for patients taking these drugs.

Glossary

Agonist – *A chemical compound (drug or neurotransmitter) that produces a biochemical response when it binds to a receptor. A receptor is a complex molecule located on a cell membrane. When an agonist binds to a receptor, this forms an agonist-receptor complex, and the formation of this complex leads to a biochemical response.*

Antagonist – *A chemical compound that blocks or reverses the effect of agonists by coupling with a receptor without triggering a physiological response. Antagonists and agonists can bind to a receptor, but they cannot do so at the same time. The degree to which an antagonist dominates an agonist depends on the binding strength and the concentration of the antagonist.*

Elimination half-life – *Time required to decrease the plasma concentration of a drug by 50%. If the half-life of a drug is shorter than 24 hours, its daily dose needs to be divided into two or three doses a day to maintain steady-state concentration in the body. It takes about five times the half-life for a drug to reach its steady state when a new drug is started or about five* *half-lives for a drug to be washed out of an individual's system after a drug is discontinued.*

Neurotransmitters – *Chemical compounds that serve as messengers in the neuronal system. Each neurotransmitter has its specific type of receptors to couple with. Common neurotransmitters for psychopharmacology include dopamine, serotonin, norepinephrine, acetylcholine, and gamma-aminobutyric acid (GABA). Others include oxytocin, growth hormone (GH), calcitonin, angiotensin, insulin, substance P, beta-endorphin, and prolactin.*

Potency – *A comparative, not absolute, measure of the strength of a drug to produce a response. The higher the potency of a drug, the lower the recommended dose will be to create a given physiological response. For example, a dose of haloperidol (Haldol) of 2 mg is thought to produce the same clinical response (antipsychotic effect) as a dose of chlorpromazine (Thorazine) of 100 mg. The potency of haloperidol is 50 times higher than that of chlorpromazine.*

Psychoeducation – *Educational intervention with a focus on skills training for managing mental health issues for patients and families to achieve behavioral changes with increased knowledge*

Psychiatric medications do not cure psychiatric disorders, but they can alleviate the symptoms caused by the disorders. The medications can minimize the disturbing impact of mental illness on a person's ability to function. The ideal treatment outcome is the removal of all the negative impact of the illness on the person's ability to achieve his or her goals in life. This is the purpose of psychopharmacological interventions when augmented with psychoeducation and rehabilitation. Both pharmacological and nonpharmacological interventions are effective because they work in the brain to adjust its biochemical brain activity. The resulting biochemical changes in the brain enhance the process of psychiatric rehabilitation in a similar manner to that of neurological rehabilitation. To attain the best benefits from psychiatric medication, the person with a psychiatric disability must see how medications can help to eliminate roadblocks in his or her life. This is best accomplished by identifying specific and concrete target symptoms with each individual.

Because people with psychotic symptoms are not aware of the difference between reality and symptoms, it is often difficult for them to see a need for the use of medication. Even if they are aware of their need for medication, it can still be difficult for them to assess a medication's efficacy because they cannot clearly distinguish what is reality and what is a symptom. Medication education, which is usually provided only at the beginning of a particular treatment, is not sufficient. Giving written information about a medication may only make the person feel more anxious. Psychoeducational support should be an ongoing process that helps to maximize the efficacy and safety of the medication regimen. With this support, the people with psychiatric disabilities will be able to value the pharmacological therapies in relation to their life goals.

This chapter provides the essential information on the psychiatric medications and their safety issues (Table 21–1). This can be used in psychoeducational interventions to clarify the value of the medications in terms of the difference they can make in the lives of people with psychiatric disabilities. This information is presented in the following order:

- Basic Concepts
- Medications for Symptoms of Anxiety Disorders
- Medications for Mood Symptoms
  - Antidepressants
  - Mood Stabilizers
- Medications for Psychotic Symptoms
  - Typical Agents
  - Atypical Agents
- Managing Side Effects of Antipsychotic Agents
- Collaborative Management for Advocacy
- Charting Tips
- Community-Based Care

BASIC CONCEPTS

Pharmacokinetics and Pharmacodynamics

It is necessary to have some basic understanding on what the body does to medications (pharmacokinetics) and what medications do to the body (pharmacodynamics).

Pharmacokinetics

Once a medication is taken orally, intramuscularly, sublingually, transdermally, or intravenously into the bloodstream, it can be eliminated in many different ways. Plasma proteins bind part of the medication, making this part inactive, or not bioavailable. Some of the medication is carried to the kidney, where it may be excreted unchanged in the urine. Some of the medication is carried to the liver, where it is transformed into a more water-soluble, active or inactive metabolite. Once transformed by the liver, the medication may be excreted in the urine or in the bile (then in the feces) and out of the body. Individual differences in the biotransformation through known or unknown mechanisms contribute to the observed wide range of clinical responses to a standard dose.

Pharmacodynamics

Psychiatric drugs can produce clinical responses even when only a small portion of the medication can reach their sites of action, that is, the receptors in the synapses.

TABLE 21–1

Summary of Safety Issues on Psychiatric Medications

Type of Adverse Event	Related Medications
Dose-related toxicity	Lithium
Lowered seizure threshold	Clozapine, clomipramine, bupropion
Hepatic toxicity	Nefazodone, duloxetine, valproic acid
Agranurocytosis	Clozapine, mirtazapine, carmabazepine, phenytoin, TCAs
Myocarditis	Clozapine
Significant weight gain	Olanzapine, clozapine, quetiapine,
Type II diabetes mellitus	Olanzapine, clozapine, quetiapine
Increased mortality due to medical conditions in the elderly with dementia and psychosis	Atypical antipsychotics
Movement disorders (tardive dyskinesia, neuroleptic malignant syndrome, extrapyramidal symptoms, akathisia)	Typical and atypical antipsychotics
Increased suicidality in children and adolescents	SSRI, TCA, and MAOI antidepressants
Paralytic ileus	Benztropine, clozapine, chlorpromazine, quetiapine
Glaucoma	Benztropine, chlorpromazine, clozapine
Altered cardiac conduction	Lithium, ziprasidone, clozapine, TCAs
High blood pressure	Venlafaxine, MAOI antidepressants
Increased toxicity or decreased efficacy due to drug interactions with other drugs, food	SSRIs, MAOIs, lithium, cimetidine, carbamazepine, phenytoin, erythromycin, ketoconazole, nicotine, caffeine, grapefruits

The drug molecules can facilitate or inhibit the effect of neurotransmitters by inter-acting with receptors on neuronal cells in different neurotransmitter systems. These systems are often described by the predominant neurotransmitter present. Examples include the dopamine, serotonin, norepinephrine, acetylcholine, hista-mine, and gamma-aminobutyric acid (GABA) systems.

The dopamine system in the brain has been thought to play a major role in causing psychotic symptoms. Blockade of certain types of dopamine receptors has been associated with alleviation of psychotic symptoms. It is recognized that blockade of other types of dopamine receptors causes neurological or endocrine side effects, as discussed later.

The serotonin system has been thought to be associated with symptoms of depression, anxiety, and hallucinations. It is also postulated that blocking of cer-tain serotonin receptors may be associated with controlling negative symptoms of schizophrenia, as discussed later. However, blocking of other types of sero-tonin receptors is associated with such side effects as hypotension, sedation, and ejaculatory dysfunction.

The norepinephrine system may be associated with mood and motivation. Some of the new antidepressants target this system. Blockade of certain norepi-nephrine receptors is thought to be associated with such adverse effects as pos-tural hypotension, dizziness, tachycardia, and sexual dysfunction.

The acetylcholine system may be associated with memory and smooth muscle functions.

Different types of pharmacological interactions with the muscarinic type of acetylcholine receptors have been associated with alleviating parkinsonian symp-toms or causing such side effects as dry mouth, constipation, blurred vision, uri-nary retention, electrocardiographic (ECG) changes, and memory impairment.

The histamine system is thought to be associated with the sedative effects of medications that interact with the histamine receptors. It is also postulated that postural hypotension and weight gain can be caused by pharmacological manip-ulation of the histamine system.

The GABA system in the brain is an inhibitory network that lowers the activ-ity levels of all other neurotransmission systems. The efficacy of the benzodi-azepine (BZ) family of medications is associated with their effect of blocking the activity of this system.

Major Categories of Common Psychiatric Medications

Major advances in psychopharmacology include discoveries of psychiatric uses of chloral hydrate (1860s), barbiturates (1900s), antipsychotic medications (1950s), nonselective (tricyclic) and monoamine oxidase inhibitor (MAOIs) antidepres-sants (1950s), BZs (1960s), lithium (1970s), selective serotonin reuptake inhibitors (SSRIs, 1980s), atypical antipsychotics (1990s), serotonin and norepi-nephrine reuptake inhibitors (SNRIs, 1990s), and selective BZ receptor agonists (1990s). Most of these categories of medications are currently in use except the barbiturates, most of which were replaced by relatively safer agents such as BZs and SSRIs.

Commonly used psychiatric medications for adults can be identified under the following conventional categories: antianxiety agents (anxiolytics, sedatives, and hypnotics), antidepressants (older and newer agents), mood stabilizers, antipsychotic agents, and medications to control side effects. The generic and trade names for the medications are listed in boxes in each section. The possible daily dosage ranges (usually in milligrams per day) are also provided for each drug.

Target Symptoms

When the pharmacological interventions are considered, the treatment team and the patient or family should specifically define the psychiatric symptoms that the drugs of each category are treating.

Refer to the appropriate chapters to review common psychiatric symptoms as targets for pharmacological treatment. After defining specific target symptoms with the patient or family, each symptom may be rated on a 10-point scale before the therapy is started and periodically afterward. This way, both the treatment team and the patient or family can keep better track of changes in reactions to medications over time.

Patient and Family Education

Educational needs of patients and their families should be assessed in the following areas in relation to psychopharmacological treatments:

- Names of the medications
- When and how to take them
- What are the target symptoms
- Skills to identify expected benefits
- Time it takes to be able to identify the beneficial effects
- Possible adverse effects
- What to do if the adverse effects are too disturbing to tolerate
- How long the medication or medications should be taken
- Possible drug interactions with alcohol, other medications, nutritional supplements, and food
- What to do if the target symptoms worsen

GENERAL CONSIDERATIONS FOR VULNERABLE POPULATIONS

Children

Children are generally more prone to serious disruptions by psychiatric medications that may interfere with development. Their livers and kidneys may not be developed enough to efficiently eliminate the drugs out of the body, although the opposite is generally the case when relatively higher doses are required for efficacy, partly because of children's faster metabolic capacity. However, few controlled studies have been done to obtain data on the efficacy and safety of psychiatric medications in children (Birmaher & Axelson, 2005). In addition, how these drugs effect growth and development with long-term use has not been well studied.

Adolescents

Adolescents often fall in between children and adults in terms of proper dosing based on body size. As with children, long-term effects and efficacy for adolescents have not been well studied. Teens may also be particularly concerned with drug side effects that negatively affect body image like weight gain and hair loss.

Older Adults

Older adults may be vulnerable to side effects of the medications in general for the following reasons:

- Decreased body water may lead to higher concentrations of medications.
- Decreased plasma proteins may lead to increased serum level of a drug that is not bound to proteins in the bloodstream.
- Increased portion of fat in the body may cause retention of a fat-soluble psychiatric medication and prolong its elimination half-life.
- Decreased liver and kidney function may also prolong elimination half-life of a medication.
- In addition, complex drug regimens which may be from multiple prescribers may be associated with poor compliance.

MEDICATIONS FOR SYMPTOMS OF ANXIETY DISORDERS

Certain clusters of anxiety symptoms can suggest various anxiety disorders (Table 21–2). However, anxiety symptoms are also common in most other psychiatric disorders such as schizophrenia, major depression, and bipolar disorders. In these cases, the primary conditions need to be treated as well. The same is true for anxiety symptoms that are secondary to other medical disorders such as mitral valve prolapse, hyperthyroidism, arrhythmia, inner ear infection, asthma, or to use of substances such as cocaine, caffeine, methamphetamines.

The most common antianxiety medications are in the categories of anxiolytics, sedatives, and hypnotics. These can be classified into two groups of BZs and non-BZs (Box 21–1). Other categories of medications for anxiety include antidepressants and beta blockers.

TABLE 21–2

Common Symptoms of Anxiety

Origin	Symptom
Physical symptoms of brainstem origin	Fatigue, cold chills, headaches, difficulty breathing, difficulty sleeping, dizziness, shaking, sweating, muscle tension, restlessness, GI disturbances, numbness in fingers and toes, and palpitations
Emotional symptoms of limbic system origin	Nervousness, fear, panic, apprehension, feeling detached from part of own body, or feeling that the surroundings are unreal
Cognitive symptoms of neocortical system origin	Intrusive thoughts or concerns about losing one's mind, losing control, frightening scenes, having physical illnesses, being inadequate, being disapproved, fainting, difficulty concentrating

BOX 21–1

Most Common Antianxiety Medications

Benzodiazepines	Dosage
Chlordiazepoxide (Librium)	15–100 mg/day
Diazepam (Valium)	2–60 mg/day
Lorazepam (Ativan)	0.5–6 mg/day
Oxazepam	30–90 mg/day
Temazepam (Restoril)	7.5–30 mg hs
Alprazolam (Xanax)	0.25–10 mg/day
Flurazepam (Dalmane)	15–30 mg hs
Clonazepam (Klonopin)	0.25–10 mg/day
Non-Benzodiazepines	
Zolpidem (Ambien)	5–15 mg hs
Zaleplon (Sonata)	5–20 mg hs
Eszopiclone (Lunesta)	2–3 mg hs
Antihistamines and Anticholinergics	
Diphenhydramine (Benadryl)	25–50 mg hs
Serotonin Antagonist	
Buspirone (BuSpar)	15–60 mg/day

HYPOTHESES OF MECHANISMS OF ACTION

The mechanisms of action of anxiety medications are unknown. However, two hypotheses on how medications alleviate anxiety symptoms involve the serotonin and GABA-BZ neurotransmission systems.

The serotonin system is supposed to be one of the mediators of a "fear network," which involves the brainstem, the hypothalamus, and the amygdala. The amygdala is a critical temporal lobe structure associated with the expression of anxiety and mammalian stress responses. It is hypothesized that medications influencing the serotonin system desensitize the "fear network" (Gorman, Kent, Sullivan, & Coplan, 2000).

The GABA system has an inhibitory function on the brain. When its function is enhanced by coupling of the BZs with the GABA-BZ receptors on surfaces of neurons, neurotransmissions are inhibited in most parts of the brain. Thus, some overexcitation can be leveled off to aid relaxation.

EFFICACY IN TREATING SYMPTOMS

Anxiety Symptoms

Anxiety symptoms respond well to BZs such as lorazepam (Ativan), clonazepam (Klonopin), chlordiazepoxide (Librium), diazepam (Valium), and alprazolam (Xanax). However, if it is expected that the symptoms will require treatment for more than several weeks, antidepressants or buspirone (BuSpar) will become the first drugs of choice. BZs can be used on an as-needed basis or only for the first several weeks until the antidepressant or buspirone takes effect because of the possible development of dependence on BZs.

Among the antidepressants used for anxiety, serotonergic agents such as paroxetine (Paxil), fluoxetine (Prozac), sertraline (Zoloft), and fluvoxamine (Luvox) are thought to be the best choices as primary medications for long-term treatment of most anxiety symptoms. Other medications for anxiety include some beta-adrenergic blockers such as propranolol (Inderal) or anticonvulsants such as gabapentin (Neurontin) (Pollack, Mathews, & Scott, 1998).

Anxiety-Related Insomnia

BZs used as central nervous system (CNS) depressants reduce anxiety (anxiolytic effect) at lower doses and produce sedative effects at slightly higher doses. Most BZs also induce sleep (hypnotic effect) at higher doses. However, unlike the case with barbiturates, the central nervous system depressant effect of BZs does not increase to cause coma or death, even if the doses are further increased, as long as they are not used with other CNS depressants such as alcohol.

BZs generally have rapid onsets (i.e., 15–60 minutes after oral administration) except temazepam (Restoril) which may take 45 to 120 minutes to begin taking effect. The long half-life (48–150 hours) of flurazepam (Dalmane) is associated with morning hangover.

OTHER USES

Dual-Diagnosis Patients Who Have Both Psychiatric Disorders and Substance Abuse Problems

BZs and tricyclic antidepressants (TCAs) should not be used in this population. BZs tend to be abused by this population (Schatzberg & Nemeroff, 2004). TCAs may have additive cardiotoxicity when they are taken with cocaine. Better choices are SSRI antidepressants or anticonvulsants (e.g., gabapentin) for anxiety symptoms.

Use of SSRIs for Obsessive-Compulsive Disorder (OCD)

Higher doses of SSRIs such as fluoxetine (Prozac) 40 to 80 mg/day, fluvoxamine (Luvox) 150 to 300 mg/day, sertraline (Zoloft) 100 to 200 mg/day, or paroxetine (Paxil) 40 to 60 mg/day can be useful. Clomipramine (Anafranil), which is also a serotonin reuptake inhibitor in the class of TCAs, can be the second-line option for SSRI nonresponders. Its poor side effect profile includes dose-related risk of seizures.

COMMON SIDE EFFECTS OF ANXIOLYTICS, SEDATIVES, AND HYPNOTICS

Disinhibition BZs can cause behavioral dysfunction, including irritability and personality changes. Children, adolescents, and elderly people may be more prone to this paradoxical side effect.

Cognitive Deficits High-potency BZs such as lorazepam (Ativan), clonazepam (Klonopin), and alprazolam (Xanax) are associated with memory impairment. These BZs may exacerbate preexisting cognitive impairment.

Dependence The use of BZs as hypnotics for temporary insomnia should be for a maximum of 2 to 4 weeks only. Continued efficacy may last as long as 5 weeks, but there is no guarantee of efficacy afterward. For persistent insomnia, regular or intermittent use of BZs as hypnotics should be re-evaluated every 2 to 4 months. In the case of zolpidem (Ambien) or zaleplon (Sonata), the duration of use should be 7 to 10 days with re-evaluation if the use exceeds 2 to 3 weeks.

Withdrawal Symptoms Anxiety symptoms, delirium, seizures.

Overdose Ataxia, hypotonia, nystagmus, coma. BZ antagonist is flumazanil.

Respiratory Depression Use of BZs for sleep disturbance caused by sleep apnea can worsen the respiratory condition. Concomitant use with alcohol, TCAs, anticonvulsants, or clozapine (Clozaril) may increase sedative effects or cause respiratory depression.

RELATED CLINICAL CONCERNS

Children

BZs have been known to have a paradoxical effect on children contributing to personality changes and irritability. The use of any kind of sedatives in sleep disturbances is not well investigated in controlled studies in children.

Adolescents

Anxiolytics may interfere with common teen activities including school, driving and sports contributing to safety and compliance issues.

Older Adults

The best choices for antianxiety medications in elderly persons are short-acting, low-potency agents without active metabolites, such as oxazepam. The minimum effective dose is 50% of the usual adult dose. This should be given as needed only for 1 to 2 weeks. Paradoxical reactions from BZs are more common in the elderly contributing to agitation rather than the desired effect.

Pregnancy

The association of fetal damage with BZs is controversial (Barki, Kravitz, & Barkin, 1998). However, it is recommended that BZs be tapered off sufficiently before delivery to minimize neonatal and infant withdrawal. Lorazepam (Ativan) and oxazepam have less potential for accumulation in neonates. BZs at relatively low doses are not contraindicated in nursing mothers (Rubey & Lydiard, 1999).

PATIENT AND FAMILY EDUCATION

- Advise patient to avoid discontinuing BZs abruptly to avoid rebound or withdrawal symptoms.
- Advise patient to avoid adjusting dosing of BZs without consulting prescriber for the above-mentioned reason.
- Teach patient that, unlike BZs, buspiron (BuSpar) has no tolerance or dependence effects.
- Teach patient that beta blockers can cause bradycardia or exercise intolerance.
- Tell patient not to take BZs with alcohol or over-the-counter medications for insomnia.
- Teach patient to avoid making important decisions if BZs disturb concentration.

MEDICATIONS FOR MOOD SYMPTOMS

There are two categories of medications for mood symptoms: antidepressants and mood stabilizers.

ANTIDEPRESSANTS

The newer antidepressants (SSRIs and SNRIs) are gradually replacing the older agents like tricyclics and MAOIs as the treatment of choice for various symptoms of depressive and anxiety disorders (Boxes 21–2 and 21–3). This change occurred because the newer agents have better side effect profiles. Owing to the broader mechanism of action of SNRIs on more than one neurotransmitter (e.g., norepinephrine and dopamine) they can be effective when SSRIs are not.

BOX 21–2
Target Symptoms of Depression

- **Apparent/reported sadness:** Sad mood reflected in speech, posture, and facial expressions. Depressed mood reported nonverbally regardless of the verbal messages (e.g., looks distressed but brightens up at times; appears miserable all the time).

- **Anhedonia or inability to experience pleasure:** Reduced interest in surroundings or activities that used to give pleasure (e.g., failure to feel any positive emotions).

- **Change in appetite:** Reduced desire for food or increased need to force oneself to eat (e.g., slightly reduced interest in food; eating because one has to).

- **Change in sleep pattern:** Reports experience of reduced duration or depth of sleep (e.g., slight dissatisfaction with sleep; sleep less than 3 hours a night).

- **Inner tension:** Feelings of vague discomfort, restlessness, or edginess leading to dread or panic (e.g., occasional edginess, irritability, restlessness; overwhelming panic).

- **Difficulty getting started:** Slowness initiating or performing daily activities (e.g., some sluggishness; unable to do anything without help).

- **Negative thoughts:** Representing thoughts of guilt, remorse, or inferiority (e.g., ideas of low self-esteem, failure, self-accusations; absurd and unshakable pessimism).

- **Poor concentration:** Representing difficulties in comprehending messages (e.g., difficulties in reading; inability to follow a conversation).

- **Thoughts of death:** Stating that a natural death would be welcome, that life is not worth living (e.g., weary of life; ending own life is considered as a possible option; active preparation for suicide).

BOX 21–3
Antidepressants

Older Agents	
Tricyclic Antidepressants (TCAs) and their derivatives	**Dosage**
Imipramine (Tofranil)	50–300 mg/day
Amitriptyline (Elavil)	50–300 mg/day
Clomipramine (Anafranil)	50–250 mg/day
Doxepin (Sinequan)	25–300 mg/day
Amoxapine (Ascendin)	50–300 mg/day
Desipramine (Norpramin)	50–300 mg/day
Nortriptyline (Pamelor/Aventyl)	25–150 mg/day
Monoamine Oxidase Inhibitors (MAOIs)	
Phenelzine (Nardil)	15–90 mg/day
Tranylcypromine (Parnate)	10–60 mg/day
Selegiline transdermal patch (EMSAM)	6–12 mg/day
Newer Agents	
Selective Serotonin Reuptake Inhibitors (SSRIs)	
Fluoxetine (Prozac)	20–80 mg/day
Fluvoxamine (Luvox)	50–300 mg/day
Paroxetine (Paxil)	10–60 mg/day
Sertraline (Zoloft)	50–200 mg/day
Citalopram (Celexa)	20–60 mg/day
Escitalopram (Lexapro)	10–20 mg/day
Non-SSRIs	
Serotonin and Norepinephrine Reuptake Inhibitor (SNRI)	
Venlafaxine (Effexor)	75–375 mg/day
Duloxetine (Cymbalta)	40–60 mg/day
Serotonin 2A Blocker	
Nefazodone (Serazone)	50–600 mg/day
Trazodone (Desyrel)	200–600 mg/day
Serotonin 2A/C and Norepinephrine (alpha-2) Blocker	
Mirtazapine (Remeron)	15–45 mg/day
Dopamine and Norepinephrine Reuptake Inhibitor	
Bupropion (Wellbutrin, Zyban)	75–450 mg/day

HYPOTHESES ON MECHANISMS OF ACTION

The exact mechanisms of action of antidepressants are unknown, but the following are hypotheses concerning the various types of antidepressants.

> **Tricyclic Antidepressants** TCAs may work by affecting serotonin, norepinephrine, and dopamine neurotransmitter systems. Their major side effects may be caused by interacting with muscarinic cholinergic receptors.

Monoamine Oxidase Inhibitors MAOIs potentiate neurotransmitters by inhibiting the function of the enzyme monoamine oxidase (MAO), which inactivates neurotransmitters. Inhibition of MAO, which is present in the central nervous system, gut, and platelets, may lead to increased absorption of tyramine, which can act as a false neurotransmitter and elevate blood pressure. Therefore, a tyramine-free diet is required with the use of MAOIs.

Selective Serotonin Reuptake Inhibitors SSRIs enhance serotonergic transmission, increasing serotonin in the synaptic clefts between neurons. This is caused by accumulation of serotonin in the cleft as the drug blocks the reuptake of serotonin back into the neuron.

Newer Agents (Non-SSRIs) Bupropion (Wellbutrin) is thought to work by inhibiting norepinephrine reuptake in addition to its effect on dopaminergic transmission. Venlafaxine (Effexor) and Duloxetine (Cynbalta) are selective inhibitors of serotonin and norepinephrine reuptake. Nefazodone (Serzone), which can be associated with liver failure, is thought to work by antagonizing serotonergic and alpha-1 adrenergic receptors.

EFFICACY IN TREATING SYMPTOMS

All antidepressants have equal efficacy on symptoms of depressive episodes. Improvement of mood may not be observed for 2 to 6 weeks. Selection of agents is based on the agents' different side effect profiles and the patient's tolerance to them. There is no reliable method to predict which patients will respond better to a specific agent. The factors to consider for agent selection include the patient's age, suicide potential, concurrent use of medications, and coexisting diseases. For example, SSRIs are safer in patients with a history of cardiac diseases or suicidal ideations. If the patient or a first-degree relative has had a good response to a certain agent in the past, another trial of the same agent is an option because the agent may be compatible with the individual's metabolic capacity.

COMMON SIDE EFFECTS OF ANTIDEPRESSANTS

Tricyclic Antidepressants and Monoamine Oxidase Inhibitors The major side effects of TCAs and MAOIs are lethargy, orthostatic hypotension, and anticholinergic symptoms (Table 21–3). These side effects tend to increase during the first month of treatment but usually subside with time. The anticholinergic side effects include dry mucosa (mouth, nose, or vagina), blurred vision, urinary retention, poor memory, and impaired concentration. These can be caused by TCAs, MAOIs; low-potency antipsychotics such as thioridazine (Mellaril) and chlorpromazine (Thorazine), clozapine (Clozaril) (except dry mouth). These disturbing side effects must be managed to enhance compliance with the treatment (Table 21–4).

Selective Serotonin Reuptake Inhibitors and Non-SSRIs The common side effects of SSRIs include insomnia, sexual dysfunction, and agitation or restlessness. These are mediated by their interactions with the serotonin neu-

TABLE 21–3

Comparing Side Effects of SSRIs and TCAs/MAOIs

Side Effects	SSRIs	TCAs/MAOIs
Orthostatic hypotension	Low	High
Sedation, weight gain	Low	High
Anticholinergic effects	Low	High

TABLE 21–4

Managing Anticholinergic and Other Common Side Effects of Antidepressants

Anticholinergic Side Effects	Management
Dry mouth	Use sugarless gums or candies. Carry a bottle of water and sip it frequently. Emphasize need for extra good dental and oral hygiene. Worse during the initial period of treatment.
Urinary retention	Report any problem on urination (e.g., dribbling, urgency, hesitancy, retention). Monitor urinary patterns, especially for confused patients. Consult prescriber if the disturbance is persistent.
Constipation	Monitor bowel movement patterns. Encourage high fiber diet, maintain sufficient fluid intake, and exercise regularly. Consult prescriber for possible use of stool softeners or laxatives.
Blurred vision	If persistent and disturbing, consult prescriber for possible medication adjustment.
Poor memory and concentration	If persistent and disturbing, consult prescriber for possible medication adjustment.
Sedation	Symptom will usually subside with time. Monitor sleep patterns and related habits to eliminate factors adversely affecting sleep hygiene. May need to avoid driving.

Continued

TABLE 21–4

Managing Anticholinergic and Other Common Side Effects of Antidepressants—*cont'd*

Other Side Effects	Management
Weight gain	Weigh patient monthly. Monitor diet patterns. Help patient to incorporate regular exercise in daily routines. Consult prescriber if weight gain is persistent despite application of practical measures as above.
Sexual dysfunction	Assess baseline sexual activity level and deviation from it. Consult prescriber if the deviation is too disturbing to tolerate.
GI upset	Take medications with or after meals.
Orthostatic hypotension	Monitor orthostatic BP regularly. Instruct patient to rise slowly when changing positions and to take sufficient fluid. Consult prescriber if BP is less than 90/60.

rotransmission system. The newer non-SSRI agents (bupropion, nefazodone, and mirtazapine) are associated with lower risks of sexual dysfunction. In akathisia-like restlessness, the dose may need to be reduced. Switching to another agent may be needed if the symptom is severe and persistent.

SSRI Withdrawal Syndrome Abrupt discontinuation of paroxetine or fluvoxamine can result in dizziness, nausea, irritability, headaches, or cholinergic rebound symptoms (e.g., salivation, loose stools).

Serotonin syndrome Mental status changes, agitation, myoclonus, and hyperreflexia may result from the concomitant use of two or more drugs that may increase CNS serotonin level through different mechanisms. This can occur when SSRIs are taken along with other drugs that increase serotonin levels including sumatriptan, L-tryptophan, and TCAs.

OTHER SIDE EFFECTS OF SPECIFIC ANTIDEPRESSANTS

Agranulocytosis Mirtazapine (Remeron) can cause agranulocytosis or neutropenia in 1 in 1000 patients. It should not be used with bone marrow–suppressing agents such as carbamazepine (Tegretol), phenytoin (Dilantin), or clozapine (Clozaril)

Priapism The incidence of priapism with trazodone (Desyrel) is rare. If the erection persists longer than 1 hour, emergency room treatment is required. If not treated promptly, priapism may result in permanent impotence.

Hypertension Venlafaxine (Effexor) is associated with higher risks of hypertension.

Seizure Bupropion (Wellbutrin) and clomipramine (Anafranil) have been associated with higher risks.

Liver Damage Duloxetine (Cymbalta) is not generally recommended with pre-existing liver disease or alcohol abuse.

RELATED CLINICAL CONCERNS

Children and Adolescents

In 2004, the Food and Drug Administration (FDA) added a black box warning to antidepressants for children and adolescents with major depressive disorder of a potential increased risk for suicide. This action has contributed to a reduction in prescribing these medications (Schatzberg, Cole, & DeBattista, 2005; Leckman & King, 2007). This action may also have contributed to more untreated depression and possible increased suicide risk (American Psychiatric Association, 2006). More studies need to be done about the potential risks and benefits of antidepressants in this age group. In 2006 the FDA increased the age range on this warning to age 24. SSRIs are the most frequent type of antidepressants used in children due to side effect profile, although TCAs have been used for enuresis and attention deficit-hyperactivity disorder.

Pregnancy

TCAs and SSRIs have shown no statistically significant evidence of increased risks for congenital defects or teratogenicity except for paroxetine (Paxil), which is associated with increased risk of cardiac birth defects when exposed in the first trimester. MAOIs are associated with higher risks. Discontinuing antidepressants in pregnancy can be associated with relapse of depression. So close monitoring must be maintained.

Older Adults

TCAs are of particular concern because of their anticholinergic side effects in this age group. Anticholinergics are a major contributor to delirium in the elderly (Schatzberg, Cole, & DeBattista, 2005). Urinary retention is a concern for men with enlarged prostates. Orthostatic hypotension can contribute to falls.

Other Clinical Concerns

QRS Prolongation A 1-week supply of TCAs may be fatal if taken all at once to reach two to six times therapeutic levels in blood (i.e., 500–1000 ng/mL).

Depressive Episodes Caused by Medical Conditions Psychiatric symptoms of depression can be part of the clinical presentation of non-psychiatric illnesses such as Addison's disease, AIDS, asthma, heart failure, Cushing's disease, diabetes, hyperthyroidism and hypothyroidism, infectious hepatitis, and malnutrition. Psychiatric medications may be tried to manage the symptoms while the underlying medical conditions are being treated.

Mania All antidepressants can cause mania in patients with bipolar disorder.

Monoamine Oxidase Inhibitors and Food Interactions MAOIs can cause high blood pressure, nausea, vomiting, and headaches as reactions with foods containing tyramine (Table 21–5). All perishable foods (vegetables, fruits, and meats) should be as fresh as possible. The special diet needs to be continued for 4 weeks after the medicine is discontinued.

Use of St. John's Wort (Hypericum) St. John's Wort is an herbal product used for treatment of depression. Its mechanism is unclear. Randomized controlled trials have not supported its efficacy, but anecdotal reports have shown that it is helpful for some patients. It is contraindicated in pregnancy, lactation, and cardiovascular disease. Because of its possible MAOI-like activity, caution is required regarding its adverse reactions with serotonergic or sympathomimetic agents and foods containing tyramine.

PATIENT AND FAMILY EDUCATION

- Teach patient that it may take several weeks before alleviation of target symptoms can be identified.

TABLE 21–5
Foods To Avoid When Using MAOIs

Food Categories	Foods to Avoid
Bread, cereals, pasta	Yeast extracts Brewer's yeast
Fruits	Overripe and spoiled fruits
Vegetables, beans	Broad bean pods. sauerkraut, Italian green beans
Meats, fish	All aged, dried, fermented, salted, smoked, and pickled meats and fish All processed meats
Milk, yogurt, and cheese	All aged cheese Soybean products (e.g., tofu, soybean milk)
Sweets, condiments, beverages	Meat and yeast extracts Sherry, vermouth, beer, ale, red wine Soy sauce

- Teach patient that the side effects tend to subside with time. The patient needs to work closely with the treatment team to minimize the discomfort during the early phase of treatment.
- Teach patient that the prescriber should be consulted before starting any other medications or dietary supplements while taking SSRIs or MAOIs.
- Advise patient that dietary precaution is crucial to avoid hypertensive crises while taking MAOIs.
- Teach patient that persistent symptoms such as headaches, nausea, insomnia, agitation, and rashes should be reported to the prescriber.
- Advise patient and family to report increased suicidality to their treatment team.
- Advise patient to avoid alcohol while taking Bupropion (Wellbutrin) because of increased seizure risk.

MOOD STABILIZERS

Lithium is still the first-line choice for symptoms of manic episodes, although other agents are available from the category of anticonvulsants. When lithium is not tolerated because of its side effects, divalproex (Depakote) or carbamazepine (Tegretol) can be tried (Box 21–4). Other newer anticonvulsants such as gabapentin (Neurontin) or lamotrigine (Lamictal) are being tested.

HYPOTHESES ON MECHANISMS OF ACTION

Lithium (Eskalith, Lithobid) Lithium's exact mechanisms of action are unknown. It appears to enhance the serotonergic transmissions. It also affects the norepinephrine system by increasing its function in some parts of the brain and decreasing it in others. It also affects membrane permeability and ionic transport. Its inhibition of intracellular enzymes is also studied as a possible mechanism of action.

BOX 21–4
Mood Stabilizers and Anticonvulsants

Mood Stabilizers	Dosage
Lithium (Eskalith, Lithobid)	900–2100 mg/day
Anticonvulsants	
Carbamazepine (Tegretol), Equetro (extended release)	600–1200 mg/day
Divalproex (Depakote)	1500–2500 mg/day
Gabapentin (Neurontin)	900–3000 mg/day
Lamotrigine (Lamictal)	100–400 mg/day
Pregabalin (Lyrica)	100–600 mg/day

Carbamazepine (Tegretol) The mechanism of action of carbamazepine is unknown. It may be related to GABA level changes.

Divalproex (Depakote) Divalproex decreases GABA metabolism to result in increased GABA in the CNS.

EFFICACY IN TREATING SYMPTOMS

Lithium (Eskalith, Lithobid) The therapeutic effect of lithium may take 4 to 8 weeks to achieve. Serum levels of 0.5 to 1.2 mEq/L are recommended.

Carbamazepine (Tegretol) The therapeutic effect of carbamazepine may take 2 to 4 weeks. The correlation between clinical responses and serum levels is not established, although plasma levels of 8 to 12 mcg/ml are suggested.

Divalproex (Depakote) The therapeutic effect of divalproex may take 2 to 4 weeks after plasma levels of 50 to 120 mcg/ml are reached.

COMMON SIDE EFFECTS

Lithium (Eskalith, Lithobid) Toxic reactions to lithium can occur even within the therapeutic range (Box 21–5). It may produce toxic effects in patients who use diuretics or who have renal failure, hyponatremia, diarrhea, and/or dehydration. Long-term toxic effects can include diabetes insipidus, hypothyroidism, leukocytosis, hypotension.

Carbamazepine (Tegretol) Toxic effects with carbamazepine include leukopenia, aplastic anemia, gastrointestinal (GI) disturbances, sedation, blurred vision, vertigo, rash, arrhythmia, and hepatitis.

BOX 21–5
Possible Side Effects and Toxic Effects of Lithium

- **Initial adjustment period of several weeks:** Increased thirst, dry mouth, increased urination, mild nausea, worsening of acne or psoriasis, metallic taste, weight gain, occasional loose stools, mild dizziness, decreased sexual desire, slight muscular weakness, sleepiness, fine tremor in hands, mild stomach cramps.
- **Long-term:** Hypothyroidism with swelling of the gland, sleepiness, feeling cold, unusual weight gain, headache, tiredness, cold fingers and toes, menstrual changes, dry puffy skin, constipation, muscle aches, slow thinking.
- **Toxic effect from elevated blood level:** Persistent diarrhea, vomiting, coarse trembling of hands or legs, frequent muscle twitching in the arms or legs, blurred vision, confusion, severe discomfort, weakness, severe dizziness, seizure, coma, death.

Divalproex (Depakote) Toxic effects with divalproex include sedation, nausea, vomiting, tremor, GI upset, weight gain, ataxia, headache, hair loss, rash, clotting abnormalities, transient transaminase elevation, and false abnormality in thyroid function test.

RELATED CLINICAL CONCERNS

Children

Divalproex therapy for children younger than 2 years of age is associated with increased risk of hepatotoxicity. Safety and effectiveness of lithium therapy in patients younger than the age of 12 have not been established.

Adolescents

Divalproex, lithium, carbamazepine are contraindicated in pregnancy, so sexually active teens need to be advised about this risk. Side effects of acne, weight gain, tremors, and polyuria may be particularly upsetting for this age group.

Older Adults

Divalproex may increase the risk of somnolence and dehydration. Risk of side effects with lithium are pronounced in this population as excretion may be reduced due to impaired kidney function. Signs of toxicity may be exhibited within normal therapeutic ranges.

Other Clinical Concerns

Managing Safety in Lithium Therapy Lithium use must be monitored closely to prevent complications. Patients need an initial laboratory screening including complete blood count (CBC), thyroid levels, creatinine, blood urea nitrogen (BUN), electrolytes, glucose level, and an ECG. For the first month on lithium, blood levels are drawn weekly, then biweekly, and then every 2 to 3 months for maintenance once a stable level is achieved.
Causes of increased lithium levels include the following:

- Decreased intake of dietary sodium
- Sweating or dehydration
- Concurrent medications such as thiazides, amiloride, furosemide, ibuprofen, tetracyclines, methyldopa, and metronidazole

Additional contraindications include pregnancy, lactation, and history of myocardial infraction.

Managing Safety in Carbamazepine Therapy For patients starting on carbamazepine therapy, the initial work-up should include CBC with platelets, liver function tests, electrolytes and BUN, and an ECG in patients older than 40 years of age or with a history of cardiac problems.

Dosing should not increase by more than 200 mg/day until 800 mg/day is reached. These patients need to be monitored for possible blood dyscrasias with periodic CBCs, liver function tests, and drug level tests. Many drugs contribute to increased blood levels of carbamazepine. Concurrent medications need to be reviewed with the treatment team. MAOIs should not be prescribed for 2 weeks before or after carbamazepine. Monitor closely for signs of infection.

Contraindications include a history of bone marrow suppression; glaucoma; cardiac, hepatic, or renal impairment; pregnancy and breast-feeding; and a history of allergic reactions to TCAs.

Managing Safety in Divalproex Therapy Initial screening should include CBC, liver function tests, and prothrombin time/partial thromboplastin time. A major concern is the risk for hepatic failure; therefore, the patient needs to have periodic liver function tests and be monitored for symptoms such as jaundice and weakness during the first 6 months of therapy. Because clotting problems can also occur, patients need to be advised to avoid aspirin products and warfarin. In addition, some drugs such as cimetidine, fluoxetine, and amitriptyline can increase the blood levels of this drug. Divalproex is contraindicated during pregnancy and lactation and in the presence of any liver disease.

PATIENT AND FAMILY EDUCATION

- Teach patient to adhere strictly to lithium or carbamazepine therapy regimen.
- Advise patient to consult prescriber before starting any new medications or nutritional supplements.
- Teach patient how to avoid possible adverse interactions.
- Advise patient and family that lithium should be taken with food or milk to avoid GI irritation.
- Teach patient the lithium side effects that should be reported to the treatment team.
- Teach patient to avoid any significant changes in diet patterns or salt intake when taking lithium.
- Teach patient how to replace loss of fluids and electrolytes after diarrhea or vigorous exercise.
- Teach patient that over-the-counter analgesics (e.g., ibuprofen and other non-steroidal anti-inflammatory agents) should be avoided while taking lithium.
- Advise pregnant patient that no mood stabilizers should be taken during pregnancy because of the risk of birth defects.
- Teach patient that flu-like symptoms that occur while taking carbamazepine should be reported to the treatment team.
- Teach patient that easy bruising or bleeding, pallor, or weakness should be reported to the treatment team.

MEDICATIONS FOR PSYCHOTIC SYMPTOMS

Antipsychotic medications can be divided into two primary categories: typical and atypical agents (Box 21–6).

The typical agents include older antipsychotics that have been available since the late 1950s. The atypical include newer antipsychotics that became available in the U.S. market after 1990.

BOX 21–6
Antipsychotic Medications

Typical Agents	Dosage
Chlorpromazine (Thorazine)	200–800 mg/day
Thioridazine (Mellaril)	200–800 mg/day
Fluphenazine (Prolixin)	10–40 mg/day
Trifluoperazine (Stelazine)	5–60 mg/day
Haloperidol (Haldol)	5–20 mg/day
Perphenazine (Trilafon)	4–60 mg/day
Fluphenazine decanoate (Prolixin decanoate)	12.5–75 mg/2 wks
Haloperidol decanoate (Haldol decanoate)	50–300 mg/4 wks
Pimozide (Orap)	1–10 mg/day (Note: Pimozide is indicated for suppression of severe motor and phonic tics in Tourette's syndrome.)
Loxapine (Loxitane)	50–250 mg/day
Molidone (Moban)	50–225 mg/day
Thiothixene (Navane)	5–60 mg/day
Atypical Agents	
Clozapine (Clozaril). Also available in oral dissolving tablet (FazaClo)	300–900 mg/day
Risperidone (Risperdal). Also available in oral dissolving tablet (M-tab) and long-acting injection (Risperdal Consta)	2–8 mg/day 25–50 mg/2wks (Consta)
Olanzapine (Zyprexa). Also available in oral dissolving tablet (Zydis)	5–30 mg/day
Quetiapine (Seroquel)	300–800 mg/day
Ziprasidone (Geodon)	40–160 mg/day
Aripiprazole (Abilify)	5–30 mg/day
Paliperidone (Invega)	3–12 mg/day

Even though both groups are effective to alleviate the positive symptoms of schizophrenia, such as delusions and hallucinations, the atypical agents have greater efficacy to manage negative symptoms or deficits in function, such as social withdrawal and blunted affect. Even though typical and atypical agents have different side effect profiles, the general rules in relation to potency may apply as shown in Table 21–6.

Most people respond to one of the typical or atypical agents to a degree at the first psychotic episode. However, some patients may go through a period of trials and errors for months or years to find the best available medication and dosage

TABLE 21–6

Potency of Typical Antipsychotics and Side Effects

		Side Effects			
Potency	Drug	EPS	Anticholinergic	Sedation	Seizure
Low	Chlorpromazine (Thorazine) (400–1000 mg/day)	Low	High	High	High
Low	Thioridazine (Mellaril) (400–800 mg/day)	Low	High	High	High
Low	Quetiapine (Seroquel) (100–800 mg/day)	Low	High	High	Low
Low	Clozapine (Clozaril) (100–900 mg/day)	Low	High	High	High
High	Fluphenazine (Prolixin) (10–60 mg/day)	High	Low	Low	Low
High	Haloperidol (Haldol) (10–60 mg/day)	High	Low	Low	Low
High	Risperidone (Risperdal) (0.5–8 mg/day)	High	Low	Low	Low

for them. A trial of any one medication should last for a substantial period, usually 6 to 8 weeks, unless intolerable side effects occur early. Even though the atypical agents have a better side effect profile for long-term treatment, the typical or older agents may be chosen for short-term management of psychosis or long-term management of symptoms that do not respond to the atypical agents.

TYPICAL AGENTS

Typical antipsychotics treat the positive symptoms of schizophrenia (Box 21–7).

HYPOTHESES ON MECHANISM OF ACTION

The effects of typical antipsychotics on positive symptoms have been thought to be associated with interactions with different types of dopamine receptors in the brain. The medications' interactions with one type of dopamine receptor may be associated with their antipsychotic efficacy, and those with another type may be associated with side effects such as movement disorders. However, it is now hypothesized that other neurotransmitter systems than the dopamine are also involved in psychoses.

EFFICACY IN TREATING SYMPTOMS

All of the typical antipsychotic agents are supposed to be equally effective. However, the amounts of the medications required to exert a certain level of antipsy-

---

BOX 21–7
Seven Categories of Positive Symptoms in Patients With Schizophrenia

1. **Hallucinations:** Perception of internal stimuli in auditory, visual, olfactory, or tactile forms.
2. **Delusions:** Beliefs that are groundless, idiosyncratic, and unreal.
3. **Conceptual disorganization:** Non-goal-directed flow of thinking process, loose associations.
4. **Excitement:** Excessive responsiveness to environment, accelerated motor behavior, hypervigilance.
5. **Hostility:** Verbal abuse, assaultive, sarcastic; nonverbal expression of anger or resentment.
6. **Grandiosity:** Unrealistic sense of superiority such as belief in extraordinary abilities, knowledge, power, wealth, or moral righteousness.
7. **Suspiciousness:** Excessive ideas of persecution resulting in guardedness, distrustful attitude, or verbalization of concern about being harmed.

chotic effect vary according to their potency or the degree of interaction with different types of dopamine receptors in each individual. A high-potency agent such as haloperidol (Haldol) in a dose of 2 mg may elicit the same level of antipsychotic effect as a low-potency agent such as thioridazine (Mellaril) in a dose of 100 mg.

Long-acting agents with average half-lives of 3 weeks (Haldol decanoate) and 2 weeks (Prolixin decanoate) are available in intramuscular forms. These lipophilic agents are injected into fatty tissues in muscles of the deltoid or gluteus maximus. In the case of Haldol decanoate, a daily oral dose of 10 mg or 300 mg/month can be replaced by a monthly injection of Haldol decanoate with one third to one-half of the monthly oral dose (100 to 150 mg). The dosages for Prolixin decanoate can generally range from 12.5 to 75 mg every 2 weeks.

COMMON SIDE EFFECTS

The low-potency typical agents have more risks of sedation and lowered seizure threshold than the high-potency agents (see Table 21–6) in general because of the greater antagonism of cholinergic, adrenergic, and histaminergic receptor systems in the brain. However, high-potency agents have more risks for the development of extrapyramidal side effects (EPS) (Table 21–7) because of the potent antagonism of the dopamine receptors that are associated with movement disorders.

The other common adverse effects of antipsychotic drugs may be minimized by the considerations listed in Table 21–8.

RELATED CLINICAL CONCERNS

Children

Children may be particularly vulnerable to the side effects of antipsychotics. In general, low doses of antipsychotic medications are found to be effective for many children with psychotic symptoms, autism, and vocal or motor tics.

Adolescents

Dosing of antipsychotics may be similar to that of adults based on the individual's body size. Side effect management becomes very important in this age group so the individual will not feel embarrassed.

Older Adults

Start with low doses of high-potency agents, which have less anticholinergic side effects than those with low potency. Bedtime dosing may reduce the risk of problems associated with orthostatic hypotension, such as falling. Anticholinergics that treat EPS may contribute to delirium.

Other Clinical Concerns

Psychotic Disorders Caused by Medical Conditions Psychiatric symptoms of psychoses can be part of nonpsychiatric disorders such as Addison's disease,

TABLE 21–7

Signs of Extrapyramidal Side Effects

Sign	Onset	Manifestations
Akathisia (motor restlessness)	Sudden or gradual	Pacing, shifting from one foot to another when standing, tapping feet while sitting, inability to sit still, rocking, feeling something jumping out of skin, feeling anxious, feeling physically tense, tossing and turning in bed, feeling wired up
Dystonia (involuntary muscle contraction with rigidity)	Sudden	Neck twisting (torticollis), back arching or head pulling backward (opisthotonos), clenched jaw (trismus), eyes fixed upward (oculogyral crisis), difficulty speaking and swallowing with hypersalivation, inability to close eyes (blepharospasm), protruding tongue
Tardive dyskinesia (muscle spasms with late onset)	After months or years of antipsychotic use	Rapid blinking of the eyes; wormlike tongue; chewing with nothing in mouth; lip puckering; facial grimacing; rhythmic involuntary movements of jaws, face, extremities, and trunk
Pseudoparkinsonism (signs similar to those of Parkinson's Disease)	Sudden or gradual	Shuffling gait; coarse tremor; drooling; fixed facial expression; apathy; slowness of voluntary movement; cogwheel rigidity in arms, shoulders, and neck; lead-pipe rigidity in torso and extremities, which become unmovable; rabbit syndrome (tremor of the lips and mouth)

pernicious anemia, AIDS, CNS infection or neoplasms, Cushing's disease, delirium, dementias, lupus, and other conditions. It may be necessary to use antipsychotic medications to manage the symptoms while the underlying medical conditions are being corrected.

Reverse Epinephrine Effect Certain antipsychotics such as clozapine, fluphenazine enanthate, chlorpromazine, and thioridazine can cause epinephrine reversal and a hypotensive response when epinephrine is used to increase blood pressure.

TABLE 21–8

Minimizing Side Effects From the Typical and Atypical Agents

Type of Side Effect	Action
Cardiac problems	Use high-potency agents except pimozide (Orap) to avoid conduction abnormalities.
Hematological disorder	Monitor CBC weekly for the first 6 months of clozapine treatment, then biweekly for additional 6 months, and every 4 weeks thereafter.
Parkinsonism	Low-potency agents may minimize parkinsonism because of their built-in anticholinergic property. The same is true of clozapine.
Prostatic hypertrophy	Avoid low-potency agents and clozapine (Clozaril), which exert high anticholinergic effects.
Seizure	Avoid loxapine (Loxitane) and clozapine (Clozaril) in clients with a history of seizure. Molidone (Moban) may have lower seizure risk than other antipsychotics.
Pregnancy	Avoid use of low-potency agents. Increased risk of anomalies is associated with use of the phenothiazines group, including chlorpromazine (Thorazine) and thioridazine (Mellaril). High-potency agents such as fluphenazine (Prolixin), haloperidol (Haldol), trifluoperazine (Stelazine), and perphenazine (Trilafon) are associated with lower risk during pregnancy. Clozapine has been used during pregnancy without short term adverse effects on the fetus
Weight gain	Loxapine (Loxitane), molidone (Moban), ziprasidone (Geodon), and aripiprazole (Abilify) are associated with lower risks.
Sexual side effects	Clozapine (Clozaril) and quetiapine (Seroquel) are associated with lower risks.

Photosensitivity The skin needs to be protected from exposure to sunlight. The eyes may be more bothered by sunlight.

Heart Block Overdoses of pimozide (Orap) or thioridazine (Mellaril) are associated with higher risk.

Blindness High doses of thioridazine (Mellaril) can cause pigmentation of the retina, which could lead to blindness.

ATYPICAL AGENTS

The medications in this category are used to treat both positive and negative symptoms of schizophrenia (Boxes 21–7 and 21–8). However, they can also be used to treat psychotic symptoms of other psychiatric disorders (schizoaffective disorders, major depression with psychotic features, and bipolar disorders).

HYPOTHESES ON MECHANISMS OF ACTION

The mechanisms of action of atypical antipsychotics are not defined. It has been hypothesized that the atypical agents are more selective than the typical ones when they interact with different types of dopamine receptors. For instance, the dopamine receptors, which are associated with movement disorders, are less affected by atypical agents such as clozapine (Clozaril) or quetiapine (Seroquel). However, the atypical agents also affect multiple neurotransmitter systems, making it difficult for their exact mechanisms of action to be understood.

EFFICACY IN TREATING SYMPTOMS

The positive symptoms respond faster to antipsychotics than the negative symptoms in general. Changes in negative symptoms or regaining of affect, social activities, or motivation may be observed over months and years of treatment when these agents are used along with psychosocial rehabilitation interventions.

BOX 21–8
Seven Categories of Negative Symptoms in Patients with Schizophrenia

1. **Difficulty with abstract or logical thinking:** Difficulty in classification, generalization, conceptualization beyond concrete thinking.

2. **Lack of spontaneity and flow of conversation:** Diminished flow of productivity in verbal interaction with others.

3. **Blunted affect:** A reduction in nonverbal communicative cues or facial expressions.

4. **Social withdrawal:** Reduced activities of daily living or neglected interpersonal involvement.

5. **Poor rapport:** Inability to show interpersonal empathy, interest, sense of closeness or openness during conversation.

6. **Emotional withdrawal with difficulty identifying own feelings:** Lack of interest or involvement in life.

7. **Stereotyped thinking:** Rigid repetitious thought content.

A new long-acting agent, risperidone (Risperdal Consta), with average half-life of 2 weeks is also available in intramuscular forms. The active agent (risperidone) in white microspheres needs to be mixed gently with the water-based diluent right before the administration every 2 weeks. The vials of 25 mg, 37.5 mg, and 50 mg come with a syringe with the diluent in it. They need to be stored in a refrigerator.

COMMON SIDE EFFECTS

The atypicals are generally less associated with EPS than the typical agents, but there are a wide range of other side effects.

Clozapine (Clozaril/FazaClo) Excessive salivation during sleep, orthostatic hypotension, sedation, tachycardia, anticholinergic effects (constipation, blurred vision, urinary retention), seizure, agranulocytosis (seen in 0.4%–1.0% of patients), myocarditis, respiratory depression, weight gain with increased appetite, urinary incontinence, diabetes mellitus type II, excessive sweating, nausea, dizziness, and low-grade fever.

Risperidone (Risperdal/Consta) Orthostatic hypotension, tachyarrhythmia, akathisia, dysmenorrhea, reduced libido, rhinitis, insomnia, headaches, weight gain, EPS, and prolactinemia.

Olanzapine (Zyprexa/Zydis) Weight gain with increased appetite, diabetes mellitus type II, tachycardia, sedation, orthostatic hypotension. EPS, akathisia.

Quetiapine (Seroquel) Sedation, weight gain with increased appetite, dry mouth, constipation, diabetes mellitus type II, orthostatic hypotension, tachyarrhythmia.

Ziprasidone (Geodon) Akathisia, EPS, orthostatic hypotension, prolonged QT interval, tachyarrhythmia

Aripiprazole (Abilify) Insomnia, nausea, akathisia, weight gain, bradyarrhythmia, tachyarrhythmia.

RELATED CLINICAL CONCERNS

Children

Because of the lack of studies on long-term effects of antipsychotics in children, a drug-free period may be periodically considered. Antipsychotic medications could contribute to cognitive blunting, leading to school problems. Atypicals have been used with some success in treatment of behavioral symptoms of autism.

Adolescents

Side effect of weight gain often affects compliance. Long-term use of antipsychotics in the presence of a serious psychiatric disorder like schizophrenia has not been well studied.

Older Adults

Use of atypical antipsychotics for dementia-related psychosis may be associated with increased risk of mortality from infection, heart failure, and other medical conditions. Orthostatic hypotension side effect can be a safety concern.

Other Clinical Concerns

Management Systems for the Patient Taking Clozapine Because of the possibility of granulocytosis, clozapine has been marketed under unique systems set up by the pharmaceutical companies. All patients to be started on clozapine must be cleared through one of the systems before the treatment begins. The therapy can be initiated if the patient has:

- White blood cell count (WBC) 3500 or greater and Absolute Neutrophil Count (ANC) of 2000 or greater
- No history of clozapine-induced agranulocytosis
- No uncontrolled seizures

The physician and pharmacist are responsible for obtaining weekly WBC and ANC. Only a week's supply of clozapine will be dispensed after the WBC/ANC counts are reported every week to the pharmacy. After 6 months of treatment with no hematological problems, a 2-week supply of clozapine can be dispensed as the acceptable WBC/ANC counts are reported biweekly (Table 21–9). After 12 months of established clozapine treatment without any abnormal hematological data, monitoring of WBC/ANC and dispensing of clozapine can be done every 4 weeks.

MANAGING SIDE EFFECTS OF ANTIPSYCHOTIC AGENTS

Extrapyramidal symptoms are the major side effect of typical antipsychotic medications. The symptoms are very distressing and uncomfortable. Their presence will affect patient's adherence with antipsychotic medications. Prevention and treatment of EPS is essential to keep patients on their medications. In addition, the side effects of the medications should be monitored, for example anticholinergic side effects from benztropine (Cogentin).

Parkinsonism and dystonia (see Table 21–7 for description of symptoms) can be treated by antiparkinsonian drugs such as benztropine (Cogentin) or trihexyphenidyl (Artane), which are acetylcholine (muscarinic) receptor antagonists (anticholinergics). Akathisia can be resolved with beta blockers such as propranolol (Inderal) and metoprolol (Lopressor). Antihistamines and benzodiazepines are also used. No medication is available to treat tardive dyskinesia. High doses of vitamin E (1600–2000 IU) have been tried. See Table 21–10 for a list of the medications that treat these symptoms.

TABLE 21–9

Monitoring Granulocyte Counts During Clozapine Therapy

WBC and Granulocyte/Neutrophil Count	Action Plan

I. Reduced WBC within normal range:
  A. WBC count drops 3000 cells from previous test
  OR
  B. Three or more consecutive drops regardless of their counts
	I. (A) Monitor for infection; (B) CBC with differentials if ordered by physician; (C) continue clozapine.

II. Mild leukopenia: WBC = 3000–3500	II. (A) Monitor for infection; (B) CBC with differentials; (C) continue clozapine.
III. Granulocytopenia: WBC = 2000–3000 Granulocytes/neutrophil = 1000–1500	III. (A) Interrupt clozapine at once; (B) start daily CBC with differentials; (C) observe closely for infection; (D) resume clozapine after normalization of granulocyte counts.
IV. Severe granulocytopenia: WBC < 2000 OR Agranulocytosis: Granulocytes/neutrophil <500	IV. (A) Discontinue clozapine at once; (B) consult with hematologist to consider protective isolation in a medical unit; (C) daily CBC with differentials; (D) clozapine must NOT be restarted at all.

Other Side Effects from Antipsychotic Medications

Neuroleptic Malignant Syndrome

Neuroleptic malignant syndrome (NMS) can develop over a few days. This syndrome is uncommon yet potentially fatal. The signs include elevated temperature (>39°C [102°F]), severe EPS, autonomic instability, delirium, and elevation of CPK, WBCs, and liver enzymes. Medical interventions are required. Cooling measures and hydration are needed.

Autonomic Dysfunction

• *Tachycardia:* Beta blockers may be used if pulse exceeds 100 beats per minute (bpm).

TABLE 21–10

Medications For Extrapyramidal Symptoms (EPS)

Drug Type	Drug and Dosage (mg/day)
Antiparkinsonian	Benztropine (Cogentin) (1–6 mg) Trihexyphenidyl (Artane) (1–15 mg)
Antihistamine	Diphenhydramine (Benadryl) (25–100 mg)
Beta-adrenergic blocker	Propranolol (Inderal) (10–80 mg) Atenolol (Tenormin) (50–100 mg) Metoprolol (Lopressor) (25–400 mg)
Alpha-2 adrenergic blocker	Clonidine (Catapres) (0.2–2.4 mg)

- *Sialorrhea (excessive salivation):* Can be excessive with clozapine (Clozaril). No anticholinergic agents are recommended to control excessive salivation.
- *Dry mouth:* Extra care of the mouth and teeth is required because of higher risk of developing cavities.
- *Orthostatic hypotension:* Patients should be cautioned about the possibility of falling on abrupt change of posture.
- *Low-grade fever:* The homeostasis for body temperature may be affected by clozapine (Clozaril)

Other Categories of Side Effects

- *Elevated cholesterol and triglycerides:* Tends to occur in patients on any antipsychotic agents. Type II diabetes may develop in association with the use of antipsychotics.
- *Weight gain:* Many psychiatric medications are associated with the risk of weight gain.
- *Sedation:* Common with most psychiatric medications. This can be used for sleep problems.
- *Endocrine dysfunction:* Most antipsychotic agents (except clozapine and quetiapine) can elevate prolactin levels. This may lead to amenorrhea.
- *Liver enzyme elevation:* This elevation may be asymptomatic.
- *Hematologic dysfunction:* All antipsychotic agents can affect CBC values.

PATIENT AND FAMILY EDUCATION

- Review signs of EPS and reinforce the idea that treatment is available to minimize risks.

- Advise carrying water and hard candies to reduce dry mouth.
- Advise against stopping medications without consulting the prescriber.
- Encourage physical activities and healthy eating habits to avoid weight gain and metabolic syndromes.
- Teach patient to report muscle stiffness or restlessness to the prescriber.
- Teach patient to report development of flu-like symptoms while taking clozapine.
- Review specific plans to manage side effects with patient, family, and care-givers.
- Advise female patients to avoid pregnancy.
- Prepare patient and family that medications take 2–12 weeks to show improvements.

COLLABORATIVE MANAGEMENT FOR ADVOCACY FOR PATIENTS TAKING PSYCHIATRIC MEDICATIONS

Patients, families, psychiatrists, nurses, family physicians, pharmacists, and other related clinicians need to work as a team in the management of the patient's medications. The patient and family can provide information on real-life experiences of the illness and the medication. Psychiatric clinicians can provide patients and families with updated clinical information on the efficacy and safety of the medications. The other clinicians and caretakers who are working with the patient can provide the data that can be used to assess the efficacy and safety.

One of the most common obstacles to advocacy is the patient's nonadherence to the treatment (Box 21–9). The patient may not admit the illness that requires medication treatment. The specific reasons for this denial need to be addressed to develop a support team with the patient/family/caretakers in the center.

BOX 21–9
Factors that Contribute to Nonadherence to Pharmacological Treatment

- Medication side effects.
- Medication not as effective as expected.
- Need to continue medication without patient sensing immediate improve-ment.
- Complicated drug regimens.
- Cost of medication.
- Patient feels worse when first starts medication; feels better when first stops medication.

BOX 21–10
Use of Psychosocial Rehabilitation Process for Medication Management

1. **Mutual Understanding** (Diagnosis): Identifying symptoms and/or needs for help from a client's and/or family's perspectives.

2. **Collaborative Mapping** (Planning): Identifying a client's and/or family's strength or coping skills to manage symptoms that are interfering with their pursuit of life goals. The client or family can move faster for adjustment when their strength is acknowledged.

3. **Negotiated Support** (Intervention): Helping a client to clarify his or her concerns about medications and providing resources for decision making to choose pharmacological therapy. Convey the idea that the medication can work only when the client or family takes charge of it.

4. **Interactive Appraisal** (Evaluation): Appraisal of pharmacological therapy with client and family in terms of balancing benefits and adverse experiences.

5. **Guided Exploration** (Assessment): Identifying factors for possible nonadherence. Identifying possibility of better balance between benefits and adverse experiences with new knowledge on available medications. The value of the medications for the client needs to be recreated at all times because it can become unclear during the life-long treatment course.

Source: Adapted from Groenwold, L. (1996). *Decreasing Readmission: The Comprehensive Role of Nursing in Psychsocial Rehabilitation.* Presented at Contemporary Forums Psychiatric Nursing Conference in Hollywood, CA.

The process of psychosocial rehabilitation (Box 21–10) provides the essential strategies to advocate for patients in the area of psychopharmacological support. The minimum data set in this chapter on the psychiatric medications can be applied for interventions with these strategies to develop partnership with patients/families and achieve the goal of valuing their medication in relation to their life goals.

CHARTING TIPS

The documentation should include information on the following elements:

1. Target symptoms
2. The patient's understanding of the efficacy of the medication
3. The patient's adherence to the medication
4. Presence of side effects

BOX 21–11
Sound/Look Alike Medications

- Clozapine/Klonopine
- Zyban/Zydis
- Celebrex/Celexa/Cerebxy
- Clonidine/clonazepam
- Lamisil/Lamictal
- Serzone/Seroquel

- Zyprexa/Zyrtec
- Wellbutrin SR/Wellbutrin XL
- Zantac/Xanax
- Prilosec/Prozac
- Chlorpropamide/chlorpromazine

---

5. Current mental status
6. Response to treatment of side effects

COMMUNITY-BASED CARE

- The patient should be given a written list of all the medications that have been tried, the current medications, the dosages, and the clinical responses. Make sure that the patient or family can verbalize the names of the medications, the dosages, and the schedule for administration. If they cannot, instruct them to carry a card with all the information on it.
- With the number of new drugs and with many look alike/sound alike medications, precautions must be taken to ensure that the correct medications are provided. See Box 21-11 for a list of common sound/look alike psychotropic medications. Clinical programs need to have mechanisms in place to prevent drug errors.
- The clinicians of all disciplines who are seeing new patients need to assess the psychiatric medication they are currently taking to avoid its interruption.
- When a patient on psychiatric medication is admitted to an acute hospital, assessment of psychiatric medication must be included in the overall nursing assessment. Then if a patient is unable to take them for some reason while in the hospital (NPO, contraindications), appropriate alternatives can be prescribed.

References

AARP. (2007). *Sexuality at midlife and beyond*. Retrieved June 16, 2007 from aarp.typepad.com/socialsecurity/2005/05/aging_in_america.html

Agency for Health Care Policy and Research (AHRQ). (1992). *Acute pain management: Operative or medical procedures and trauma. Clinical practice guideline*. Rockville, MD: Public Health Service, US Department of Health and Human Services (DHHS).

Agency for Health Care Policy and Research. (1993). *Depression in primary care*, vols 1 and 2. Rockville, MD: Public Health Service, US Department of Health and Human Services (DHHS).

Agency for Health Care Policy and Research. (1994). *Management of cancer pain. Clinical practice guideline*. Rockville, MD: Public Health Service, US Department of Health and Human Services (DHHS).

Agency for Healthcare Quality and Research. (2001). *Outcomes for 19 mental diseases and disorders*. Retrieved September 30, 2001 from http//hcup.ahrq.gov/hcupnet.asp.

Agency for Healthcare Quality and Research. (2000). *Improving quality of care for people with depression: Translating research into practice fact sheet*. Agency for Healthcare Research and Quality, Rockville, MD.

Agency for Healthcare Research and Quality. (2006). *Report on Review of Current Available Research On Eating Disorders*. Retrieved June 15, 2006 from ahrq.gov.

Agency for Healthcare Research and Quality (AHRQ). (2007). *Newer class of antidepressants similar in effectiveness but side effects differ*. AHRQ Electronic Newsletter. January 26, 2007, Issue #219. Available at www.ahrq.gov.

Agency for Healthcare Research and Quality. (2007). *One in four hospital patients is admitted with a mental health or substance abuse disorder*. AHRQ Electronic Newsletter. April 13, 2007, Issue #225. Available at www.ahrq.gov.

Aguilera, D. C. (1998). *Crisis intervention theory and methodology* (8th ed.). St. Louis: Mosby.

Alcoholics Anonymous. (1953). *Twelve steps and twelve traditions*. New York: Alcoholics Anonymous World Services Inc.

Alzheimers Association. (2006). *Statistics about Alzheimer's Disease*. Retrieved December 22, 2006, from www.alzheimers.org.

American Academy of Pediatrics. (2000). Clinical practice guideline: Diagnosis and evaluation of the child with attention-deficit/hyperactivity disorder. *Pediatrics, 105,* 1158–1170.

American Association of Suicidology. (2004). *Suicide in the U.S.A.* Retrieved January 18, 2007, from www.suicidology.org/associations/1045/files/suicideintheus.pdf.

American Association of Suicidology. (2005). *Recommendations for inpatient and residential patients known to be at elevated risk for suicide.* Retrieved January 15, 2007, from www.suicidology.org/association/045/files/finalrec.pdf.

American Association of Suicidology. (2007). *Survivors of suicide facts.* Retrieved January 18, 2007, from www.suicidology.org/associations/1045/files/survivorfactsheet.pdf.

American Hospital Formulary Service (AHFS). (2000). *Drug information.* Bethesda, MD: American Society of Hospital Pharmacists.

American Nurses Association. (2006). *Code of ethics.* Retrieved September 2, 2006, from www.nursingworld.org/ethics/code.

American Nurses Association. (2002). *Preventing workplace violence.* Retrieved April 9, 2006, from www.nursingworld.org/osh/wp5.htm.

American Pain Society. (2003). *Principles of analgesic use in treatment of acute pain and cancer* (5th ed.). Glenview, IL: American Pain Society.

American Psychiatric Association (APA). (2000). *Diagnostic and statistical manual of mental disorders—text revision (TR.)* Washington, DC: American Psychiatric Association (DSM-IV-TR).

American Psychiatric Association (APA). (1994). *Diagnostic and statistical manual of mental disorders* (4th ed.). Washington, DC: American Psychiatric Association (DSM-IV).

American Psychiatric Association. (2004). *Disaster psychiatry handbook.* Retrieved February 22, 2007 from www.psych.org/disaster.

American Psychiatric Association. (1995). Practice guidelines for treatment of patients with substance abuse disorders. *American Journal of Psychiatry, 15* (Supplement), 1–59.

American Psychiatric Association. (2006). APA Lauds FDA Findings that Antidepressants Protect Against Suicide 12/13/06. Retrieved January 10, 2007 from www.psych.org/news.

American Psychiatric Association Work Group on Eating Disorders. (2000). Practice guidelines for treatment of patients with eating disorders. *American Journal of Psychiatry, 157,* 1–39.

Anandarajah, G. & Hight, I. (2001). Spirituality and medical practice: Using the HOPE questions as a practical tool for spiritual assessment. *American Family Physician, 63,* 81–88.

Anderson, C. (2002). Past victim, future victim? *Nursing Management, 33(3),* 26–32.

Andrews, M. M. & Boyle, J. S. (2002). *Transcultural concepts in nursing care* (4th ed.). Philadelphia: Lippincott.

Antai-Otong, D. (1995). *Psychiatric nursing: Biological and behavioral concepts.* Philadelphia: WB Saunders.

Antai-Otong, D. (1995). Helping the alcoholic patient recover. *American Journal of Nursing, 22(8),* 22–30.

Antai-Otong, D. (2000). The neurobiology of anxiety disorders. Implications for psychiatric nursing practice. *Issues in Mental Health Nursing, 21,* 71–89.

Barki, Z. K., Kravitz, H. M., & Berki, T. M. (1998). Psychotropic medications in pregnancy. *Psychiatric Annals 28*(9), 486–500.

Barkin, R. L., Barkin, S. J., & Barkin, D. S. (2005). Perception, assessment, treatment and management of pain in the elderly. *Clinics in Geriatric Medicine, 21,* 465–490.

Barnum, B. S. (2006). *Spirituality in nursing: From traditional to new age.* New York: Springer.

Barry, P. D. (1996). *Psychosocial nursing assessment and intervention* (3rd ed.). Philadelphia: Lippincott-Raven.

Beattie, M. (1992). *Codependent no more.* New York: Harper Collins.

Beck, A. (1979). *Cognitive therapy and emotional disorder.* New York: New American Library.

Beck-Little, R., & Weinrich, S. P. (1998). Assessment and management of sleep disorders in the elderly. *Journal of Gerontological Nursing, 24,* 21–29.

Belcher, A. & Griffiths, M. (2005). The spiritual care perspectives and practices of hospice nurses. *Journal of Hospice and Palliative Nursing, 7,* 271–279.

Bergh, I., & Sjostrom, B. (1999). A comparative study of nurses' and elderly patients' ratings of pain and pain tolerance. *Journal of Gerontological Nursing, 25,* 30–36.

Berkow, R. (1992). *Merck manual.* Rahway, NJ: Merck Research Laboratories.

Berlinger, J. S. (2001). Domestic violence. How you can make a difference. *Nursing, 31,* 58–63.

Bernardo, M. L. (2007). Social anxiety disorder restricts lines. *Nurseweek,* August 13, 18–20.

Bernstein, S. B. (1989). Breaking the vicious cycle of noncompliance. *Nursing, 19(1),* 74–75.

Bezchlibnyk-Butler, K. Z., & Virani, A. S. (Eds.). (2004). *Clinical handbook of psychotropic drugs for children and adolescents.* Toronto: Hogrefe & Huber.

Birmaher, B. & Axelson, D. (2005). Pediatric psychopharmacology. In B. J. Sadock & V. A. Sadock (Eds.), *Kaplan & Sadock's comprehensive textbook of psychiatry* (8th ed.) (pp. 3363–3376). Philadelphia: Lippincott Williams & Wilkins.

Black, C. (1987). *It will never happen to me.* New York: Ballantine.

Blair, D. T., & New, S. A. (1991). Assaultive behavior: Know the risks. *Journal of Psychosocial Mental Health Service, 29,* 25.

Bond, S. M., Neelon, V. J., & Belyea, M. J. (2006). Delirium in hospitalized older patients with cancer. *Oncology Nursing Forum, 33,* 1075–1083.

Borsook, D., McPeek, B., & Lebel, A. A. (1996). *The Massachusetts General Hospital Handbook of pain management.* Philadelphia: Lippincott-Raven.

Bottomley, J. M. (2001). Politics of health care and the needs of the older adult: The social context of changes in delivery. *Geriatric Rehabilitation, 16,* 28–44.

Bowen, M. (1978). *Family therapy in clinical practice.* New York: Aronson.

Brady, K. T., & Malcolm, R. J. (2006). Substance use disorders and co-occuring axis I psychiatric disorders. In M. Galanter & H. D. Kleber (Eds.), *The Amer-*

ican Psychiatric Publishing textbook of substance abuse treatment (3rd ed.) (pp. 529–538). Washington DC: American Psychiatric Publishing.

Brauner, D. J., Muir, J. C., & Sachs, G. A. (2000). Treating nondementia illnesses in patients with dementia. *Journal of the American Medical Association, 283(24),* 3230–3235.

Breitbart, W., & Holland, J. C. (Eds.), (1993). *Psychiatric aspects of symptom management in cancer patients.* Washington, DC: American Psychiatric Press.

Brentin, L., & Sieh, A. (1991). Caring for the morbidly obese. *American Journal of Nursing, 91,* 40–43.

Brink, T. L., Yesavage, J. A., Lum, O., Heersema, P. H., Adey, M., & Rose, T. L. (1982). Screening tests for geriatric depression. *Clinical Gerontologist, 1,* 37–44.

Brown, T. M., & Stoudemire, A. (1998). *Psychiatric side effects of prescription and over-the-counter medications—recognition and management.* Washington, DC: American Psychiatric Press, Inc.

Brownell, K. D., & Wadden, T. A. (2000). Obesity. In B. J. Sadock & V. A. Sadock (Eds.), *Kaplan and Sadock's Comprehensive textbook of psychiatry* (7th ed.) (pp. 1787–1797). Philadelphia: Lippincott Williams & Wilkins.

Burke, M. M., & Walsh, M. B. (1992). *Gerontologic nursing: care of the frail elderly.* St. Louis: Mosby.

Buttriss, G., Kuiper, R., & Newbold, B. (1995). The use of a homeless shelter as a clinical rotation for nursing students. *Journal of Nursing Education, 34,* 375–377.

Caine, E. D., & Lyness, J. M. (2000). Delirium, dementia, amnestic and other cognitive disorders. In B. J. Sadock & V. A. Sadock (Eds.), *Kaplan and Sadock's comprehensive textbook of psychiatry* (7th ed.) (pp 852–924). Philadelphia: Lippincott Williams & Wilkins.

Cameron, D. R. & Braunstein, G. D. (2004). Androgen replacement therapy in women. *Fertililty & Sterility, 82,* 273–289.

Campbell, J., & Humphreys, J. (1993). *Nursing care of survivors of family violence.* St. Louis: Mosby.

Campinha-Bacote, J. (1994). Cultural competence in psychiatric mental health nursing. A conceptual model. *Nursing Clinics of North America, 29(1),* 1–8.

Captain, C. (2006). Is your patient a suicide risk? *Nursing, 36(8),* 43–47.

Carpenito-Moyet, L. (2006). *Nursing diagnosis: application to clinical practice* (11th ed.). Philadelphia: Lippincott Williams & Wilkins.

Carroll-Johnson, R. M., Gorman, L. M., & Bush, N. J. (1998). *Psycohosocial nursing care along the cancer continuum.* Pittsburgh: Oncology Nursing Press.

Carroll-Johnson, R. M., Gorman, L. M. & Bush, N. J. (2006). *Psychosocial nursing care along the cancer continuum* (2nd ed). Pittsburgh: Oncology Nursing Press.

Carson, V. B. & Varcarolis, E. M. (2006). Family therapy. In E. M. Varcarolis, V. B. Carson, & N. C. Shoemaker (Eds.), *Foundations of psychiatric mental health nursing* (5th ed.) (pp. 730–748). Philadelphia: Saunders.

Carson, V. B. & Smith-Dijulio, K. (2006). Family violence. In E. M. Varcarolis, V. B. Carson, & N. C. Shoemaker (Eds.), *Foundations of psychiatric mental health nursing* (5th ed.) (p. 512). Philadelphia: Saunders.

Casper, L. M., & Haaga, J. G. (2005). Family and health demographics. In S. M. Harmon Hanson, V. Gedaly-Duff, & J. Rowe Kaakinen (Eds.), *Family health care nursing* (3rd ed.) (pp. 39–68). Philadelphia: FA Davis.

Cassidy, K. (1999). How to assess and intervene in a domestic violence situation. *Home Health Nurse, 17,* 664–672.

Cassileth, B. R. (1998). *The alternative medicine handbook.* New York: WW Norton and Co.

Catlette, M. (2005). A descriptive study of perception of workplace violence and safety strategies of nurses working in Level I trauma centers. *Journal of Emergency Nurses 31,* 519–525.

Cauthorne-Burnette, T., & Estes, M. (2006). *Clinical companion to accompany health assessment and physical examination.* (3rd ed.). Clinton Park, NY: Thompson/Delmar Learning Edition.

Center for Advancement of Palliative Care (CAPC). *Hospital Palliative Care Programs continue Rapid Growth.* Retrieved July 11, 2007 from www.Capc.org.

Center for Disease Control and Prevention. (2000). *National Health and Nutrition Examination Survey.* Retrieved June 1, 2006, from cdc.gov/nchs/about/major/nhanes/questions.html.

Centers for Disease Control and Prevention (CDC). (2004). *Methods of suicide among persons aged 10-19 years.* Retrieved January 15, 2007, from www.cdc.gov/mmwrpdf/wk/mm5322.pdf.

Centers for Disease Control and Prevention (CDC). (2006). *Self-inflicted injuries/suicide.* Retrieved January 2, 2007, from cdc.gov/nchs.fastfacts/suicide.htm.

Center for Disease Prevention and Control. (2006). *Fact sheets on domestic violence.* Retrieved July 15, 2006, from www.cdc.gov.

Center of Budget and Policy Priorities. (2004). *"What does the safety net accomplish."* Retrieved June 1, 2007, from www.cbpp.org

Centers for Disease Control and Prevention. (2002). *Violence: occupational hazards in hospitals.* Retrieved June 2, 2006, from www.cdc.gov/niosh/2002

Centers for Medicare and Medicaid Services (CMS). (2006). CMS publishes final patients' rights rules on use of restraints and seclusion. Retrieved May 29, 2007, from cms.hhs.gov/apps/media/press/release.asp?counter=2057&intNumPerPage=10

Chenvevert, M. (1994). *STAT: Special techniques in assertiveness training for women in health professions* (4th ed.). St. Louis: Mosby.

Chez, N. (1994). Helping the victim of domestic violence. *American Journal of Nursing, 94(7),* 32–37.

Chien, W. (2000). The use of physical restraints on hospitalized psychogeriatric patients. *Journal of Psychosocial Nursing and Mental Health Services, 38(2),* 13–22.

Child and Adolescent Bipolar Foundation. (2007). *About pediatric bipolar disorder.* Retrieved January 15, 2007, from www.bpkids.org.

Chung-Park, M., Hatton, D., Robinson, L., & Kleffel, D. (2006). RN-to-MSN students' attitudes toward women experiencing homelessness: A focus group study. *Journal of Nursing Education, 45(8)*, 317–322.

Cochrane, C. E. (1998). Eating regulation responses and eating disorders. In G. W. Stuart & M. T. Laraia (Eds.), *Stuart and Sundeen's principles and practices of psychiatric nursing* (6th ed.) (pp. 523–543). St. Louis: Mosby.

Collins, C. E. (1994). Intervetions with family caregivers of persons with Alzheimer's disease. *Nursing Clinics of North America, 29(1)*, 195–207.

Collins, J. J., & Walker, S. (2006). Pain: An introduction. In A. Goldman, R. Hain, & S. Liben (Eds.), *Oxford textbook of palliative care in children* (pp. 268–280). New York: Oxford University Press.

Contillo, C. (2007). Health literacy. *Working Nurse*. February 26, 24-5.

Copeland, L. G. (1993). Caring for children with chronic conditions. Model of critical times. *Holistic Nurse Practice, 8(1)*, 45–55.

Corbin, J. (2004). Chronic illness. In S. C. Smeltzer & B. G. Bare (Eds.), *Brunner and Suddarth's textbook of medical-surgical nursing* (pp. 146–157). Philadelphia: Lippincott Williams & Wilkins.

Cotter, V. T. (2005). Alzheimer's disease: Issues and challenges in primary care. *Nursing Clinics of North America, 41*, 83–94.

Coward, D. D. (1997). Self-transcendence: Constructing meaning from the experience of cancer. *Seminars in Oncological Nursing, 13*, 248–251.

Curtis, C. P. (2006). The psychosocial impact of the pain experience. In R. M. Carroll-Johnson, L. M. Gorman, & N. J. Bush (Eds.), *Psychosocial nursing care along the cancer continuum* (2nd ed.) (pp. 143–154). Pittsburgh: Oncology Nursing Press.

Czeisler, C. A.,Winkelman, S. W., & Richardson, G. S. (2005). Sleep disorders. In D. L. Kasper, E. Braunwald, A. S. Fauci, S. L. Hauser, D. L. Longo, L. Jameson, et al (Eds.), *Harrison's internal medicine* (16th ed.) (pp. 153–162). New York: McGraw-Hill.

Daudet, A. (2002). *In the land of pain*. New York: AA Knopf.

Davidizar, R. (1999). Meeting a client's spiritual needs. *Caring, 18*, 3–6.

Davis, K. L. (2005). Delirium, dementia, and amnestic and other cognitive disorders and mental disorders due to general medical conditions. In B. J. Sadock & V. A. Sadock (Eds.), *Kaplan and Sadock's comprehensive textbook of psychiatry* (8th ed.) (pp. 1053–1054). Philadelphia: Lippincott Williams & Wilkins.

de Rond, M. E., deWit, R., vanDam, F., vanCampen, B., denHartag,Y., Klievink, R., et al (1999). Daily pain assessment: Value for nurses and patients. *Journal of Advanced Nursing, 29(12)*, 436–444.

de Rond, M. E., deWit, R., vanDam, F. S., & Muller, M. J. (2000). A pain monitoring program for nurses: Effect on the administration of analgesics. *Pain, 89*, 25–38.

Decker, G. M. (1999). *An introduction to complementary and alternative therapies*. Pittsburgh, PA: Oncology Nursing Press.

Deeny, P. & McFetridge, B. (2005). The impact of disaster on culture, self, and identify: Increased awareness by health care professionals is needed. *Nursing Clinics of North America, 40(3)*, 431–444.

DeLaune, S. C. (1991). Effective limit setting: How to avoid being manipulated. *Nursing Clinics of North America, 26(13)*, 757–764.

Denkins, B. A. (2005). My side: Are we really helping? The problem of dual diagnoses, homes and hospital hopping. *Journal of Psychosocial Nursing and Mental Health Services, 43(11)*, 48–50.

Devlin, B. K., & Reynolds, E. (1994). Child abuse. *American Journal of Nursing, 94(3)*, 26–32.

Doenges, M. E., Townsend, M. C., & Moorhouse, M. F. (1998). *Psychiatric care plans: guidelines for individualizing care* (3rd ed.). Philadelphia: FA Davis.

Domrose, C. (2007). Listening to voices. *Nurseweek*, August 13, 12–13.

Dowd, M. D. (1998). Consequences of violence. *Pediatric Clinics of North America, 45*, 333–340.

Dubovsky, S. L., Davies, R. & Doboxsky, A. N. (2003). Mood disorders. In R. E. Hales & S. C. Yodofsky (Eds.), *Textbook of clinical psychiatry* (4th ed.) (pp. 439–542). Washington, DC: American Psychiatric Press.

Duffy, J. (2005). Brokenhearted—the biology and health consequences of grief. *American Academy of Hospice and Palliative Medicine Bulletin*, Summer, pp. 1–3.

Dunn, H. (2001). Hard choices for loving people. Herndon, VA: A&A Publishers.

Ebersole, P., & Hess, P. (1997). *Toward healthy aging* (5th ed.). St. Louis: Mosby.

Eisenberg, D. M., Davis, R. B., Ettner, S. L., Appel, S., Wilkeys, S., vanRompay, M., et al. (1998). Trends in alternative medicine use in the US: 1990–1997. *Journal of the American Medical Association, 280(11)*, 1569–1575.

Ellis, J. A., Blouin, R., & Lockett, J. (1999). Patient-controlled analgesia: Optimizing the experience. *Clinical Nursing Research, 8(3)*, 283–294.

Elsayem, A., Driver, L., & Bruera, E. (2003). *The MD Anderson symptom control and palliative care handbook* (2nd ed.). Houston, TX: University of Texas Health Science Center at Houston.

Emergency Mental Health and Traumatic Stress. Retrieved December 4, 2006 from http://mentalhealth.samhsa.gov/cmhs/EmergencyServices/after.asp.

Emergency Nurses Association. (2006). *Position statement on violence in emergency care settings*. Retrieved May 29, 2007 from ena.org/about/position/

Epstein, S. A. & Hicks, D. (2005). Anxiety disorders. In J. L. Levenson (Ed.), *Textbook of psychosomatic medicine* (pp. 251–270). Washington, DC: American Psychiatric Association Publications.

Everly, G. S., Lating, J. M., & Mitchell, J. T. (2000). Innovations in group crisis intervention: Critical incident debriefing and critical incident stress management. In A. R. Roberts (Ed.), *Crisis intervention handbook* (2nd ed.) (pp. 77–100). New York: Oxford University Press.

Everson-Rose, S. A. & Lewis, T. T. (2005). Psychosocial factors and cardiovascular diseases. *Annual Review of Public Health, 26*, 469–500.

Falvo, D. R. (1999). *Medical and psychosocial aspects of chronic illness and disability* (2nd ed.). Gaithersburg, MD: Aspen Publishers.

Falvo, D. R. (2004). *Effective patient education* (3rd ed). Sudbury, MA: Jones & Bartlett.

Fava, M. & Rosenbaum, J. F. (1999). Anger attacks in patients with depression. *Journal of Clinical Psychiatry,* suppl 15, 21–24.

Fein, M. L. (1993). I.A.M.: *A common sense guide to coping with anger.* Westport, CT: Prager Press.

Fergusson, D. (1999). Is sexual orientation related to mental health problems and suicidality in young people? *Archives of General Psychiatry, 56,* 876–880.

Ferrell, B. J., Virani, R., Grant, M., Coyne, P., & Uman, G. (2000). Beyond the Supreme Court decision: Nursing perspectives on end of life care. *Oncology Nursing Forum, 27,* 445–455.

Ferszt, G. G. (2006). How to distinguish between grief and depression? *Nursing, 36,* 60–61.

Feske, U., Frank, E., Mallinger, A. G., Houck, P. R., Fagiolini, A., Shear, M. K., et al. (2000). Anxiety as a correlate of response to the acute treatment of bipolar 1 disorder. *American Journal of Psychiatry, 157,* 956–962.

Fillingham, R. B. (2000). *Sex gender, and pain. Progress in pain research and management.* Seattle, WA: International Association for the Study of Pain Press.

Fincannon, J. L. (1995). Analysis of psychiatric referrals and interventions in an oncology population. *Oncology Nursing Forum, 22,* 87–92.

Finger, W. W., Lund, M., & Slagle, M. A. (1997). Medications that may contribute to sexual disorders. *Journal of Family Practice, 41,* 33–43.

Fischer, C., & Hegge, M. (2000). The elderly woman as risk. *American Journal of Nursing, 100(6),* 54–55.

Fitchett, G. (2002). *Assessing spiritual needs: A guide for caregivers.* Lima, OH: Academic Renewal Press.

Fochtmann, L. J. & Gelenberg, A. J. (2005). *Guideline watch: Practice guideline for the treatment of patients with major depressive disorder* (2nd ed.). Arlington, VA: American Psychiatric Association. Retrieved April 14, 2007 from http://psych.org/psych_pract/treatg/pg/prac_guide.cfm

Folstein, M. F., Folstein, F. E., & McHugh, P. R. (1975). Mini-mental state: A practical method for grading the cognitive state of patients for the clinician. *Journal of Psychiatric Research, 12,* 189–198.

Ford, D. E., & Kamerow, D. B. (1989). Epidemiological study of sleep disturbances and psychiatric disorders. *Journal of the American Medical Association, 262,* 1479–1484.

Forrest, J., Willis, L., Holm, K., Kwan, M. S., Anderson, M. A., & Foreman, M. D. (2007). Recognizing quiet delirium. *American Journal of Nursing, 107(4),* 35–39.

Fraser, K., & Gallop, R. (1993). Nurses' confirming/disconfirming responses to patients diagnosed with borderline personality disorder. *Archives of Psychiatric Nursing, (6),* 336–341.

Freedman, N. S., Kotzer, N., & Schwab, R. J. (1999). Patient perception of sleep quality and etiology of sleep disruption in the intensive care unit. *American Journal of Respiratory Critical Care Medicine, 159(4),* 1155–1162.

Friedman, M. M. (1998). *Family therapy: Theory and practice* (4th ed.). Norwalk, CT: Appleton & Lange.

Galanter, M., & Kleber, H. D. (1994). *Textbook of substance abuse therapy*. Washington, DC: American Psychiatric Press.

Gallagher, S. (1999). Tailoring care for obese patients. *RN, 625*, 43–47.

Gates, D. M. (2004). The epidemic of violence against healthcare workers. *Occupational and Environmental Medicine, 61*, 649–650.

Gauthier, S., Reisberg, B., Zaudig, M., Petersen, R. C., Ritchie, K., Broich, K., et al. (2006). Mild cognitive impairment. *Lancet, 367*, 1262–1270.

Gelazis, R. S., & Kempe, A. (1988). Therapy with clients with eating disorders. In Beck, C. K., Rawlins, R. P., & Williams, S. R. (Eds.), *Psychiatric nursing* (pp. 662–680). St. Louis: CV Mosby.

Geary, S. M. (1994). Intensive care unit psychosis revisited: Understanding and managing delirium in the critical care unit. *Critical Care Nursing Quarterly, 179*, 51–63.

Geriatric Depression Scale. Retrieved January 29, 2007, from www.stanford.edu/-yesavage/testing.htm.

Giger, J. N., & Davidhizar, R. E. (2004). *Transcultural nursing assessment and intervention* (4th ed.). St. Louis: Mosby.

Glod, C. A. (1993). Long-term consequences of childhood physical and sexual abuse. *Archives of Psychiatric Nursing, 7*, 163–173.

Goff, D. C., Freudenreich, O., & Henderson, D. C. (2004). Psychotic patients. In T. A. Stern, G. L. Friccione, N. H. Cassem, M. S. Jellinek, & J. F. Rosenbaum (Eds.), *Massachusetts General Hospital Handbook of general hospital psychiatry* (5th ed) (pp. 155–174). St. Louis: Mosby.

Goldberg, T. (2006). Undermining drug safety. *Washington Times*, December 18.

Goldenberg, I., & Goldenberg, H. (2004). *Family therapy: An overview* (16th ed.). Pacific Grove, CA: Brooks/Cole.

Goldsmith, C. (2000). Obesity: Epidemic of the 21st century? *Newsweek*, May 8.

Goldsmith, C. (2007). Insomnia: Sleepless in America. *Nurseweek*, Feb. 26, 16–18.

Goldsmith, R. J. & Garlapai V. (2004). Behavioral interventions for dual-diagnosis patients. *Psychiatric Clinics of North America, 27*, 709–726.

Goodwin, F. K., & Jamison, K. R. (1990). *Manic-depressive illness*. New York: Oxford University Press.

Gorman, J. M., Kent, J. M., Sullivan, G. M., & Coplan, J. D. (2000). Neuroanatomical hypothesis of pain disorder, revised. *American Journal of Psychiatry, 157(4)*, 493–505.

Gorman, L., Sultan, D., & Luna-Raines, M. (1989). *Psychosocial nursing handbook for the nonpsychiatric nurse*. Baltimore, MD: Williams & Wilkins.

Gorman, L. M., Raines, M. R., & Sultan, D.M. (2002). *Psychosocial nursing for the nonpsychiatric nurse* (2nd ed). Philadelphia: FA Davis.

Gorman, L. M. (2006). The close of life. In R. M. Carroll-Johnson, L. M. Gorman, & N. J. Bush (Eds.), *Psychosocial nursing care along the cancer continuum* (2nd ed.) (pp. 450–463). Pittsburgh, PA: Oncology Nursing Press.

Grant, M. S., Cordts, G. A., & Doberman, D. J. (2007). *Acute pain management in hospitalized patients with current opioid abuse*. Medscape. Retrieved June 13, 2007 from www.medscape.com/viewarticle/557043

Gray-Vickery, P. (2000). Combating abuse, Part 1: Protecting the older adult. *Nursing, 30,* 34–38.

Greene, J. M., Ennett, S. T., & Ringwalt, C. L. (1999). Prevalence and correlates of survival sex among runaway and homeless youth. *American Journal of Public Health,* 89(9), 1406–1409.

Groves, J. E. (2004). Difficult patients. In T. A. Stern, G. L. Friccione, N. H. Cassem, M. S. Jellinek, & J. F. Rosenbaum (Eds.), *Massachusetts General Hospital handbook of general hospital psychiatry* (5th ed.) (pp. 293–312). St. Louis: Mosby.

Groenewold, D. (1996). *Decreasing readmission: The comprehensive role of nursing in psychosocial rehabilitation.* Presented at Contemporary Forums Psychiatric Nursing Conference in Hollywood, CA.

Grossman, D. (1994). Enhancing your cultural compentence. *American Journal of Nursing,* 94, 58–62.

Gunderson, J. G. (2001). *A borderline personality disorder brief.* Retrieved January 26, 2007, from www.bpdresourcecenter.org.

Haber, J., et al. (1997). *Comprehensive psychiatric nursing* (5th ed.). St. Louis: Mosby.

Hamolia, C. C. (1998). Preventing and managing aggressive behavior. In G. W. Stuart & M. T. Laraia (Eds.), *Stuart and Sundeen's principles and practices of psychiatric nursing* (6th ed.) (pp. 618–640). St. Louis: Mosby.

Hanna, V. M., & Smith, J. A. (1992). Helping a dependent patient help himself. *Nursing,* 92, 22, 32c–32f.

Harmon Hanson, S. M. (2005). Family health care nursing: An introduction. In S. M. Harmon Hanson, V. Fedaly-Duff, & J. Rowe Kaakinen (Eds.), *Family health care nursing* (3rd ed.) (pp. 3–37). Philadelphia: FA Davis.

Harper-Jaques, S., & Reimer, M. (2005). Management of aggression and violence. In M. A. Boyd (Ed.), *Psychiatric Nursing: Contemporary Practice* (3rd ed) (pp. 802–822). Philadelphia: Lippincott Williams & Wilkins.

Harvath, T. A., Palsdaughter, C. A., Bumbalo, J. A. & McCane, M. K. (1995). Dementia-related behaviors. *Journal of Psychosocial Nursing and Mental Health Services, 3(1),* 35–39.

Hatton, C., & Valente, S. (1984). *Suicide: assessment and interventions.* Norwalk, CT: Appleton, Century, and Crofts.

Haven, E., & Piscitello, V. (1989). The patient with violent behavior. In S. Lewis, R. D. Grainger, W. A. McDowell, R. J. Gregory, & R. L. Messner (Eds.), *Manual of psychosocial nursing inverventions* (pp. 187–204). Philadelphia: WB Saunders.

Hebert, L. E., Scheer, P. A., Bienias, J. L., Bennett, D. A., & Evans, D. A. (2003). Alzheimers disease in US population: Prevalence estimates using 2000 census. *Archives of Neurology, 60(8),* 119–122.

HELP. (2006). *Information about the issues of homelessness.* Retrieved September 19, 2006 from http://www.agrm.org/help.html.

Highfield, M. E. F. (2000). Providing spiritual care to patients with cancer. *Clinical Journal of Oncology Nursing,* 4, 115–120.

Himelstein, B. P. (2006). Palliative care for infants, children, adolescents, and their families. *Journal of Palliative Medicine, 9,* 163–181.

Hingson, R., & Howland, J. (1993). Alcohol and nontraffic unintended injuries. *Addiction, 88,* 877–893.

Hirschfeld, R. M. A. (2005). *Guideline watch: Practice guideline for the treatment of patients with bipolar disorder.* Arlington, VA: American Psychiatric Association. Retrieved July 6, 2007 from http://www.psych.org/psych_pract/treatg/pg/prac_guide.cfm

Hirschfeld, R. M. A., Bowden, C. I., Gidian, M. J., Keck, P. E., Suppes, T., Thase, M. E., et al. (2002). *Practice guidelines for the treatment of patients with bipolar disorders* (2nd ed). Arlington, VA: American Psychiatric Association, Retrieved July 6, 2007 from http://www.psych.org/psych_pract/treatg/pg/prac_guide.cfm

Hockenberry, M. J., Wilson, D., & Winkelstein, M. L. (2005). *Wong's essentials of pediatric nursing* (7th ed). St Louis: Mosby.

Hollander, E. & Simeon, D. (2003). Anxiety disorders. In R. E. Hales & S. C. Yodofsky (Eds.), *Textbook of clinical psychiatry* (4th ed.) (pp. 543–630). Washington, DC: American Psychiatric Publishing.

Hollinworth, H., Clark, C., Harland, R., Johnson, L., & Partington, G. (2005). Understanding the arousal of anger: A patient-centered approach. *Nursing Standard, 19,* 41–47.

Horgas, A. L., & Elliott, A. F. (2004). Pain assessment and management in persons with dementia. *Nursing Clinics of North America, 39,* 593–606.

Hospice and Palliative Nurses Association. (2000). *Hospice and Palliative Nurses Association Statement on the Scope and Standards of Hospice and Palliative Nursing Practice.* Dubuque, IA: Kendall Hunt Publishing Co.

Huart, S., & O'Donnel, M. (1993). The road to recovery from grief and bereavement. *Caring, 13,* 71–75.

Hudelson, E. (1992). Points to remember when caring for an obese patient. *Nursing, 22,* 62–63.

Iowa University Injury Previous Research Center. (2000). *Workplace violence: a report to the nation.* Iowa City, IA: Iowa University Injury Previous Research Center.

Irving, K., Fick, D., & Foreman, M. (2006). Delirium: A new appraisal of an old problem. *International Journal of Older People Nursing, 1(2),* 106–1112.

Jacob, S. R. (1993). An analysis of the concept of grief. *Journal of Advanced Nursing, 18,* 1787–1794.

Jacobs, D. G. (1999). *The Harvard Medical School guide to suicide assessment and intervention.* San Francisco: Jossey-Bass Publishers.

Jacobs, D. G., Baldessarini, R. J., Conwell, Y., Fawcett, J. A., Horton, L., Meltzer, H., et al. (2003). *American Psychiatric Association practice guidelines for assessment and treatment of patients with suicide disorders.* Washington, DC: American Psychiatric Association. Retrieved July 15, 2007 from www.psych.org/psych_pract/treatg/pg/prac_guide.cfm

Jefferson, L. V. (1998). Chemically mediated responses and substance-related disorders. In G. W. Sundeen & M. T. Laraia (Eds.), *Stuart and Sundeen's principles and practices of psychiatric nursing* (6th ed.) (pp. 485–522). St. Louis: Mosby.

Jensen, D. P., & Herr, K. A. (1993). Sleeplessness. *Nursing Clinics of North America, 28*, 385–405.

Jimerson, D. C., Wolfe, B. E., Brotman, A. W., & Metzger, E. D. (1996). Medication in the treatment of eating disorders. *Psychiatric Clinics of North America, 19*, 739–754.

Johnston, J. E. (1994). Sleep problems in the elderly. *Journal of the American Academy of Nurse Practitioners, 15(6)*, 161–166.

Joint Commission on Accreditation of Health Care Organizations (JCAHO). (2005, 2006, 2007). *Accreditation manual for hospitals*. Chicago: Joint Commission on Accreditation of Health Care Organizations.

Joint Commission on Accreditation of Heath Care Organizations. (2007). *What did the doctor say? Improving health literacy to protect patient safety.* Retrieved February 8, 2007 from jointcommission.org.

Kagawa-Singer, M., & Blackhall, L. J. (2001). Negotiating cross-cultural issues at the end of life: "You got to go where he lives." *Journal of the American Medical Association, 286*, 2993–3001.

Kahn, D. M., Cook, T. E., Carlisle, C. C., Nelson, D. L., Kramer, N. R., Millman, R. P. (1998). Identification and modification of environmental noise in an ICU setting. *Chest, 114*, 535–540.

Karasu, T. B., Gelengerg, A., Merriam, A., & Wang, P. (2000). *American Psychiatric Association practice guidelines for treatment of patients with major depressive disorders* (2nd ed). Washington, DC: American Psychiatric Association Retrieved July 15, 2007 from www.Psych.org/psych_pract/treatg/pg/prac_guide.cfm.

Kelly, G. L. (1991). Childhood depression and suicide. *Nursing Clinics of North America, 26*, 545–558.

Kellehear, A. (2000). Spirituality and palliative care: a model of needs. *Palliative Medicine, 14*, 149–155.

Kemp, C. (1999). *Terminal illness: A guide to nursing care* (2nd ed.). Philadelphia: Lippincott Williams & Wilkins.

Kerfoot, K. (1995). Keeping spirituality in managed care: The nurse manager's challenge. *Nursing Economics, 18*, 49–51.

Kessler, R. C., Berglund, P., Demler, O., Jin, R., Merikanges, K. R., & Walters, E. E. (2005). Lifetime prevalence and age of onset distributions of DSM-IV disorders in the national comorbidity survey replication. *Archives of General Psychiatry, 62*, 593–602.

King, C. J., VanHasselt, V. B., Siegal, D. L. & Hersen, M. (1994). Diagnosis and assessment of substance abuse in older adults: Current strategies and issues. *Addictive Behavior, 19*, 41–55.

Kirsh, K. L., & Passik, S. D. (2006). Palliative care of terminally ill drug addict. *Cancer Investigation, 24*, 425–431

Kluger, J. (2000). The battle to save your memory. *Time,* June 12, 46.

Knowles M. A. (1970). *The modern practice of adult education.* Englewood Cliffs, NJ: Prentice-Hall.

Koenig, H. (2005). *Faith and mental health: Religious resources for healing.* West Conshohocken, PA: Templeton Foundation Press.

Koenig, H. (2006). *In the wake of disaster: religious responses to terrorism and catastrophe.* West Conshocken, PA: Templeton Foundation Press.

Kowatch, R. A., Fristad, M., Birmaher, B., Wagner, K. D., Findling, R. L., Hellander, M., et al. (2005). Treatment guidelines for children and adolescents with bipolar disorder. *Journal of the American Academy of Child and Adolescent Psychiatry, 44,* 213–235.

Krach, P. (1993). Nursing implications: Functional status of older persons with schizophrenia. *Journal of Gerontological Nursing, 19,* 21–27.

Kreisman, J. J., & Straus, H. (1989). *I hate you—don't leave me: understanding the borderline personality.* New York: Avon Books.

Kübler-Ross, E. (1969). *On death and dying.* New York: MacMillan.

Kuebler, K. K., Heidrich, D. E., Vena, C., & English, N. (2006). Delirium, confusion, and agitation. In B. F. Ferrell & N. Coyle (Eds.), *Textbook of palliative nursing* (2nd ed.) (pp. 401–420). New York: Oxford University Press.

Kurlowicz, L. H. (2003). Depression in older adults. In M. Mesey, T. Fulmer, I. Abraham, & D. A. Zwicker (Eds.), *Geriatric nursing protocol for best practice* (2nd ed.) (pp. 185–206). New York: Springer.

Kushel, M. B., Perry, S., Bangsberg, D., Clark, R., & Moss, A. R. (2002). Emergency department use among the homeless and marginally housed: Results from a community-based study. *American Journal of Public Health, 92,* 778–784.

Lamb, M. A. (2006). Sexuality. In B. Ferrell & N. Coyle (Eds.), *Textbook of palliative nursing* (2nd ed.) (pp. 421–428). New York: Oxford University Press.

Lamb, H. R. (n.d.). *Deinstitutionalization and the homeless mentally ill.* Retrieved August 14, 2006 from http://www.interactivist.net/housing/deinstitutionalization_1.html.

Laraia, M. T., & Sundeen, S. J. (2001). Cognitive responses and organic mental disorders. In G. W. Stuart & M. T. Laraia (Eds.), *Stuart and Sundeen's principles and practices of psychiatric nursing* (7th ed.) (pp. 460–484). St. Louis: Mosby.

Laumann, E., Park, A., & Rosen, R. C. (1999). Sexual dysfunction in the US.: Prevalence and predictors. *Journal of the American Medical Association, 281(6),* 542–544.

Leach McMahon, A. (1997). The nurse-client relationship. In J. Haber, B. Krainovich-Miller, A. Leach McMahon, & P. Price-Hoskins (Eds.), *Comprehensive psychiatric nursing* (5th ed.) (pp. 143–161). St. Louis: Mosby.

Leckman, J. F., & King, R. A. (2007). A developmental perspective on the controversy surrounding the use of SSRIs to treat pediatric depression. *American Journal of Psychiatry, 164(9),* 1304–1306.

Ledray, L. E., & Arndt, S. (1994). Examining the sexual assault victim: A new model for nursing care. *Journal of Psychosocial Nursing and Mental Health Services, 32(2),* 7–12.

Lego, S. (1990). Borderline personality disorders. In E. Varcarolis (Ed.), *Foundations in mental health nursing* (pp. 408–420). Philadelphia: WB Saunders.

LeMone, P., & Jones, D. (1997). Nursing assessment of altered sexuality: A review of salient factors and objective measures. *Nursing Diagnosis, 8,* 120–128.

Levenkron, S. (1978). *The best little girl in the world.* New York: Warner Books.

Levine, S. (1999). The newly revised standards of care for gender identity disorders. *Journal of Sex Education Therapy, 24,* 121–125.

Lewis, A., & Levy, J. (1982). *Psychiatric liaison nursing.* Reston, VA: Reston Publishing.

Lewis, S. (1993). Verbal intervention. In Blumenreich, P. E., & Lewis, S. (Eds.), *Managing the violent patient* (pp. 41–52). New York: Brunner/Mazel.

Lewis, J. H., Andersen, R. M., & Gelberg, L. (2004). Health care for homeless women: Unmet needs and barriers to care. *Journal of General Internal Medicine, 18,* 921–928.

Levetown, M., Barnard, M. U., Hellstein, M. B., Byock, I. R., Cater, B. S., Connor, S. R., et al. (2001). *A Call to Change: Recommendations to improve care for children living with long term conditions.* Alexandria, VA: National Hospice and Palliative Care Organization.

Liken, M. A., & Collins, C. D. (1993). Grieving: Facilitating the process for dementia caregivers. *Journal of Psyochosocial Nursing and Mental Health Services, 31,* 21–26.

Lilley, L. L., & Aucker, R. N. (1999). *Pharmacology and the nursing process* (2nd ed.). St. Louis: Mosby.

Lindemann, E. (1944). Symptomatology and management of acute grief. *American Journal of Psychiatry, 101,* 141–148.

Lipson, J. G., & Steiger, N. J. (1996). *Self-care nursing in a multi-cultural context.* Thousand Oaks, CA: Sage Publications.

Lipson, J. G., Dibbie, S. L., & Minarik, P. A. (Eds.), (1996). *Culture and nursing care.* San Francisco: University of California San Francisco Nursing Press.

Liptzen, B. & Jacobson, S. A. (2006). Delirium. In B. J. Sadock & V. A. Sadock (Eds.), *Kaplan & Sadock's comprehensive textbook of psychiatry* (8th ed.) (pp. 3693–3700). Philadelphia: Lippincott Williams & Wilkins.

Lo, B., Rushton, D., Kotes, L. W., Arnold, R. M., Cohen, C. B., Faber-Langendoen, K., et al. (2003). Discussing religious and spiritual issues at the end of life. *Journal of American Medical Association, 287,* 749–754.

Luckman, J. (1999). *Transcultural communication in nursing.* Albany, NY: Delmar Publishers.

Lynch, S. H. (1997). Elder abuse: What to look for, how to intervene. *American Journal of Nursing, 97(1),* 27–33.

Mace, N. L., & Rabins, P. V. (2001). *The 36-hour day* (revised ed.). Baltimore, MD: Johns Hopkins University Press.

Manos, P. J., & Braun, J. (2006). *Care of the difficult patient*. New York: Routledge.

Maciejewski, P. K., Zhang, B., Block, S. D., & Prigerson, H. G. (2007). An empirical examination of the stage theory of grief. *Journal of the American Medical Association*, 297(7), 716–723.

McCaffery, M. (1999). Pain management: problems and progress. In M. McCaffery & C. Pasero (Eds.), *Pain: Clinical manual* (2nd ed.) (pp. 1–14). St. Louis: Mosby.

Mariani, S. (2004). *Origin and neuropathology of schizophrenia*. Medscape. Retrieved October 20, 2006, from www.medscape.com.

Maintaining a Healthy State of Mind: for Parents and Caregivers. Retrieved December, 2006 from www.redcross.org/preparedness/cdc.htm.

Marks, R. M., & Sachar, E. J. (1994). Undertreatment of medical inpatients with narcotic analgesics. *Annals of Internal Medicine, 78*, 173–181.

Markwell, S. K. (2005). Long-term restraint reduction. *Journal Nursing Care Quality, 29*, 253–260.

Maslow, A. (1954). *Motivation and personality*. New York: Harper & Row.

Matheny, K. B., & Riordan, R. J. (1992). *Stress—and strategies for lifestyle management*. Atlanta: Georgia State University Business Press.

Mayfield, D., McLeod, G., & Hall, P. (1974). The CAGE questionnaire: Validation of a new alcoholism screening instrument. *American Journal of Psychiatry, 131*, 121–133.

McAndrew, M. (1994). People who depend on substances other than alcohol. In E. M. Varcarolis (Ed.), *Foundations of psychiatric mental health nursing* (2nd ed.) (pp. 632–676). Philadelphia: WB Saunders.

McCaffery, M. (1968). *Nursing practice theories related to cognition, bodily pain and man—environmental interactions*. Los Angeles: UCLA Student Store.

McCaffery, M., & Ferrel, B. R. (1997). Nurses' knowledge of pain assessment and management: How much progress have we made? *Journal of Pain & Symptom Management, 14*, 175–188.

McCaffery, M., & Pasero, C. (1999). *Pain: Clinical manual* (2nd ed.). St. Louis: Mosby.

McCracken, A. L. (1998). Healthy people 2000: Aging and alcohol. *Journal of Gerontological Nursing, 24*, 37–43.

McDaniels, J. S., & Sharma, S. M. (2002). Mania. In M. G. Wise & J. R. Rundell (Eds.), *Textbook of consultation liaison psychiatry* (2nd ed.) (pp. 339–359). Washington, DC: American Psychiatric Press.

McGrath, P. J., & Finley, G. A. (1999). *Chronic and recurrent pain in children and adolescents. Progress in pain research and management 17*. Seattle, WA: International Association for the Study of Pain Press.

McKenry, L. M., & Salernoe, E. (2001). *Mosby's pharmacology in nursing* (21st ed.). St. Louis, Mosby.

Mendlowicz, M. V., & Stein, M. B. (2000). Quality of life in individuals with anxiety disorders. *American Journal of Psychiatry, 157(5)*, 669–692.

Merikangus, K. (2006). Anxiety disorders: Epidemiology. In B. J. Sadock & V. A. Sadock (Eds.), *Kaplan & Sadock's comprehensive textbook of psychiatry* (8th ed.) (pp. 1720–1728). Philadelphia: Lippincott Williams & Wilkins.

Miller, J. F. (2000). *Coping with chronic illness* (3rd ed.). Philadelphia: FA Davis.

Miller, N. S., & Brady, K. T. (2004). Addictive disorders. *Psychiatric Clinics of North America, 27(4),*b 627–648.

Mitchell A. M., Sakraida T. J., & Zalice K. K. (2005). Disaster care: Psychological considerations. *Nursing Clinics of North America, 40(3):*535–550

Moller, M., & Murphy, M. F. (2001). Neurobiological responses and schizophrenia and psychotic disorders. In G. W. Stuart & M. T. Laraia (Eds.), *Stuart and Sundeen's priniciples and practices of psychiatric nursing* (7th ed.) (pp. 402–437). St. Louis: Mosby.

Montano, C. B. (2003). *New frontiers in the treatment of depression.* Retrieved January 14, 2007 from http://www.medscape.com/viewprogram/2689.

Morrison, R., & Siu, A. L. (2000). Survival in end-stage dementia following acute illness. *Journal of the American Medical Association, 284,* 47–52.

Moscicki, E. K. (1999). Epidemiology of suicide. In D. G. Jacobs (Ed.), *Harvard Medical School guide to suicide assessment and intervention* (pp. 40–51). San Francisco, Jossey-Bass.

Moscicki, E. K. (1997). Identification of suicide risk factors in epidemiological studies. *Psychiatric Clinics of North America, 20,* 499–517.

Mulryan, K., Cathers, P., & Fagin, A. (2000). Combating abuse part II: Protecting the child. *Nursing, 30,* 39–45.

Mulvey, M. A. (2004). Fluid and electrolytes: balance and distribution. In S. C. Smeltzer & B. G. Bare (Eds.), *Brunner & Suddarth's textbook of medical-surgical nursing* (10th ed.) (pp. 249–294). Philadelphia: Lippincott Williams & Wilkins.

National Alliance for the Mentally Ill. (2007). *About bipolar disorder.* Retrieved January 15, 2007 from www.nami.org.

National Alliance for the Mentally Ill (NAMI). (2007). *Major depression.* Retrieved January 14, 2007 from www.nami.org.

National Association for Mentally Ill (NAMI). (2006). *Dual diagnosis and integrating treatment of mental illness and substance abuse disorders.* Retrieved December 11, 2006 from www.nami.org.

National Center for Complementary and Alternative Medicine. (2004). More than one-third of U.S. adults use complementary and alternative medicine. Retrieved May 24, 2007 from http://nccam.nih.gov/news/2004/052704.htm

National Center for Health Statistics. (2003). *Deaths/mortality.* Retrieved November 10, 2006 from www.cdc.gov/nchs/faststats/deaths/HTM.

National Center for Health Statistics. (2007). *Vital and health statistics.* Retrieved July 11, 2007 from www.cdc.gov/nchs.

National Center on Sleep Disorders Research (2006). *Insomnia.* Retrieved July 11, 2007 from www.nhibi.nih.gov/heath/dci/diseses/inso/inso_whatis.html

National Consensus Project for Quality Palliative Care. (2004). *Clinical practice guidelines for quality palliative care.* Retrieved December 1, 2006 from http://www.nationalconsensusproject.org.

National Coalition for the Homeless. (2006). *Fact sheet #12*. Retrieved June 20, 2006 from http://www.nationalhomeless.org.

National Council on Alcoholism and Drug Dependence. (2002). *America's number one health problem*. Retrieved August, 2006 from www.ncadd.org/facts/numberoneprob.html

National Council on Child Abuse and Family Violence. (2006). *Spouse/partner Abuse Information*. Retrieved July 15, 2006 from www.nccafv.org/spouse.htm.

National Council on Child Abuse and Family Violence. (2006). *Child Abuse Information*. Retrieved July 15, 2006 from www.nccafv.org/child.htm.

National Crisis Prevention Institute. (1991). *Art of setting limits: Participant manual*. Brookfield, WI: National Crisis Prevention Institute.

National Council of Child Abuse and Family Violence. (2004). *Link between childhood maltreatment and juvenile delinquency*. Retrieved June 16, 2007 from nccafv.org/maltreatmentdelinquency.htm

National Institute of Alcohol Abuse and Alcoholism. (2007). *FAQs*. Retrieved May 1, 2007 from www.niaaa.org.

National Hospice and Palliative Care Organization. (2007). *Statistics*. Retrieved July 14, 2007 from www.nhpco.org.

National Institutes of Health. (1998). *First federal obesity clinical guidelines*. Retrieved September 2000 from www.nhlbi.nih.gov.

National Institute of Mental Health (NIMH). (2001). *Borderline personality disorder*. Retrieved January 25, 2007 from www.nimh.nih.gov/publicat/bpd.cfm.

National Institute of Mental Health (NIMH). (2007a). *Depression*. Retrieved January 14, 2007 from www.nimh.nih.gov/publicat/depression.cfm.

National Institute of Mental Health (NIMH). (2007b). *Antidepressant medications for children and adolescents*. Retrieved April 14, 2007 from www.nimh.nih.gov/healthinformation/andepressants_child.cfm.

National Institute on Alcohol Abuse and Alcoholism (NIAAA). (2005). *The facts about youth and alcohol*. Retrieved December 10, 2006 from www.pubs.niaaa.nih.gov/psa/factsheet.htm.

National Institute of Neurological Disorders and Stroke. (2007). *Brain basics: understanding sleep*. Retrieved July 11, 2007 from ninds.nih.gov/disorders/brain_basics/understanding_sleep htm

National Health & Nutrition Examination Survey (NHANES). (2000). *Obesity Rates in the U.S.* Retrieved March 16, 2002 from www.cdc.gov/nhanes

National Mental Health Association. (2006). *Homelessness: reviewing the facts*. Retrieved August 8, 2006 from *National Sleep Foundation*. (2007). The Silent Killer. Retrieved July 11, 2007 from sleepfoundation.org http://home.fuse/net/mhankey/ResourceDirectory/HOMELESSNESS REVIEWINGTHEFACTS.pdf.

Neimeyer, R. A. (1997). Meaning reconstruction and the experience of chronic loss. In K. J. Doka & J. Davidson (Eds.), *Living with grief: when illness is prolonged* (pp. 159–176). Philadelphia: Taylor and Francis.

Nelson, R. (2006). Designing to heal. *American Journal of Nursing, 106*, 25–27.

Norris, W. M., Wenrich, M. D., Nielsen, E. L., Treece, P. D., Jackson, J. C., &

Curtis, J. R. (2005). Communication about end of life care between language discordant patients and clinicians: Insights from medical interpreters. *Journal of Palliative Medicine, 8,* 1016–1024.

North American Nursing Diagnosis Association (NANDA). (2001). *Nursing diagnoses: Definitions and classifications 2001.* Philadelphia: North American Nursing Diagnosis Association.

Norwood, A. E., Ursano, R. J., & Fullerton, C. S. (2007). *Disaster Psychiatry Plan of Action.* Retrieved February 11, 2007 from www.psych.org/disasterpsych/sl/principlespractice.cfm.

Novello, A. C., & Soto-Torres, L. E. (1992). Women and the hidden epidemic. *The Female Patient, 17,* 17.

O'Connell, J. J., Roncarati, J. S., Reilly, E. C., Kane, C. A., Morrison, S. K., Swain, S. E., et al (2004). Old and sleeping rough: Elderly homeless persons on the streets of Boston. *Care Management Journal, 5,* 101–106.

O'Brien, M. E. (2003). *Spirituality in nursing.* Boston: Jones and Bartlett.

Office for Civil Rights, HIPAA. (2006). Retrieved September 2, 2006 from hhs.gov.ocr/hipaa.

Oldman, J. M. (2005). *Guideline watch: Practice guideline for the treatment of patients with borderline personality disorder.* Washington, DC: American Psychiatric Association.

Oldman J. M., Gabbard, G. O., Goin, M. K., Gunderson, J., Soloff, P., Spiegel, D., et al (2001). *Practice guidelines for the treatment of patients with borderline personality disorder.* Washington, DC: American Psychiatric Association.

Oncology Nursing Society. (2006). *Position statement on use of placeboes for pain in patients with cancer.* Retrieved October 3, 2006 from www.ons.org.

Ott, C. H. (2003). The impact of complicated grief on mental and physical health at various points in the bereavement process. *Death Studies, 27,* 249–272.

Pacquette, M. (1998). Anger. In R. M. Carroll-Johnson, L. M. Gorman, & N. J. Bush (Eds.), *Psychosocial nursing care along the cancer continuum* (pp. 139–152). Pittsburgh: Oncology Nursing Press.

Paice, J., & Fine, P. (2006). Pain at the end of life. In B. Ferrell & N. Coyle (Eds.), *Textbook of palliative nursing* (2nd ed.) (pp. 131–153). New York: Oxford University Press.

Park, E. J. (2006). Telehealth technology in case/disease management. *Lippincott's Case Management, 11,* 175–182.

Parker, B., & Campbell, J. C. (1998). Care of survivors of abuse and violence. In G. W. Stuart & M. T. Laraia (Eds.), *Stuart and Sundeen's principles and practices of psychiatric nursing* (7th ed.) (pp. 830–840). St. Louis: Mosby.

Partnership for a Drug-free America. (2006). *What every parent needs to know about cough medicine.* Retrieved December 10, 2006 from www.drugfree.org.

Pasero C., Portenoy R. K., & McCaffery M. (1999). Opioid analgesics. In M. McCaffery & C. Pasero (Eds.), *Pain: Clinical manual* (2nd ed.) (pp. 161–299). St Louis: Mosby.

Perdue, B., & Piotrowski, C. (2000). A nurse's guide to mental health assessment reference sources. *Journal of Psychosocial Nursing and Mental Health Services, 38(2),* 40–49.

Phipps, W. J. (1999). Chronic illness and rehabilitation. In W. J. Phipps, J. K. Sandas, & J. F. March (Eds.), *Medical surgical nursing* (6th ed.) (pp. 129–162). St. Louis: Mosby.

Pollack, M. H., Mathews, J., & Scott, E. L. (1998). Gabapentin as a potential treatment for anxiety disorders. *American Journal of Psychiatry, 155,* 992–993.

Poorman, S. G. (2001). Sexual responses and sexual disorders. In G. W. Stuart & M. T. Laraia (Eds.), *Stuart and Sundeen's principles and practices of psychiatric nursing* (7th ed.) (pp. 548–571). St. Louis: Mosby.

Pope, H. G. & Drower, K. J. (2006). Anabolic-androgenic steroids. In M. Galanter & H. D. Kleber (Eds.), *The American Psychiatric Publishing textbook of substance abuse treatment* (3rd ed.) (pp. 257–264). Washington, DC: American Psychiatric Publishing.

Puchalski, C., & Romer, A. L. (2000). Taking a spiritual history allows clinicians to understand patients more fully. *Journal of Palliative Medicine, 3,* 129–137.

Purnell, M. L., & Paulanka, B. J. (1998). *Transcultural health care: A culturally competent approach.* Philadelphia: FA Davis.

Raia, S. (2004). The problem of impaired nurses. *New Jersey Nurse, 34,* 8–10.

Raines, M. L. (2000). Ethical decision-making in nurses: Relationships among moral reasoning, coping style and ethics stress. *Journal of Nursing Administration Healthcare Law, Ethics, and Regulation, 2,* 29–41.

Ramakrishnan, K., & Scheid, D. (2007). Pharmacologic treatments of insomnia. *American Family Physician, 76,* 517–526.

Rando, T. (1993). *Treatment of complicated mourning.* Champaign, IL: Research Press.

Rando, T. A. (2000). Anticipatory Mourning: A Review and Critique of the Literature. In T. A. Rando (Ed.), *Clinical dimensions of anticipatory mourning* (pp. 17–20). Champaign, IL: Research Press.

Rawlins, R. P., Williams, S. R., & Beck, C. K. (1993). *Mental health-psychiatric nursing: a holistic life-cycle approach* (3rd ed.). St. Louis: Mosby.

Redman, B. K. (1997). *The practice of patient education* (8th ed.). St. Louis: Mosby.

Redman, B. K. (1993). *The practice of patient education* (7th ed.). St. Louis, Mosby.

Rieckmann, N., Gerin, W., Kronish, I. M., Burg, M. M., Chaplin, W. F., Kong, G., et al. (2006). Course of depressive symptoms and medication adherence after acute coronary syndromes: An electronic medication monitoring study. *Journal of the American College of Cardiology, 48,* 2218–2222.

Ripamonti, C., Zecca, E., & Bruera, E. (1997). An update on the clinical use of methadone for cancer pain. *Pain, 70,* 109–115.

Rivara, F. B., Garrison, M. M., Ebel, B., McCarty, C. A., & Christakis, D. A. (2004). Mortality attributable to harmful drinking in U.S. *Journal of Studies on Alcohol, 65,* 530–536.

Robert Wood Johnson Foundation. (1996). *Chronic care in America: A 21st century challenge.* Princeton, NJ: Robert Wood Johnson Foundation.

Roper, J. M., & Manela, J. (2000). Psychiatric patients perceptions of waiting time in the psychiatric emergency service. *Journal of Psychosocial Nursing, 38,* 18–27.

Roscoe, J. A., Kaufman, M. E., Matteson-Rusby, S. E., Palesh, O. G., Ryan, J. L., Perlis, M. L., et al. (2007). Cancer related fatigue and sleep disorders. *The Oncologist, 12(suppl 1),* 35–42.

Ross, L. (1997). Elderly patients' perceptions of their spiritual needs and care: A pilot study. *Journal of Advanced Nursing, 26(4),* 710–715.

Rouchell, A. M., Pounds, R., & Tierney, L. (2002). Depression. In M. G. Wise & J. R. Rundell (Eds.), *Textbook of consultation—liaison psychiatry* (2nd ed.) (pp. 307–308). Washington, DC: American Psychiatric Association Press.

Rubey, R. N., & Lydiard, R. B. (1999). Management of side effects of anxiolytics. In R. Balon (Ed.), *Practical management of the side effects of psychotropic drugs* (pp. 145–168). New York: Marcell Dekker, Inc.

Russell, S. S. (2006). An overview of adult-learning processes. *Urologic Nursing, 26,* 349–352.

Saarmann, L., Daugherty, J. A., & Riegel, B. (2000). Patient teaching to promote behavioral change. *Nursing Outlook, 48,* 281–287.

Sadock, B. J. & Sadock, V. A. (2007). *Kaplan & Sadock's synopsis of psychiatry* (10th ed). Philadelphia: Lippincott Williams & Wilkins.

Sadock, V. A. (2005). Normal human sexuality and sexual and gender identification disorders. In B. J. Sadock & V. A. Sadock (Eds.), *Kaplan & Sadock's comprehensive textbook of psychiatry* (8th ed.) (pp. 902–935). Philadelphia: Lippincott Williams & Wilkins.

Saltzmann, K. B. (2006). Transforming the grief experience. In R. M. Carroll-Johnson, L. M. Gorman, & N. J. Bush (Eds.), *Psychosocial nursing care along the cancer continuum* (2nd ed.) (pp. 293–314). Pittsburgh, PA: Oncology Nursing Press.

Samuels, S. C. & Neugroschl, J. A. (2005). Delirium. In B. J. Sadock & V. A. Sadock (Eds.), *Kaplan & Sadocks's comprehensive textbook of psychiatry* (8th ed.) (pp. 1054–1068). Philadelphia: Lippincott Williams & Wilkins

Schatzberg, A. F., & Nemeroff, C. B. (Eds.), (2004). *The American Psychiatric Press textbook of psychopharmacology.* Washington, DC: American Psychiatric Press, Inc.

Schatzberg, A. F., Cole, J. O., & DeBattista, C. (2005). *Manual of clinical psychopharmacology* (5th ed). Washington, DC: American Psychiatric Publishing, Inc.

Schnelle, J. F., Alessi, C. A., Al-Samarrai, N. R., Fricker, R. D. & Ouslander, J. G. (1999). The nursing home at night: Effects of an intervention on noise, light, and sleep. *Journal of American Geriatric Society, 45,* 430–438.

Schooler, N. R. (1994). Negative symptoms in schizophrenia: Assessment of the effects of risperidone. *Journal of Clinical Psychiatry, 55(suppl),* 22–28.

Schuckit, M. A. & Tapert, S. (2004). Alcohol. In M. Galanter & H. D. Kleber (Eds.), *The American Psychiatric Publishing textbook of substance abuse treatment* (3rd ed.) (pp. 151–166). Washington, DC: American Psychiatric Publishing.

Schuckit, M. A. (2006). *Drug and alcohol abuse* (6th ed.). New York: Springer.

Schultz, J. M., & Videbeck, S. D. (2000). *Manual of psychiatric nursing care plans* (5th ed.). Philadelphia: Lippincott-Raven.

Schuster, M. A., Stein, B. D., Jaycox, L., Collins, R. L., Marshall, G. N., Elliott, M. N., et al. (2001). A national survey of stress reactions after September 11, 2001. *New England Journal of Medicine 345(20),* 1507–1512.

Schuster, P. M. (2000). *Communication: the key to the therapeutic relationship.* Philadelphia: FA Davis.

Schutte, D. L. (2006). Alzheimer disease and genetics: Anticipating the questions. *American Journal of Nursing, 106(12),* 40–47.

Seligman, M. (1975). *Helplessness: on depression, development, and death.* New York: WH Freeman.

Shea, C. A., Mahoney, M., & Lacey, J. (1997). Breaking the barriers to domestic violence interventions. *American Journal of Nursing, 97(6),* 26–34.

Shinn, M. & Weitzmann, B. (1996). Homeless families are different. In J. Baumohl (Ed.), *Homelessness in America for the National Coalition for the Homeless* (pp. 109–122). Phoenix, AZ: Oryx Press.

Shoemaker, N. C. & Varcarolis, E. M. (2006). Personality disorders. In E. M. Varcarolis, V. B. Carson, & N. C. Shoemaker (Eds.), *Foundations of psychiatric mental nursing* (5th ed.) (pp. 275–298). St Louis: Saunders Elsevier.

Shoemaker, N. C. & Varcarolis, E. M. (2006). Psychiatric mental health nursing and managed care issues. In E. M. Varcarolis, V. B. Carson, & N. C. Shoemaker (Eds.), *Foundations of psychiatric mental nursing* (5th ed.) (pp. 63–71). St Louis: Saunders Elsevier

Shoemaker, N. C. & Varcarolis, E. M. (2006). Suicide. In E. M. Varcarolis, V. B. Carson, & N. C. Shoemaker. *Foundations of psychiatric mental health nursing* (5th ed.) (pp. 473–489). St Louis: Saunders Elsevier.

Slesnick, N. & Prestopnik, J. (2005). Dual and multiple diagnosis among substance using runaway youth. *American Journal of Drug and Alcohol Abuse, 31(1),* 179–201.

Smeltzer, S. C. & Bare, B. G. (2004). *Brunner & Suddarth's textbook of medical-surgical nursing.* Philadelphia: Lippincott Williams & Wilkins.

Smith-Dijulio, K., & Hozapfel, S. K. (1994). Families in crisis: Family violence. In E. M. Varcarolis (Ed.), *Foundations of psychiatric mental health nursing* (2nd ed.) (pp. 514–525). Philadelphia: WB Saunders.

Smith-DiJulio, K. (2006). Care of the chemically impaired. In E. M. Varcarolis, V. B. Carson, & N. C. Shoemaker (Eds.), *Foundations in psychiatric mental health nursing* (5th ed.) (pp. 547–574). St Louis: Saunders Elsevier.

Smythe, E. (1984). *Surviving nursing.* Menlo Park, CA: Addison-Wesley.

Soloff, P. H., Lynch, K. G., Kelly, T. M., Malone, K. M., & Mann, J. J. (2000). Characteristics of suicide attempts of patients with major depressive episode and borderline personality disorder: A comparative study. *American Journal of Psychiatry, 157(4),* 601–608.

Spader, C. (2007). Manorexia. *Nurseweek,* August 13, 24–25.

Stanley, K. J. (2000). Silence is not golden: Conversation with the dying. *Clinical Journal of Oncology Nursing, 4,* 34–40.

Stanley, M., & Beare, P. G. (1995). *Gerontological nursing*. Philadelphia: FA Davis.

Strehlow, A. J., & Amos-Jones, T. (1999). The homeless as vulnerable population. *Nursing Clinics of North America, 34(2)*, 261–274.

Sternberg, S. (2005). Chronic pain: The enemy within. *USA Today*, May 9.

Stephenson, P. L., Draucker, C. B., & Martsolf, D. S. (2003). The experience of spirituality in the lives of hospice patients. *Journal of Hospice and Palliative Nursing, 5*, 51–58.

Stewart, J. C., Janicki, D. L., Muldoon, M. F., Sutton-Tyrrell, K., & Kamarch, T. W. (2007). Negative emotions and three year progression of subclinical atherosclerosis. *Archives General Psychiatry, 64(2)*, 225–233.

Stoner, S. C. & Dubisar, B. (2006). Psychotropics. *RN, 69*, 31–37.

Stratton, L. (1999). Evaluating the effectiveness of a hospital's pain management program. *Journal of Nursing Care Quality, 13(4)*, 8–18.

Strauss, A. L. (1984). *Chronic illness and the quality of life* (2nd ed.). St. Louis: CV Mosby.

Strehlow, A. J., & Amos-Jones, T. (1999). The homeless as vulnerable population. *Nursing Clinics of North America, 34*, 261–274.

Strohe, W., & Schut, H. (2001). Risk factors in bereavement outcome: A methodological and empirical review. In M. S. Strohe, R. O. Hanssen, W. Stroehe, & H. Schut (Eds.), *Handbook of bereavement research: Consequences, coping and care* (pp. 349–371). Washington, DC: American Psychological Association.

Stuart, G. W. (2001a). Anxiety responses and anxiety disorders. In G. W. Stuart & M. T. Laraia (Eds.), *Stuart and Sundeen's principles and practices of pschiatric nursing* (7th ed.) (pp. 274–298). St. Louis: Mosby.

Stuart, G. W. (2001b). Self-protective responses and suicidal behavior. In G. W. Stuart & M. T. Laraia (Eds.), *Stuart and Sundeen's principles and practices of psychiatric nursing* (7th ed.) (pp. 381–401). St. Louis: Mosby.

Stuart, G. W. (2001c). Emotional responses and mood disorders. In G. W. Stuart & M. T. Laraia (Eds.), *Stuart and Sundeen's principles and practices of psychiatric nursing* (7th ed.) (pp. 345–380). St. Louis: Mosby

Stuart, G. W., & Sundeen, S. J. (2001). *Stuart & Sundeen's principles and practices of psychiatric nursing* (7th ed.). St. Louis: Mosby.

Sullivan, J. T., Sykora, K., Schneiderman, J., Naranjo, C. A., & Sellers, E. M. (1989). Assessment of alcohol withdrawal: The revised Clinical Institute Withdrawal Assessment for Alcohol Scale (CIWA-Ar). *British Journal of Addiction, 84*, 1353–1357.

Surgeon General of the United States. (2000). *Mental health. A report of the Surgeon General*. Washington, DC: US Government Printing Office. Retrieved June 15, 2007 from www.nimh.nib.gov/mhsgrpt.

Tariman, J. D. (2007). Emergency preparedness for cancer care. *ONS Connect*, September, 8–12.

Taylor, B. (1999). "Coming out" as a life transition. Homosexual identity formation and its implications of healthcare practice. *Journal of Advanced Nursing, 30*, 570–576.

Taylor, E. J. (2006). Spirituality and spiritual nurture in cancer care. In R. M. Carroll-Johnson, L. M. Gorman, N. J. Bush (Eds.), *Psychosocial nursing care along the cancer continuum* (2nd ed.) (pp. 117–131). Pittsburgh, PA: Oncology Nursing Press.

Taylor, E. J., Amenta, M., & Highfield, M. (1995). Spiritual care practices of oncology nurses. *Oncology Nursing Forum, 22,* 31–39.

Teno, J. M., Clarridge, B. R., Casey, B., Welch, L. C., Wetle, L. C., Shield, R., et al. (2004). Family perspective on end of life care at last place of care. *Journal of American Medical Association, 291,* 88–93.

Thomas, S. P. (2001). Teaching healthy anger management. *Perspectives in Psychiatric Care, 37,* 41–48.

Thornton, A. & Young-DeMarcko, A. (2001). 4 decades of attitudes toward family issues in the U.S. 1960s–1990s. *Journal of Marriage & Family, 63,* 1009–1037.

Torkelson, D., & Dobal, M. (1999). Sexual rights of people with serious and persistent mental illness. *Journal of the American Psychiatric Nurses Association, 5,* 150–163.

Torrey, E. F. (1988). *Surviving schizophrenia: a family manual.* New York: Perennial Library.

Townsend, M. C. (2005). *Essentials of psychiatric mental health nursing* (3rd ed). Philadelphia: FA Davis

Townsend, M. C. (2006). *Psychiatric mental health nursing* (5th ed.). Philadelphia: FA Davis.

Traumatic Incident Stress: Information for Emergency Response Workers: Retrieved December 4, 2006 from cdc.gov/niosh/unp_trinstrs.html

Treatment Advocacy Center. (2006). *Historical view of mental illness crisis and debacle of deinstitutionalization.* Retrieved September 14, 2006 from http://www.psychlaws.org/GeneralResources/fact2.htm

Tunnessen, W. W. (2000). *Signs and symptoms in pediatrics* (3rd ed.). Philadelphia: Lippincott Williams & Wilkins.

Tweed, S. H. (1998). Intervening in adolescent substance abuse. *Nursing Clinics of North America, 33,* 29–45.

Twycross, A., Moriarity, A., & Betts, T. (1998). *Pediatric pain management: a multidisciplinary approach.* Abingdon, UK: Scovill-Patterson, Inc.

Twycross, A. (1999). Pain management: A nursing priority. *Journal of Child Health Care, 3,* 19–26.

U.S. Census Bureau. (2005). *2005 community survey.* Retrieved October 12, 2006 from www.factfinder.census.gov.

U.S. Conference of Mayors. (2005). *A status report on hunger and the homeless in America's cities.* Washington, DC: Author.

U.S. Department of Health and Human Services. (2005). National survey on drug use and health: national findings. Retrieved December 9, 2006 from www.oas.samhsa.gov.

U.S. Department of Health and Human Services (1995). *Youth with runaway, throwaway, and homeless experiences: Prevalence of drug use and other at-*

risk behaviors. Silver Spring, MD: National Clearinghouse on Families and Youth.

Valente, S., & Saunders, J. (1997). Diagnosis and treatment of major depression among patients with cancer. *Cancer Practice, 2,* 65–68.

Van Fleet, S. (2006). Crisis Intervention. In R. M. Carroll-Johnson, L. M. Gorman, & N. J. Bush (Eds.), *Psychosocial nursing care along the cancer continuum* (2nd ed.) (pp. 403–418). Pittsburgh, PA: Oncology Nursing Society.

VandWeerd, C., Paveza, G. J., & Gulmer, T. (2005). Abuse and neglect in older adults with Alzheimer's disease. *Nursing Clinics of North America, 41,* 43–56.

Varcarolis, E. M. (2006). *Foundations of psychiatric mental health nursing* (5th ed.). St. Louis: Saunders Elsevier.

Varcarolis, E. M. (1998). *Foundations of psychiatric mental health nursing* (3rd ed.). Philadelphia: WB Saunders.

Varcarolis, E. M. (1990). *Foundations of psychiatric mental health nursing,* Philadelphia: WB Saunders.

Varcarolis, E. M. (2006). Assessment strategies and the nursing process. In E. M. Varcarolis, V. B. Carson, & N. C. Shoemaker (Eds.), *Foundations of psychiatric mental health nursing* (5th ed.) (pp. 138–154). St Louis: Saunders Elsevier.

Varcarolis, E. M. (2006). Bipolar disorder. In E. M. Varcarolis, V. B. Carson, & N. C. Shoemaker (Eds.), *Foundations of psychiatric mental health nursing* (5th ed.) (pp. 359–383). St Louis: Saunders Elsevier.

Varcarolis, E. M. (2006). Mood disorders: Depression. In E. M. Varcarolis, V. B. Carson, & N. C. Shoemaker (Eds.), *Foundations of psychiatric mental health nursing* (5th ed.) (pp. 326–358). St Louis: Saunders Elsevier.

Varcarolis, E. M. (2006). The schizophrenias. In E. M. Varcarolis, V. B. Carson, & N. C. Schoemaker (Eds.), *Foundations of psychiatric mental health nursing* (5th ed.) (pp. 384–421). St Louis: Saunders Elsevier.

Videbeck, S. L. (2004). *Psychiatric mental health nursing* (2nd ed.). Philadelphia: Lippincott Williams & Wilkins.

Wadland, W. C., & Ferenchick, G. S. (2004). Medical comorbidity in addictive disorders. *Psychiatric Clinics of North America, 27,* 675–687.

Walker, L. (1979). *The battered woman.* New York: Harper & Row.

Watson, A. C. (2006). Anger and cancer. In R. M. Carroll-Johnson, L. M. Gorman, & N. J. Bush (Eds.), *Psychosocial nursing care along the cancer continuum* (2nd ed.) (pp. 223–240). Pittsburgh, PA: Oncology Nursing Press.

Weber, M. & Clevien, P. A. (2006). Bariatric surgery. *British Journal of Surgery, 93,* 259–260.

Weiner, E., Peterson, B., Ladd, K., McConnell, E., & Keefe, F. (1999). Pain in nursing home residents. An exploration of prevalence, staff perspectives, and pratical aspects of measurement. *Clinical Journal of Pain, 15,* 92–101.

Wells, A. (1997). *Cognitive therapy of anxiety disorders: A practice manual and conceptual guide.* New York: John Wiley.

Wessman, A. C., & McDonald, D. D. (1999). Nurses' personal pain experiences and their pain management knowledge. *Journal of Continuing Education Nursing, 30,* 152–157.

White, J. H. (2005). Eating disorders. In M. A. Boyd (Ed.), *Psychiatric nursing: Contemporary practice* (pp. 492–523). Philadelphia: Lippincott Williams & Wilkins.

Widom, C. S., Dumont, K., & Czaja, S. J. (2007). A prospective investigation of major depressive disorder and comorbidity in abused and neglected children grown up. *Archives of General Psychiatry, 64,* 49–56.

Williams, L. D., & Boyd, M. A. (2005). Stress, crisis, and disaster management. In M. A. Boyd (Ed.), *Psychiatric nursing* (3rd ed.) (pp. 771–780). Philadelphia: Lippincott Williams & Wilkins.

Wilmoth, M. N. (2006). Life after cancer: What does sexuality have to do with it? *Oncology Nursing Forum, 33,* 905–910.

Winkleby, M. A., & White, R. (1992). Homeless adults without apparent medical and psychiatric impairment: Onset of morbidity over time. *Hospital and Community Psychiatry, 43,* 1017–1023.

Winstanley, S., & Whittington, R. (2004). Aggression toward healthcare staff in a UK general hospital: Variations among professionals and departments. *Journal of Clinical Nursing, 13,* 3–10.

Wolfe, B. E. (1998). Eating disorders. In C. A. Glod (Ed.), *Contemporary psychiatric-mental health nursing* (pp. 460–477). Philadelphia: FA Davis.

Wong, D. L., & Hockenberry-Eaton, M. (2001). *Wong's essentials of pediatric nursing* (6th ed.). St. Louis: Mosby.

Wynne, C. F., Ling, S. M., & Remsburg, R. (2000). Comparison of pain assessment instruments in cognitively intact and cognitively impaired nursing home residents. *Geriatric Nursing, 21(1),* 20–23.

World Health Organization. (2006). *WHO Pain Relief Ladder.* Retrieved September 25, 2006 from www.who.int/cancer/palliative/painladder/en/.

Yager, J., Devlin, M. J., Halmi, K. A., Herzog, D. B., Mitchell, S. E., Powers, P., et al (2006). *Practice guidelines for treatment of patients with eating disorders* (3rd ed.). Washington, DC: American Psychiatric Association. Retrieved February 11, 2007 from www.psych.org/guidelines

Yager, J., & Andersen, A. E. (2005). Anorexia nervosa. *New England Journal of Medicine, 353,* 1481–1488.

Index

Note: Page numbers followed by f refer to figures; those followed by t refer to tables.